Whole-Body FDG PET Imaging in Oncology

Pier Francesco Rambaldi

Whole-Body FDG PET Imaging in Oncology

Clinical Reports

In collaboration with Giovanni Fontanella

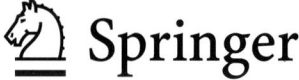 Springer

Pier Francesco Rambaldi
Dipartimento Medico Chirurgico di
  Internistica Clinica Sperimentale
  ''F. Magrassi-A. Lanzara'', Diagnostica per Immagini
Seconda Università degli Studi di Napoli
Naples
Italy

ISBN 978-88-470-5294-9   ISBN 978-88-470-5295-6   (eBook)
DOI 10.1007/978-88-470-5295-6
Springer Milan Heidelberg New York Dordrecht London

Library of Congress Control Number: 2013946884

This is the English version of the Italian edition published under the title PET-TC BODY con
FDG in ONCOLOGIA. © E.L.I. Medica srl 2012. The author particularly thanks Dr. Giovanni
Fontanella for his collaboration and for the translation of the volume.

Printed on acid-free paper

Springer is part of Springer Science+Business Media (www.springer.com)

My heart leaps up when I behold
A rainbow in the sky:
So was it when my life began;
So is it now I am a man;
So be it when I shall grow old,
Or let me die!
The Child is father of the Man;
And I could wish my days to be
Bound each to each by natural piety.

William Wordsworth

Foreword

I am particularly pleased to write a foreword for this book written by Dr. Pier Francesco Rambaldi, Assistant Professor of Nuclear Medicine at the Second University of Naples, and addressed to the medical world, students, GPs as well as Nuclear Medicine specialists.

This manual points out the need to rationalize the prescription of diagnostic tests, particularly CT- PET, which is a task of great responsibility of each doctor, framing the diagnosis of a diverse range of oncological clinical cases in a series of medical decisions, established as a logical consequence.

Its meaning for students and young newly qualified doctors is found in the fact that, starting with the history of the individual patient (history), it reaches the diagnostic question and the evaluation of the patient. The resulting conclusions and key points at the end of each clinical case not only allows the achievement of a response to the diagnostic question, but also allows to understand the diagnosis, at the same time framing it in the broader context of the therapeutic management and guidelines for the treatment and follow-up.

I also believe this book to be an excellent expression of the academic tradition of our School of Medicine, combining in Nuclear Medicine, two of the most important branches of medicine: clinical medicine and imaging.

This book is therefore evidence of the huge commitment of those who have made their experience available to future generations.

Therefore, I hope this book will achieve the deserved consensus among students and physicians and arouse interest in all readers.

Fortunato Ciardiello

Preface

This manual is a collection of clinical cases, treating total body CT imaging with FDG -PET in Oncology. The aim of this book is to suggest an integrated approach to PET–CT, an approach that includes medical history, diagnostic question, report, conclusions and key points.

The starting point of every clinical case is a detailed medical history, which includes the definition of the disease, previous hospitalizations, diagnostic tests and therapy. Here, the nuclear medicine specialist will acquire clinic and new elements, such as radiology and laboratory tests, vital for a consistent interpretation of the metabolic images.

From the experience gained in the medical history, it is clear that the radiological reports carried out in different hospitals do not follow a standard report, but are characterized by a varied terminology, sometimes questionable, that in any case can be considered an enrichment.

In fact, drawing from the clinical and radiological-wide vocabularies, nuclear medicine reaches a critical assessment that joins the two souls of modern medicine: clinical and imaging diagnostics, both having the task to suggest the right diagnosis, the best choice of treatment and prognostic definition in the context of a PET-CT standardized report.

The diagnostic question sums up the problem formulated by the prescriber, whether family doctor or specialist, which requires the PET-CT to follow an algorithm to get to the final diagnosis. PET-CT is more frequently required during follow -up of neoplastic conditions to change the treatment plan and/or define the prognosis.

The law criminalizes both the prescriber and the diagnostician (radiologist or nuclear medicine physician) if the services are not properly justified and optimized.

In this context it must be remembered that medical exposure is carried out by a specialist (radiologist and nuclear medicine physician) upon reasoned request of the prescriber. The choice of methods and techniques capable of achieving the greatest clinical benefit with minimal individual detriment is the responsibility of the specialist, who must also consider the possibility of using alternative procedures , not based on ionizing radiation. Nuclear medicine techniques are also among the health activities involving exposure to ionizing radiation and its associated risks. While remaining within acceptable limits, special attention is still required for the workers, the public and the patients.

The report is the document which defines the nuclear medicine physician as a specialist and it is its official way of communicating with the prescriber and with those who undergo diagnostic tests. For this reason it should be clearly written and understandable, in order to be defined as the orderly description of all the pathological elements detected by PET-CT.

In the report, there are references to possible clinical or instrumental elements reported in history or at least detected by CT . This stage is the focal point of each clinical case described in this manual and is strongly supported by a wide iconography of PET, CT and PET-CT fusion images.

The conclusions are a synthesis of all the above-mentioned elements, a short, clear and concise response to the clinical question. In this phase, it is essential to define the metabolic state of the neoplastic disease both in cancer patients in the follow-up stage, and in those who underwent radio-chemotherapy or biological drugs, in particular, it is crucial to indicate the presence of a complete or partial response, or metabolic progression of pathology . The findings may include specific clinical suggestions, especially the timing of the subsequent follow-up or the need to perform additional diagnostic tests in cases of doubt. At the end of each case, there is a space dedicated to the key points, in which some pathophysiological critical elements are discussed.

The key points point out the awareness that the clinical aid is essential in order to reach a correct diagnosis and to determine the timing of the chemo-radiotherapy procedures. Just in oncology, PET-CT allows prognostic stratification that has immediate, sometimes dramatic consequences, not only on the subsequent choice of treatment, but also on the quality of life of patients and their families.

Contents

Part XI Stomach

Part XII Urinary Tract

Contributors

Gioconda Argenziano Diagnostica per Immagini, Azienda Ospedaliera Santobono-Pausilipon, Naples, Italy

Alfonso Fiorelli Dipartimento di Scienze Cardio-Toraciche e Respiratorie, Seconda Università degli Studi di Napoli, Naples, Italy

Giovanni Fontanella Dipartimento Medico Chirurgico di Internistica Clinica Sperimentale "F. Magrassi- A. Lanzara", Diagnostica per Immagini, Seconda Università degli Studi di Napoli, Naples, Italy

Roberto Grassi Dipartimento Medico Chirurgico di Internistica Clinica Sperimentale "F. Magrassi- A. Lanzara", Diagnostica per Immagini, Seconda Università degli Studi di Napoli, Naples, Italy

Luigi Mansi Dipartimento Medico Chirurgico di Internistica Clinica Sperimentale "F. Magrassi- A. Lanzara", Diagnostica per Immagini, Seconda Università degli Studi di Napoli, Naples, Italy

Floriana Morgillo Dipartimento Medico Chirurgico di Internistica Clinica Sperimentale "F. Magrassi- A. Lanzara", Oncologia Medica, Seconda Università degli Studi di Napoli, Naples, Italy

Lanfranco Musto Diagnostica per Immagini, ASL di Avellino 1, Avellino, Italy

Francesca Polverino, Boston, Massachusetts, USA

Mario Polverino Dipartimento Strutturale delle Discipline, Mediche degli Ospedali Riuniti delle Tre Valli, ASL Salerno 1, Bergamo, Italy

Pier Francesco Rambaldi Dipartimento Medico Chirurgico di Internistica Clinica Sperimentale "F. Magrassi- A. Lanzara", Diagnostica per Immagini, Seconda Università degli Studi di Napoli, Naples, Italy

Antonio Rotondo Dipartimento Medico Chirurgico di Internistica Clinica Sperimentale "F. Magrassi- A. Lanzara", Diagnostica per Immagini, Seconda Università degli Studi di Napoli, Naples, Italy

Massimo Zeccolini Diagnostica per Immagini, Azienda Ospedaliera Santobono-Pausilipon, Naples, Italy

Collaborators

Paola Nargi Medicina Nucleare—Napoli
Annarita Ianniello Medicina Nucleare—Napoli
Rossella Ferrara Medicina Nucleare—Napoli
Maria Rosaria Prisco Medicina Nucleare—Napoli
Andrea Vaccaro Medicina Nucleare—Napoli
Francesco Barbato Medicina Nucleare—Napoli
Barbara Magliulo Medicina Nucleare—Napoli
Alessia Spagnuolo - Seconda Università di Napoli—Napoli

Part I

Cholecystis and Biliary Ducts

1

1.1 Clinical History

70-year-old woman with gallbladder carcinoma who underwent surgery and subsequent adjuvant chemotherapy.

The follow-up to 3 years shows a peripancreatic mass suspicious for relapse:

- FNAB: recurrent carcinoma of the gallbladder.
- CT-PET: pathological increase in the consumption of glucose in the right hypochondrium which extends in the hepatic hilum and retrocavity of epiploon, towards the uncinate process of the pancreas (SUV max 6.7). This mass shows a photopenic area inside which is probably due to colliquation.
- Markers: CA19.9 = 121 U/ml (NV < 37).

Subsequently, chemotherapy is performed.

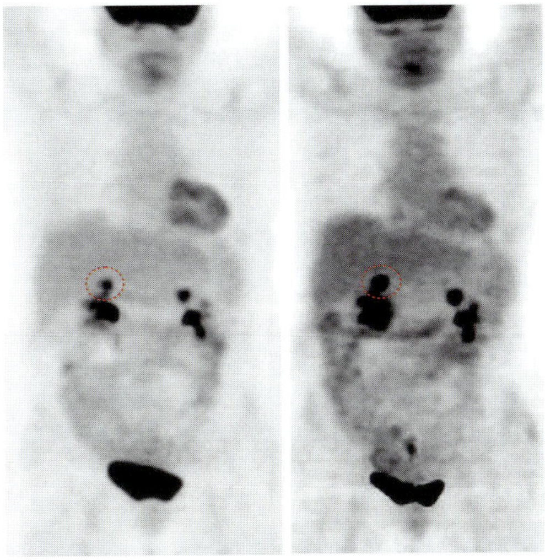

Fig. 1.1 MIP image with different intensities of printing: The pathological FDG concentration of the mass is masked by the physiological renal excretion

1.2 Diagnostic Question

Restaging after chemotherapy completed 3 weeks before, in patient with recurrent carcinoma of the gallbladder: search for lesions with a high metabolism of glucose.

1.3 Report

Presence of a mass characterized by pathological glucose consumption in the right hypochondrium which extends in the hepatic hilum and the retrocavity of epiploon, towards the uncinate process of the pancreas, SUV max 8.1. This mass shows a photopenic area inside which is probably due to colliquation. Absence of lesions characterized by abnormal metabolism in the remaining parts of the body examined.

1.4 Conclusions

Patient with recurrent carcinoma of the gallbladder treated with chemotherapy, shows persistence of high metabolism disease in today's scan (Figs. 1.1, 1.2).

P. F. Rambaldi, *Whole-Body FDG PET Imaging in Oncology*,
DOI: 10.1007/978-88-470-5295-6_1, © Springer-Verlag Italia 2014

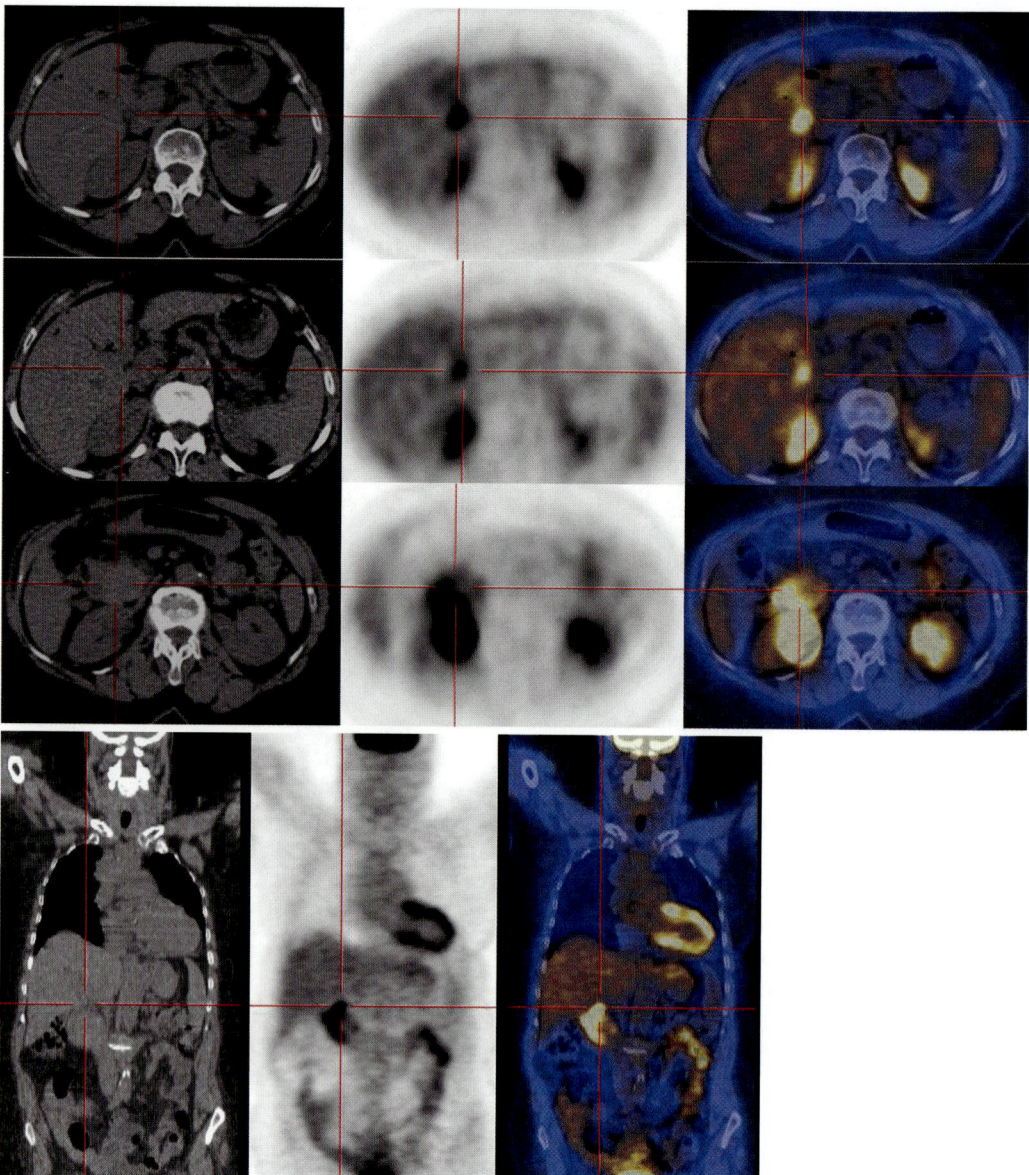

Fig. 1.2 The TC shows a *solid*, inhomogeneous mass of parenchymal density, which extends towards the hepatic hilum and retrocavity of epiploon until uncinate process of the pancreas and the kidney, from which it appears dissociable. PET has high metabolism of glucose

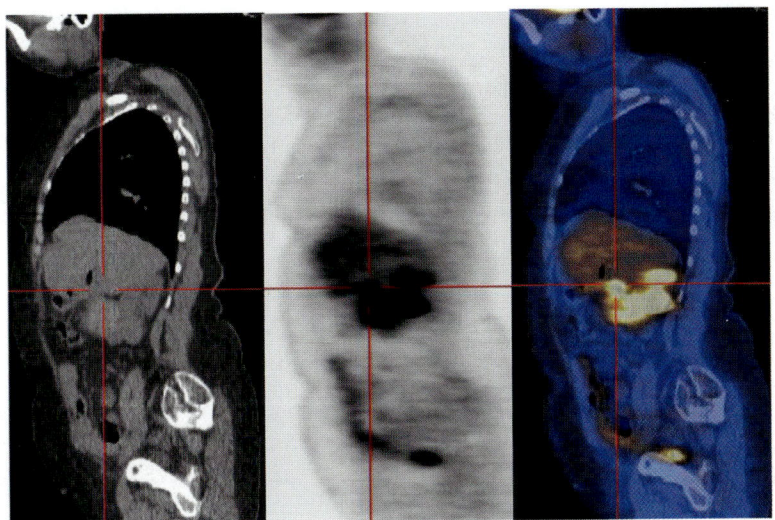

Fig. 1.2 (continued)

Recurrent Klatskin's Tumor: Peritoneal Carcinosis

2

2.1 Clinical History

67-year-old man with Klatskin's tumour, who previously underwent biliary tract resection at the common hepatic duct, with hepatic-jejunal-anastomosis and a *Roux-en-Y reconstruction* with cholecystectomy. Adjuvant chemotherapy performed.

Follow up during chemotherapy.

CT: Diffusely dishomogeneous and enlarged liver, with metallic clips in the cholecystic bed, due to previous surgery. Areas of structural dishomogeneity in the posterior portion of the VI segment, with a slightly less dishomogeneous area found in segment VIII and segment I, adjacent to the hilum, to be evaluated after contrast.

- PET-FDG: Diffusely dishomogeneous liver with focal uptake areas found in segments VI, VII and VIII.

Chemotherapy went on.

2.2 Diagnostic Question

Restaging after chemotherapy in patient with Klatskin's tumour: search for lesions with elevated glucose metabolism.

2.3 Report

Mild focal glucose uptake in two hepatic nodules, both due to local recurrence, the first in the right biliary tract, just above the site of previous surgery, SUV max 3.5 (Fig. 2.1a), the other at the hilum, adjacent to the metallic clips, SUV max 2.5 (Figs. 2.1b, 2.2).

Some abdominal centimetric nodules due to carcinosis are found, showing slight glucose uptake, SUV max 2.3 (Fig. 2.1c). Millimetric nodule at the right diaphragmatic pleura, with pathological metabolism, SUV max 1.1 (Fig. 2.3).

The left kidney is small and does not show neither uptake nor washout of the marker, due to severe obstructive hydronephrosis, as shown in CT: it's a typical morpho-functional case of 'excluded kidney' (Fig. 2.4).

2.4 Conclusions

PET scan shows a metabolic activity which could be due to local recurrence of disease, associated with peritoneal carcinosis and pleural involvement.

P. F. Rambaldi, *Whole-Body FDG PET Imaging in Oncology*,
DOI: 10.1007/978-88-470-5295-6_2, © Springer-Verlag Italia 2014

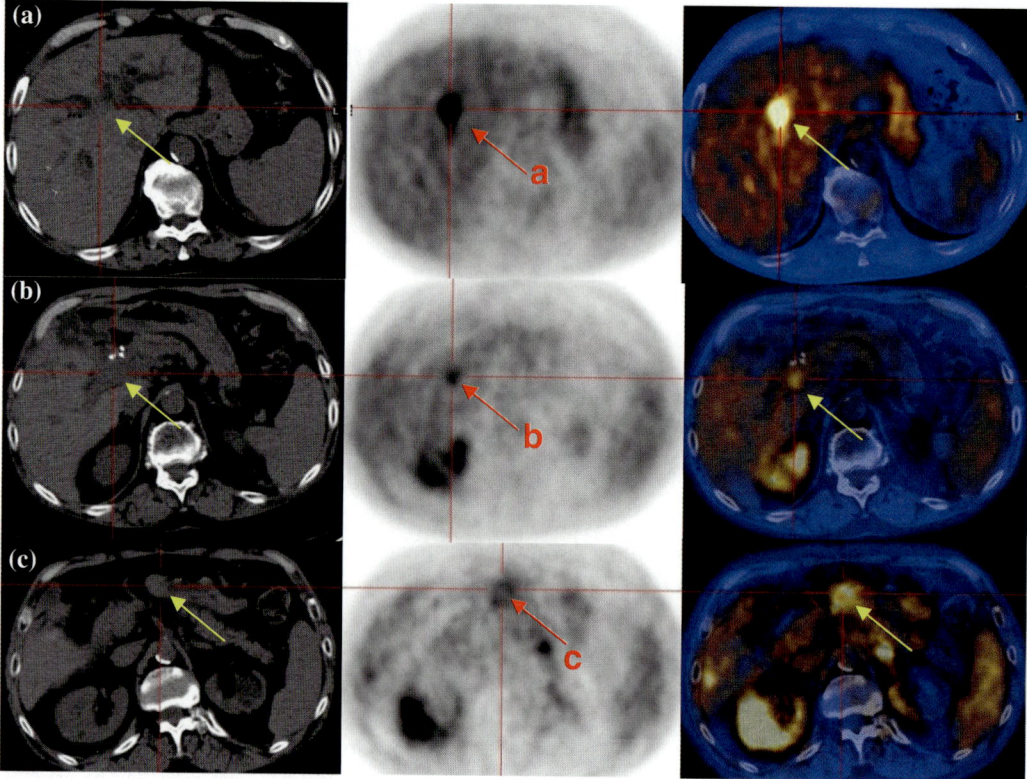

Fig. 2.1 Mild focal glucose uptake in two hepatic nodules, both due to local recurrence

In miliary carcinosis, characterized by sub-centimetric lesions, PET scan can have a limited accuracy: in this patient, the MIP image shows a modest glucose metabolism of the peritoneal and pleural nodules; only the bigger hepatic recurrence shows an increase of the FDG uptake. CT scan is then compulsory for a comprehensive understanding of the functional data.

2.5   Key Points

The scan shows severe hydronephrosis; thus, a differential is required (Fig. 2.1f):

• calcolosis,

• postoperative complications,
• congenital diseases.

When these diseases are not found in previous radiological examinations, an occult peritoneal carcinosis has to be suspected; it has to be searched for in all of the CT and PET images. Every dubious lesion, which could be part of a carcinosis, has to be reported, even when it shows low FDG metabolism.

You do not have to forget that the patient is an oncological one:

When the clinical conditions are poor and the PET scan does not show high metabolism lesions, a low metabolism recurrence of disease has to be suspected.

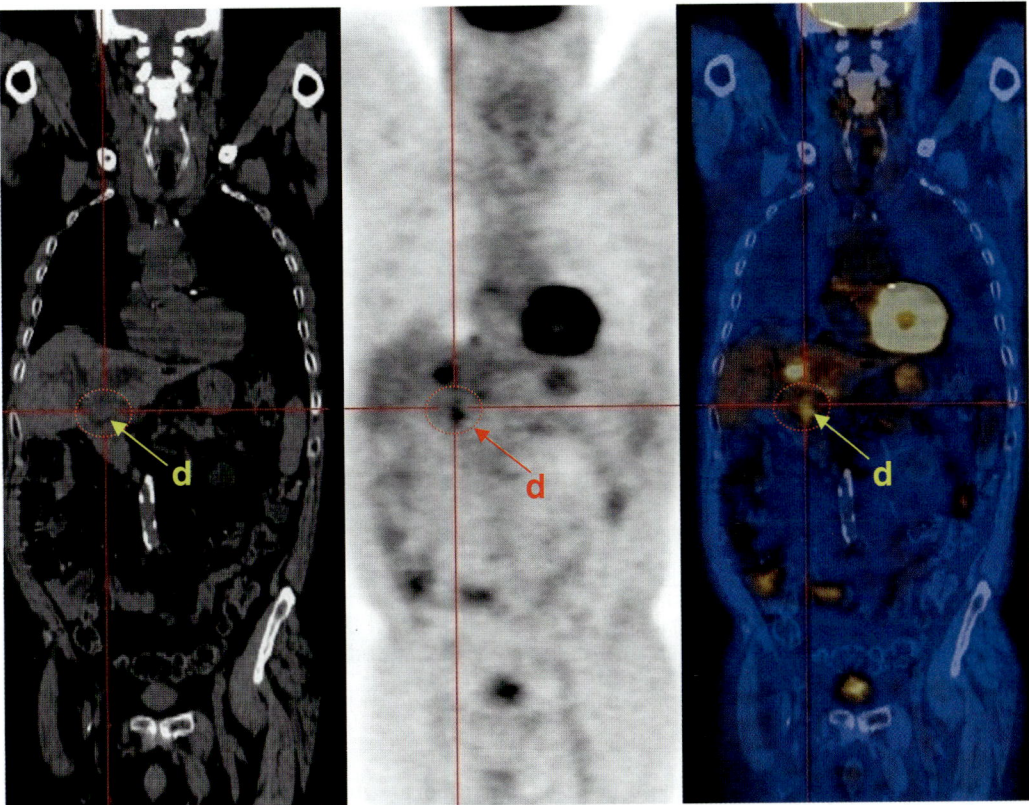

Fig. 2.2 Hepatic nodule at the hilum

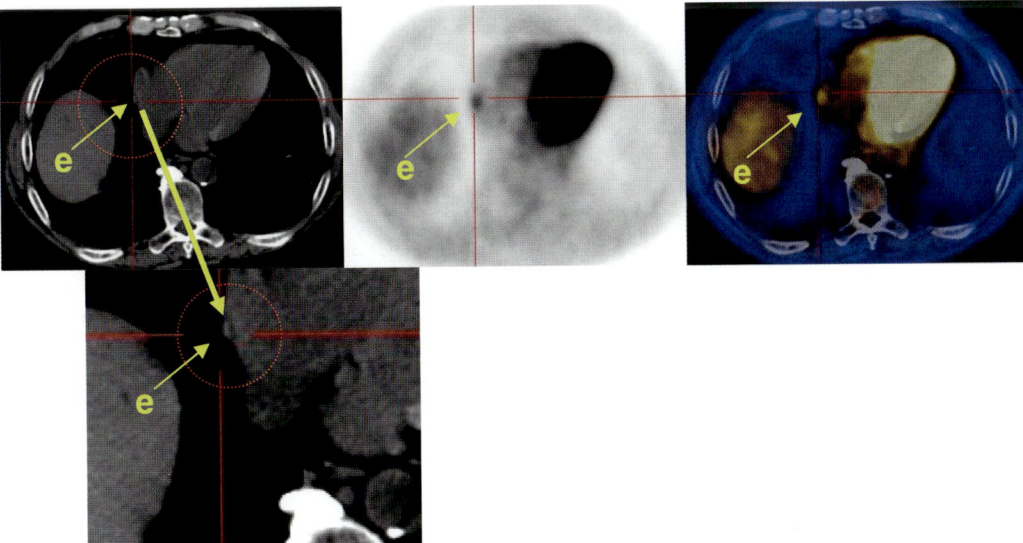

Fig. 2.3 Millimetric nodule at the right diaphragmatic pleura, with pathological metabolism, SUV max 1.1

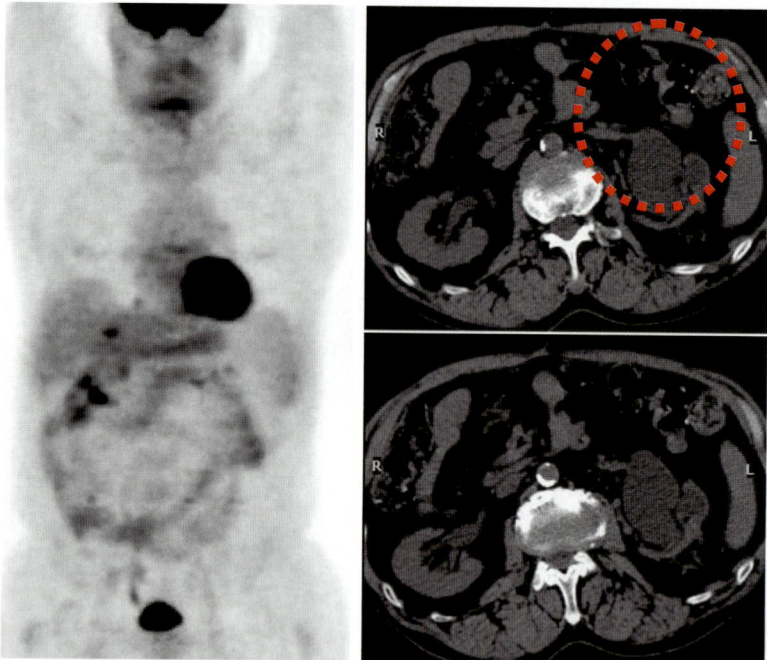

Fig. 2.4 Typical morpho-functional case of excluded kidney

- In this patient, the limited metabolism of the lesions could be due, at least in part, to the chemotherapy.

Pleural involvement is a sign of the advanced stage of disease.

Part II
Head-Neck

Parotid Cancer Recurrence and Metachronous Lung Cancer

3

3.1 Clinical History

78-year-old man who previously underwent surgery for squamous cell carcinoma of the right ear. After 6 months he underwent subtotal parotidectomy and right latero-cervical lymph node ipsilateral dissection. Adjuvant radiotherapy is then performed.

- Histology: infiltrating squamous cell carcinoma contiguous to the skin. Intermediate degree of differentiation, G2. Surgical resection margins are free. 10 lymph nodes are free of tumor localization.

   Reassessment after surgery.

- Contrast-enhanced CT: Moderate tissue thickening of the skin in the right latero-cervical area due to scarring phenomena. 2 cm-pseudonodular area behind the ipsilateral mandibular angle.

   Re-evaluation after 3 months.

- Contrast-enhanced CT: solid nodular lesion in the right parotid region, scarcely dissociable from locoregional vascular structures, associated with diffuse thickening tissue and latero-cervical adenopathy. Presence of a 3 cm-lymph node 3 at the left lung hilum and some repetitive confluent small nodules (biggest dimension 2 cm) in the context of the ipsilateral upper lobe.

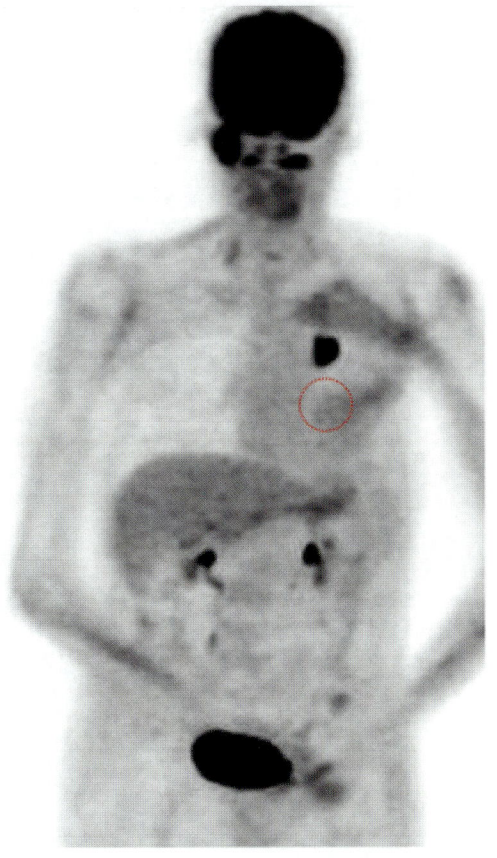

Fig. 3.1 The PET scan shows loco-regional recurrence of disease in the right parotid area with metachronous lung cancer

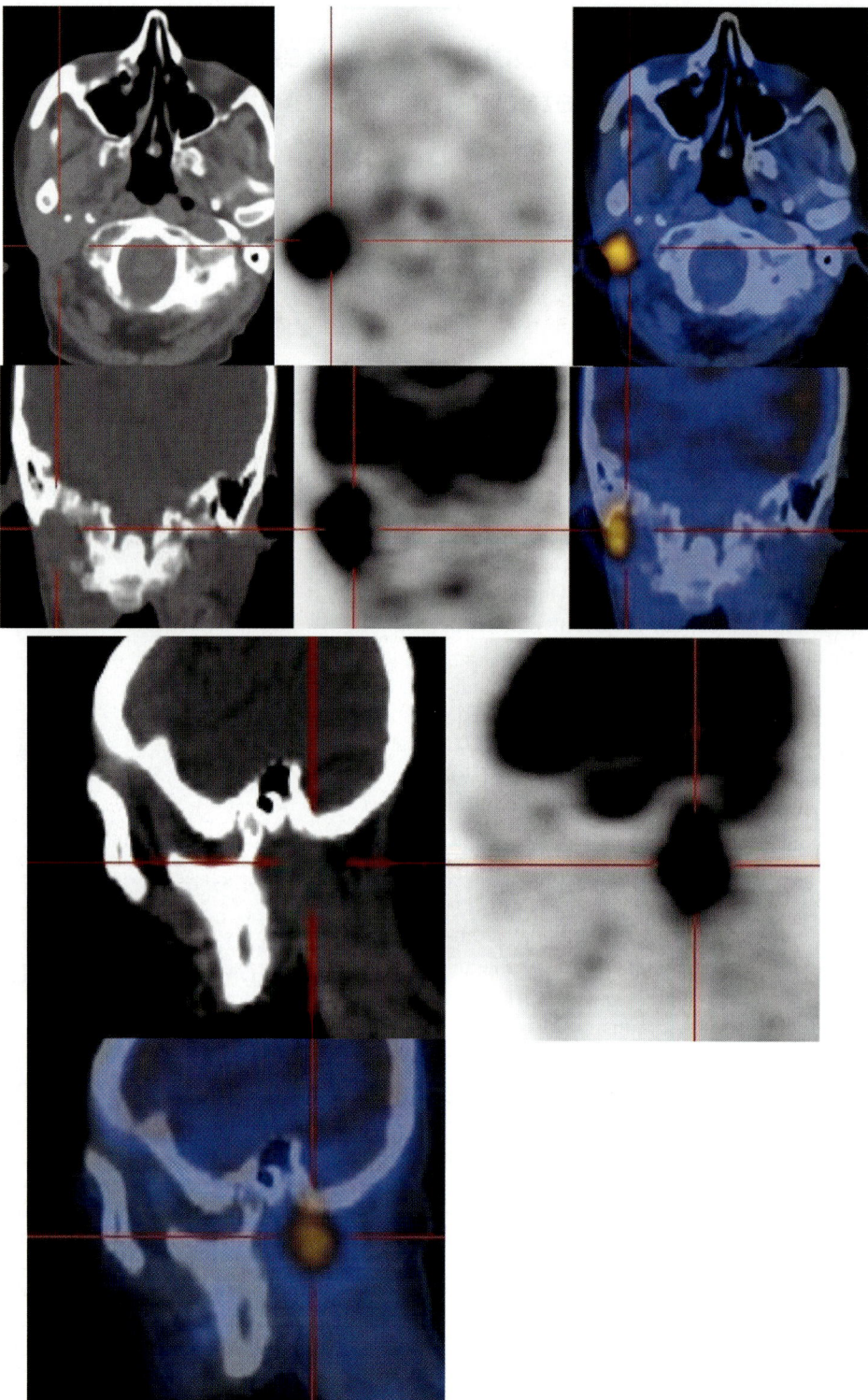

Fig. 3.2 The MIP image demonstrates the intense metabolism of the right ear-parotid nodule

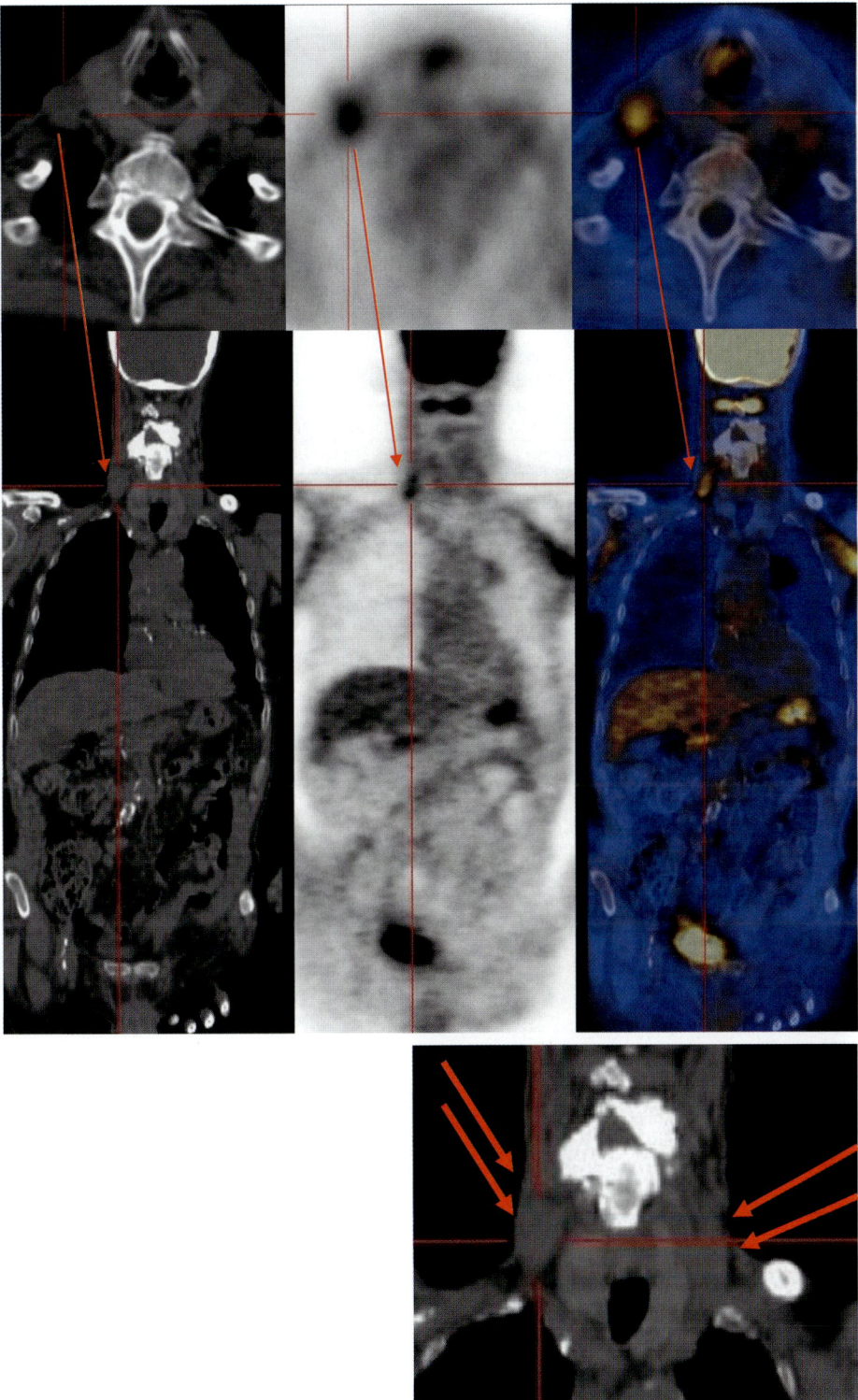

Fig. 3.3 PET: limited increase of glucose metabolism in the lower left laterocervical area

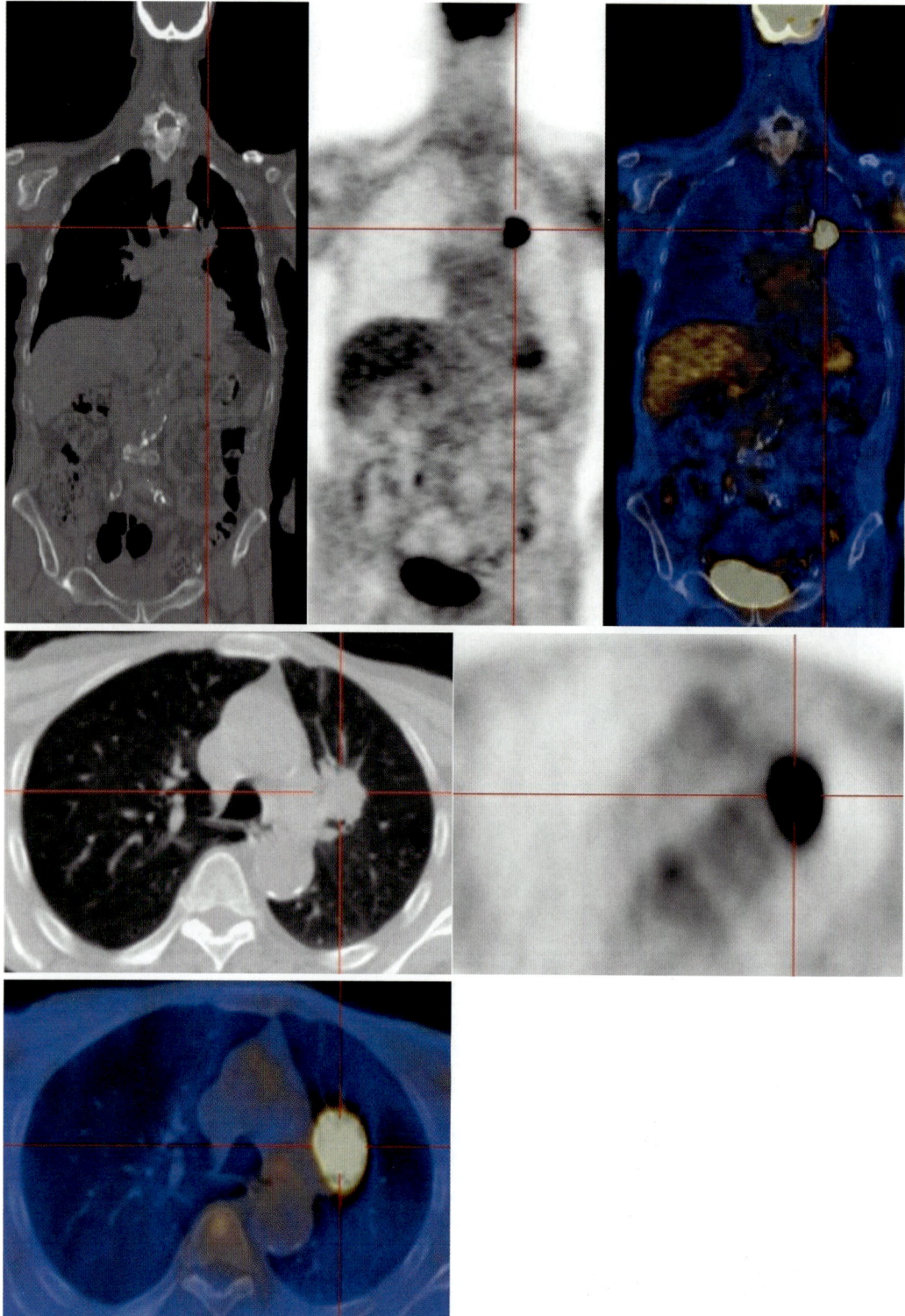

Fig. 3.4 CT-PET: at the lingula, a solid speculated mass with irregular margins, indistinguishable from the hilum, which has intense carbohydrate consumption

3.2 Diagnostic Question

Search for focal lesions with high glucose metabolism in patient with squamous cell carcinoma of the ear after surgery: restaging.

3.3 Report

Nodule with a high consumption of glucose in the ear—right parotid region extending to the temporal and sphenoid bones, which are infiltrated, SUV max 12.

Left lung mass with extensive metabolism, not clearly dissociable from the ipsilateral hilum, SUV max 16.

Limited metabolic activation in the lower right laterocervical area, indicating a muscular nonspecific concentration of FDG, SUV max 2.2.

3.4 Conclusions

The PET scan shows loco-regional recurrence of disease in the right parotid area, extending to the temporo-sphenoidal area, with metachronous lung cancer (Fig. 3.1).

The MIP image demonstrates the intense metabolism of the right ear-parotid nodule and left pulmonary mass.

Widespread activation of some muscle groups of the neck is shown, with the arms presenting an antalgic attitude.

In the right ear—parotid CT-PET a solid, uneven nodule can be seen, characterized by intense consumption of glucose (Fig. 3.2).

In the axial images it is evident the locoregional bone infiltration of the temporal and sphenoid, that appear eroded. See also (Figs 3.3, 3.4).

CT shows no focal adenopathies, so this can be considered as non-specific accumulation, caused by muscle activation.

3.5 Key points

- It is not easy to determine whether lung mass is a metastasis or metachronous cancer.
- The biopsy in these cases is not always conclusive.

You can suspect a metachronous cancer here because

- CT-PET shows a lung mass of considerable size;
- at their onset secondary injuries are multiple and smaller;
- metastases are generally mantellar, rarely involving the hilum;
- squamous tumors frequently have synchronous or metachronous localizations.

Laryngeal Squamous Carcinoma: Staging

4

4.1 Clinical History

67-year-old man with hoarseness and swelling in the left high latero-cervical area.

- Ultrasound of the neck: morpho-volumetric normal thyroid, homogeneous echotexture without focal lesions. In the left latero-cervical area presence of transonic nodule posterior to the sternocleidomastoid.
- Laryngoscopy with biopsy: squamous cell carcinoma of the larynx.
- CT: regular morphology of the nasopharynx. The left aryepiglottic fold is flattened with a swelling below that shows inhomogeneous enhancement after contrast and a contextual hypodense areola. This lesion protruding into the lumen, has contiguity/continuity with adjacent structures, in particular the lower left horn of the thyroid cartilage that is incorporated. The lesion extends caudally up to a plane passing through the true vocal cords. On the left, subcentimetric deep latero-cervical and back-submandibular lymph nodes are found. Posterior to the sternocleidomastoid muscle at the level of the thyroid cartilage, a 4 cm round formation of liquid density that displaces adjacent structures can be seen; it particularly compresses the jugular vein and slips anterior to it.

4.2 Diagnostic Question

Search for focal lesions with high glucose metabolism in patient with squamous cell carcinoma of the larynx: staging.

4.3 Report

The nodule at the left laryngeal aryepiglottic fold shows pathological consumption of FDG, SUV max 6.7.

The deep lateral cervical lymph nodes on the left and the retro-ipsilateral submandibular described in the CT scan found in the history, shows limited metabolism, SUV max 0.9.

No areas of abnormal FDG deposition in the remaining body segments examined. See Figs. 4.1, 4.2.

4.4 Conclusions

The PET scan shows high glucose consumption of the laryngeal lesion on the left.

The small groups are characterized by ipsilateral adenopathies with limited metabolism, therefore of nonspecific meaning

P. F. Rambaldi, *Whole-Body FDG PET Imaging in Oncology*,
DOI: 10.1007/978-88-470-5295-6_4, © Springer-Verlag Italia 2014

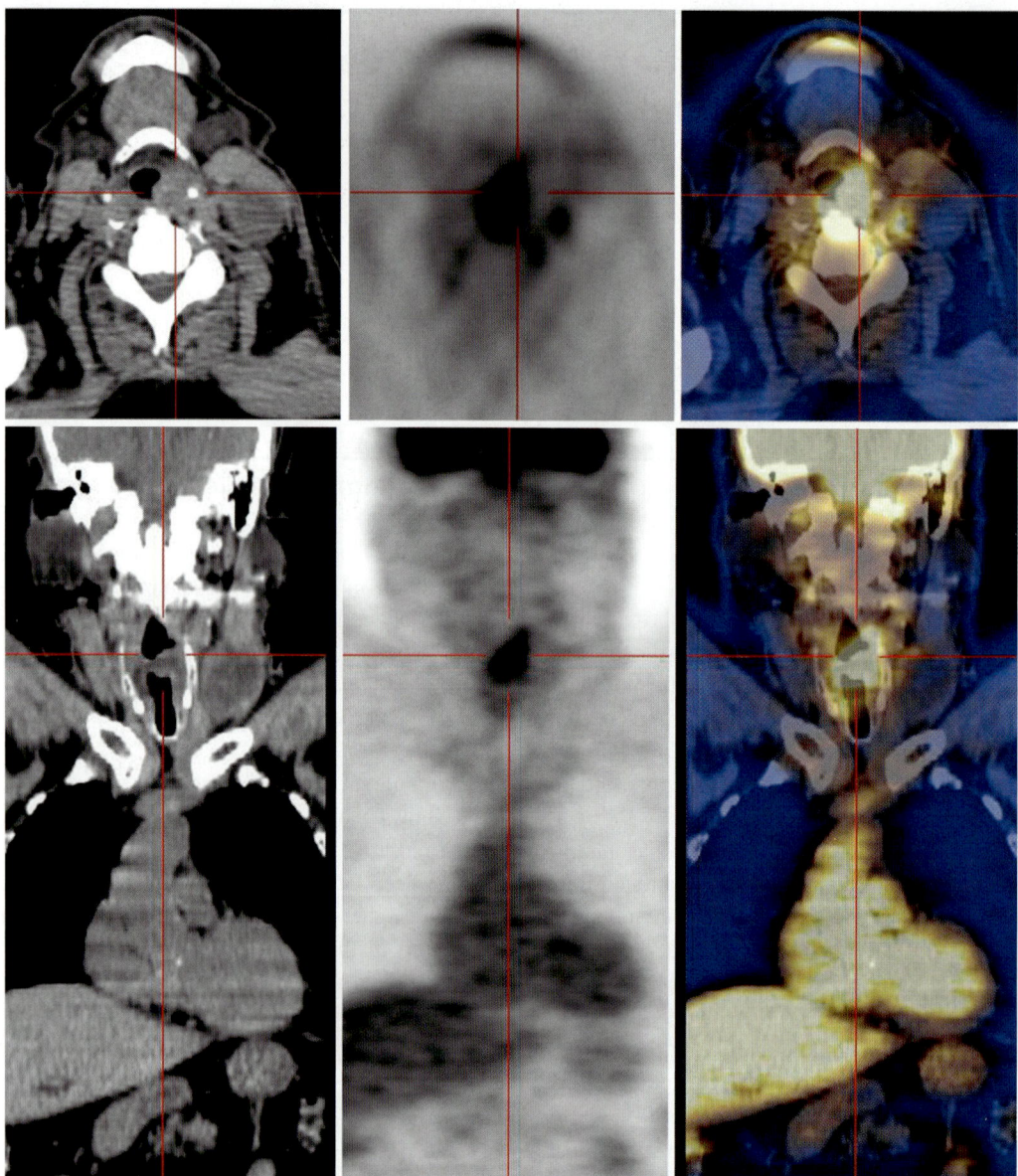

Fig. 4.1 The PET-CT scan shows a hypodense mass below the aryepiglottic fold that is expressed partly in the lumen and has relationships with the lower left horn of the thyroid cartilage, from which it is separable. The lesion drops infero-posteriorly to the true vocal cords and shows increased metabolism

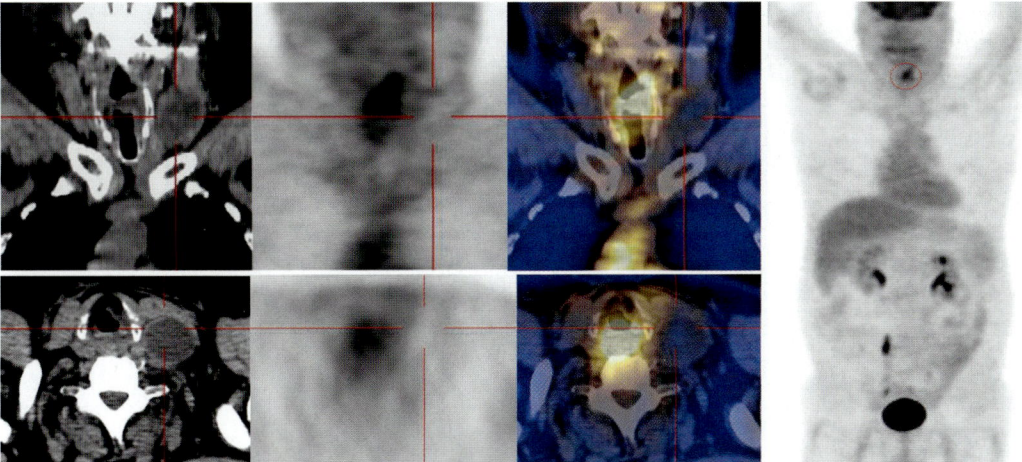

Fig. 4.2 CT-PET shows below the thyroid cartilage, behind the sternocleidomastoid, a cystic, oval image with no metabolism, displacing the jugular vein and slipping anteriorly to it

4.5   Key Points

- In patients with laryngeal cancer, PET does not provide crucial information in the diagnostic definition of the parameter T;
- However, the volume of consumption of glucose correlates with the biological aggressiveness of the disease, thus expressing the lesional grading;
- It is always important to rule out distant metastases or synchronous tumors for the obvious change in the therapeutic program that would follow.

Squamous Neoplasia of the Subglottic Region

5

5.1 Clinical History

79-year-old man with worsening dysphonia, secondary to squamous neoplasia of the subglottic region left, in staging.

5.2 Diagnostic Question

Search for focal secondary lesions with high glucose metabolism.

5.3 Report

The PET scan shows two nodules in the laryngeal subglottic, median—left paramedian area, the first measuring 1 cm and showing pathological glucose consumption, SUV max 5.8, the other measuring a millimeter with limited metabolism, probably a satellite lesion (Fig. 5.1, *arrows*).

5.4 Conclusions

The FDG PET shows high concentration of the subglottic cancer. Absence of lesions characterized by abnormal metabolism in the remaining parts of the body examined.

5.5 Key Points

- PET-CT shows high incidence of false-positives in the detection of tumors in glottis because it has limited value in diagnostic definition of the parameter T. On the other hand, tumors can be detected more accurately by determining the parameters N and M when compared to CT alone or with MRI.

P. F. Rambaldi, *Whole-Body FDG PET Imaging in Oncology*,
DOI: 10.1007/978-88-470-5295-6_5, © Springer-Verlag Italia 2014

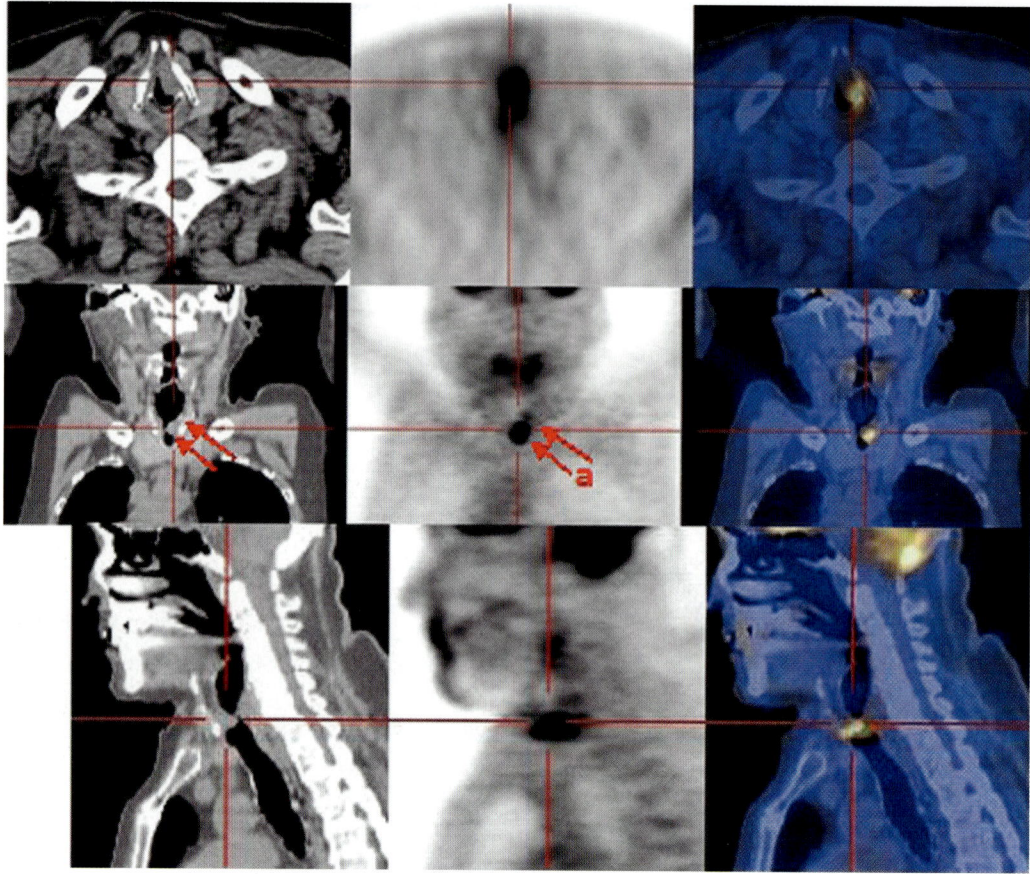

Fig. 5.1 Satellite lesion

- The high glucose consumption of the tumor shows a direct correlation with locoregional invasiveness, grading, and histology.

Squamous Ulcerated Carcinoma of the Tongue: Restaging After Chemotherapy

6

6.1 Clinical History

67-year-old ex-smoker with a diagnosis of squamous cell ulcerated carcinoma of the tongue; the patient did not undergo surgery.

- PET: hyperaccumulation in the oropharyngeal (SUV max 23) and right lateral cervical upper regions (SUV max 13.8).
- CT: voluminous ulcerated lesion of the tongue with extending to the right over the median raphe and the floor of the mouth. Presence of compressive phenomena at the level of the ipsilateral vallecula with submandibular extension. Right retromandibular adenopathy (max = 15 mm). Apparent interruption of the right mandibular margin on the vestibular side. Presence of lymph nodes in the left lateral cervical region, anterior to the neurovascular structures of the neck.

  Chemotherapy was then performed.

6.2 Diagnostic Question

Restaging of carcinoma of the tongue, 14 days after the end of chemotherapy: search for focal lesions with a high metabolism of glucose (Fig. 6.1).

6.3 Report

Compared to the previous scan, reduction of carbohydrate consumption of the paramedian right lesion of the floor of the mouth can be seen today, SUV max 8.

Retromandibular right adenopathy with limited metabolism due to chemotherapy, SUV max 0.8. No areas of abnormal glucose consumption in other parts of the body examined.

6.4 Conclusions

The PET scan shows partial response to chemotherapy, with persistence of disease with a high metabolism at the primary lesion at the level of the floor of the mouth.

6.5 Key Points

- The metabolic study is critical in restaging after chemotherapy to define the actual response determined by the treatment, the subsequent treatment plan, and prognosis.
- CT alone does not define the vitality of cancer because it does not differentiate the fibrotic share from the residual tumor.

P. F. Rambaldi, *Whole-Body FDG PET Imaging in Oncology*,
DOI: 10.1007/978-88-470-5295-6_6, © Springer-Verlag Italia 2014

Fig. 6.1 At the CT scan, a coarse solid mass extending to the right beyond the median raphe and the floor of the mouth can be seen. It is associated with retromandibular right nodal mass measuring more than a centimeter. A PET scan shows incomplete response to chemotherapy for the presence of residual lesional vitality. The right submandibular lymph node on CT scan size is increased, but has little metabolic activity, which is probably due to chemotherapy. This is also a useful element in the definition of subsequent therapeutic and prognostic strategy

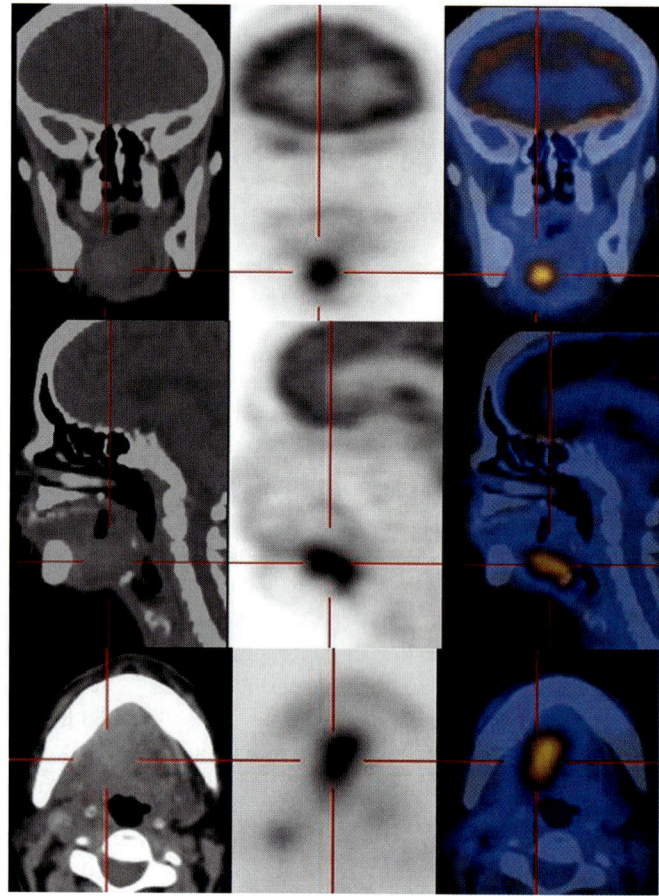

- At MRI, it is not always possible to quantify the proportion of residual vital tissue after treatment.
- Compared with CT and MRI, CT-PET alone better defines the prognosis after chemotherapy in the course of "restaging"; the persistence of metabolic activity after treatment indicates an incomplete response and suggests a worse prognosis.

- After the second cycle of chemotherapy (interim PET), the persistence of high metabolic activity correlates with a low survival rate, while a lesional reduction in the consumption of 30 % glucose compared baseline examination suggests a better prognosis.

Undifferentiated Carcinoma of the Nasopharynx: Restaging After Surgery and Radiochemotherapy

7

7.1 Clinical History

55-year-old man with undifferentiated carcinoma of the nasopharynx: restaging after surgery.
- total body CT: presence of bilateral lateral cervical lymph node swelling.
- neck MRI: latero-cervical multiple lymph nodes on both sides with a maximum diameter of 32 mm on the left.
- PET: pathological glucose consumption in lateral cervical lymph nodes indicating bilateral metastatic lesions.

  Reassessment after adjuvant chemotherapy and radiotherapy of the primary lesion.
- neck MRI: bilateral lateral cervical lymph nodes are smaller than they were in the previous scan.
- Skull, neck, chest, abdomen CT: small bilateral lateral cervical lymph node swelling.

7.2 Diagnostic Question

Search for focal lesions with high glucose metabolism in patient with undifferentiated carcinoma of the nasopharynx: restaging after radiotherapy and adjuvant chemotherapy, the latter terminated by 4 weeks.

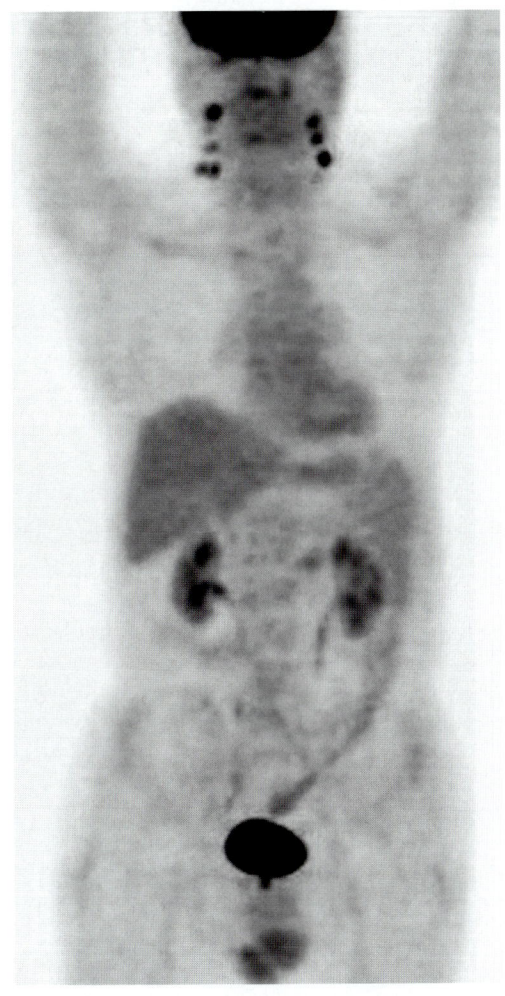

Fig. 7.1 The MIP image documents the presence of lymph node metastases. There are not secondary lesions in any other organs or systems

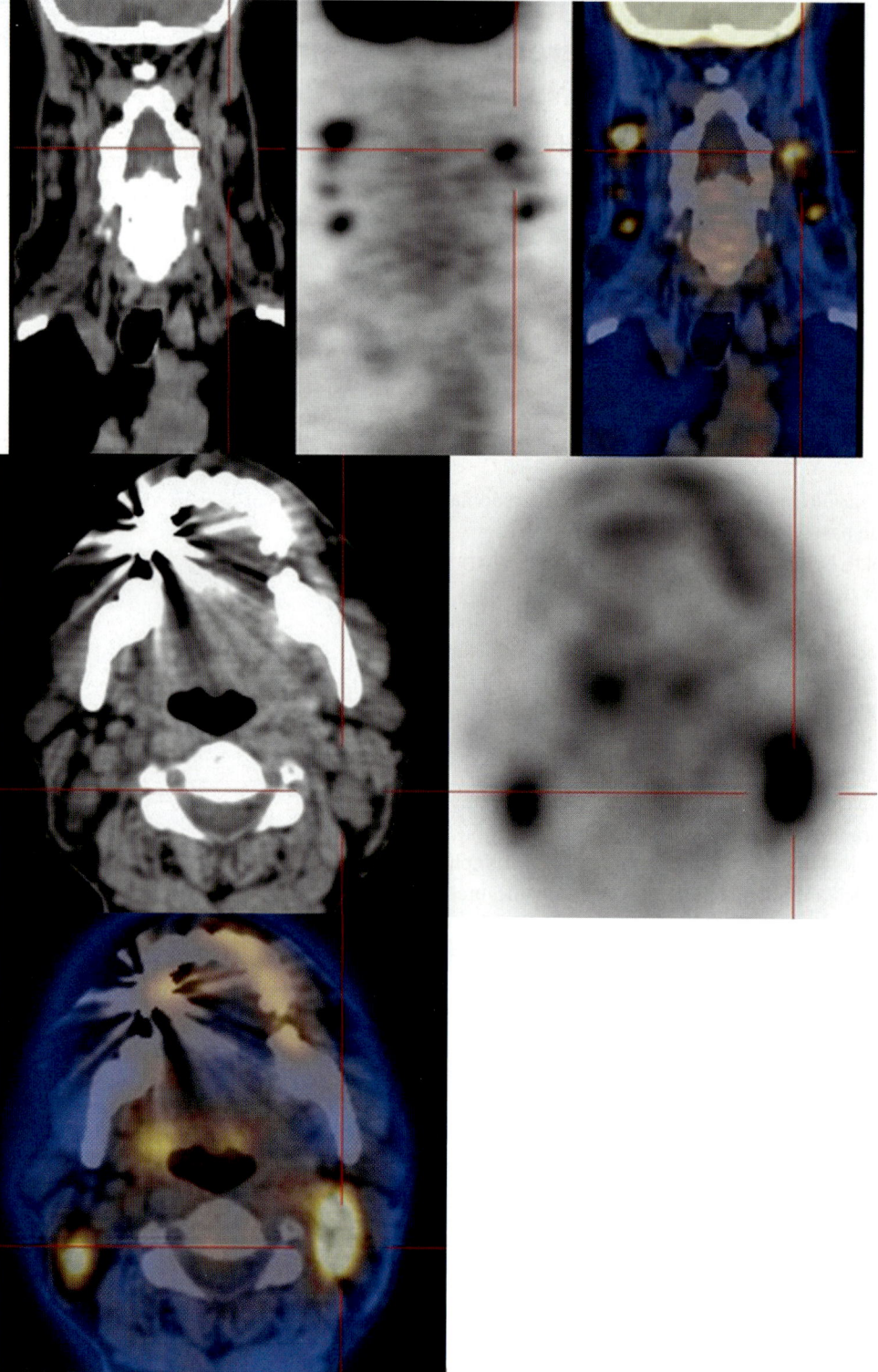

Fig. 7.2 In correspondence with the lateral triangle of the neck, CT-PET shows multiple nodes bilaterally increased in size, some, measuring more than a centimeter, characterized by intense glucose metabolism

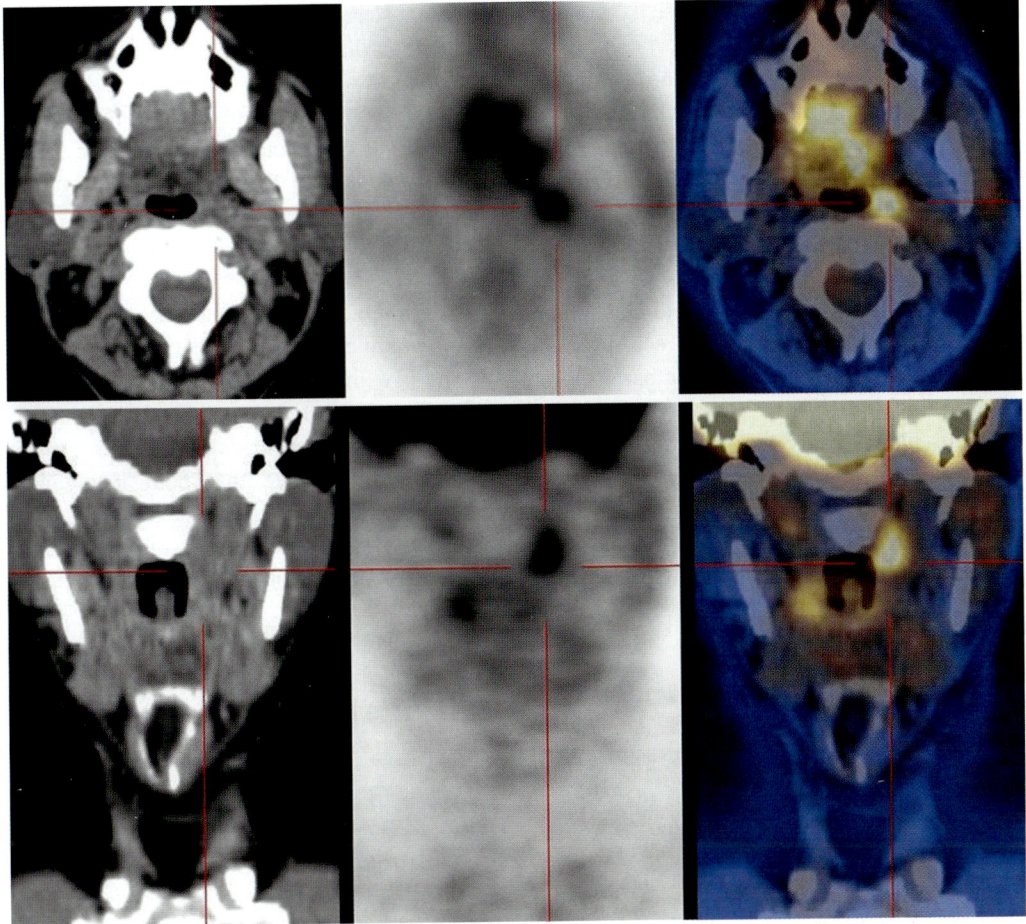

Fig. 7.3 CT-PET: presence of hypodense tissue in the left retropharyngeal region, with limited metabolism, therefore, to be attributed to post—actinic remodeling

7.3   Report

Multiple centimetric lymph nodes characterized by pathological consumption of glucose in the lateral cervical and bilateral submandibular regions, SUV max 8.5.

Mild metabolic activity in the retropharyngeal left, SUV max 2.6, and right regions, SUV max 2.2, due to actinic remodeling.

Absence of significant areas of pathological glucose consumption in the remaining body segments examined.

7.4   Conclusions

The PET scan shows persistence of disease with intense deposition of FDG due to involvement of the lateral cervical and submandibular lymph nodes on both sides.

The coronal reconstruction provides an overview of metastatic involvement of the lymph nodes on both sides. See Figures 7.1-7.3.

7.5 Key Points

CT-PET has a limited role in the staging of cancer of the head and neck, in particular in defining the extent of locoregional disease;

- it is essential in the characterization of lymph node status and the search for distant metastases;
- it is irreplaceable in the follow-up to determine cell vitality after radio- and chemotherapy to exclude locoregional recurrence or progression of disease in other parts of the body.

In this patient, only the primary tumor was radiotreated; therefore, we can say that the CT-PET scan defines:

- good response to radiotherapy in a nasopharyngeal lesion does not show high deposition of FDG,

- the presence of limited carbohydrate consumption due to actinic reaction in the radiotreated area,
- poor response to chemotherapy for the persistence of high metabolism and vitality of the lymph nodes. In these cases, some authors suggest lymphadenectomy.
- no substantial progression of the disease because:
  - the individual lesions do not show increase in volumetric and metabolic activity
  - no new metastases.

The persistence of nodal disease is a poor prognostic sign, correlates with lower survival and a higher chance that both locoregional recurrence and distant metastases could be found in the subsequent follow-up.

Zygomatic Spinalioma and Synchronous Pulmonary Neoplasm

8

8.1 Clinical History

76-year-old man with epidermoid lung cancer: staging.

- CT: 26 × 24 mm nodule in the dorsal and lateral segments of the lower lobe of the right lung. Presence of two ground-glass areas respectively in the upper lobe of the right lung and the posterior segment of the ipsilateral lower lobe.

- Bronchoscopy: Chronic inflammation of the larynx. Presence of protruding lesion in the lower right lobar bronchial lumen.
- Biopsy: epidermoid carcinoma.

8.2 Diagnostic Question

NSCLC in staging: research for focal lesions with a high glucose metabolism.

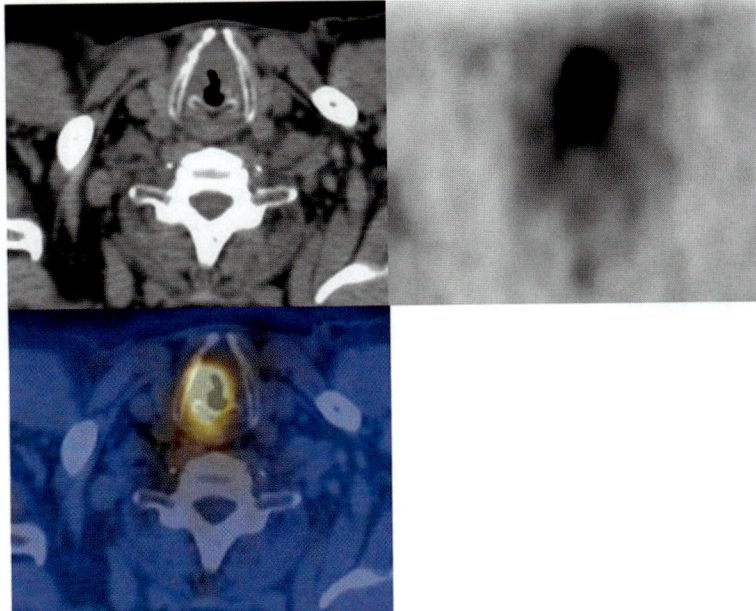

Fig. 8.1 Diffuse thickening of the laryngeal mucosa, with no solid focal nodular lesions seen

P. F. Rambaldi, *Whole-Body FDG PET Imaging in Oncology*,
DOI: 10.1007/978-88-470-5295-6_8, © Springer-Verlag Italia 2014

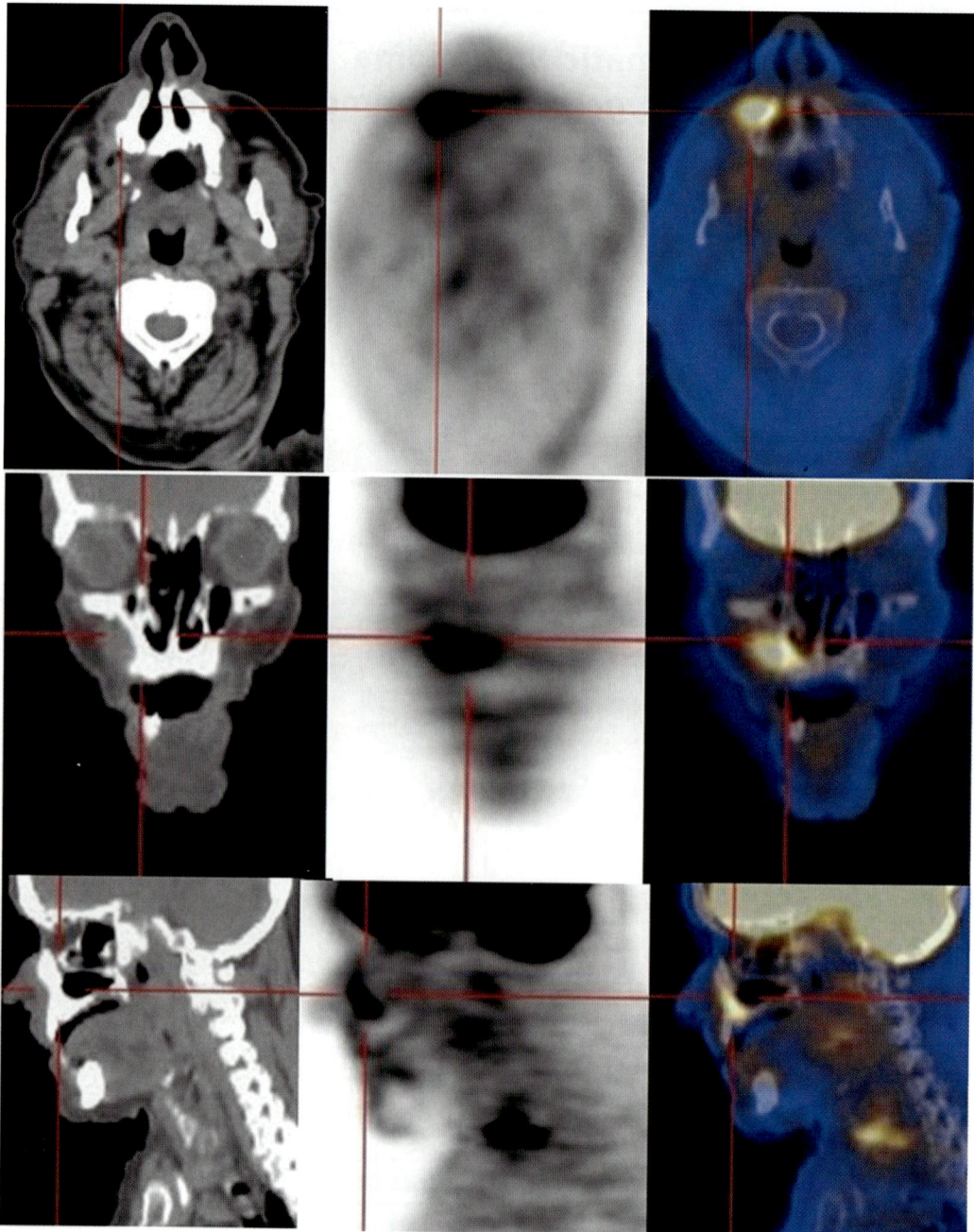

Fig. 8.2 CT scans show a diffuse thickening of the laryngeal mucosa, with no solid focal nodular lesions seen

8.3   Report

Pulmonary nodule with a high metabolism of glucose in the dorsal segment of the lower lobe of the right lung, SUV max 11.8.

Pathological glucose consumption in the region under the right-orbital superficial cutaneous and subcutaneous planes, in correspondence of a palpable mass of hard-wood consistency, SUV max 9. (See Figs. 8.1, 8.2).

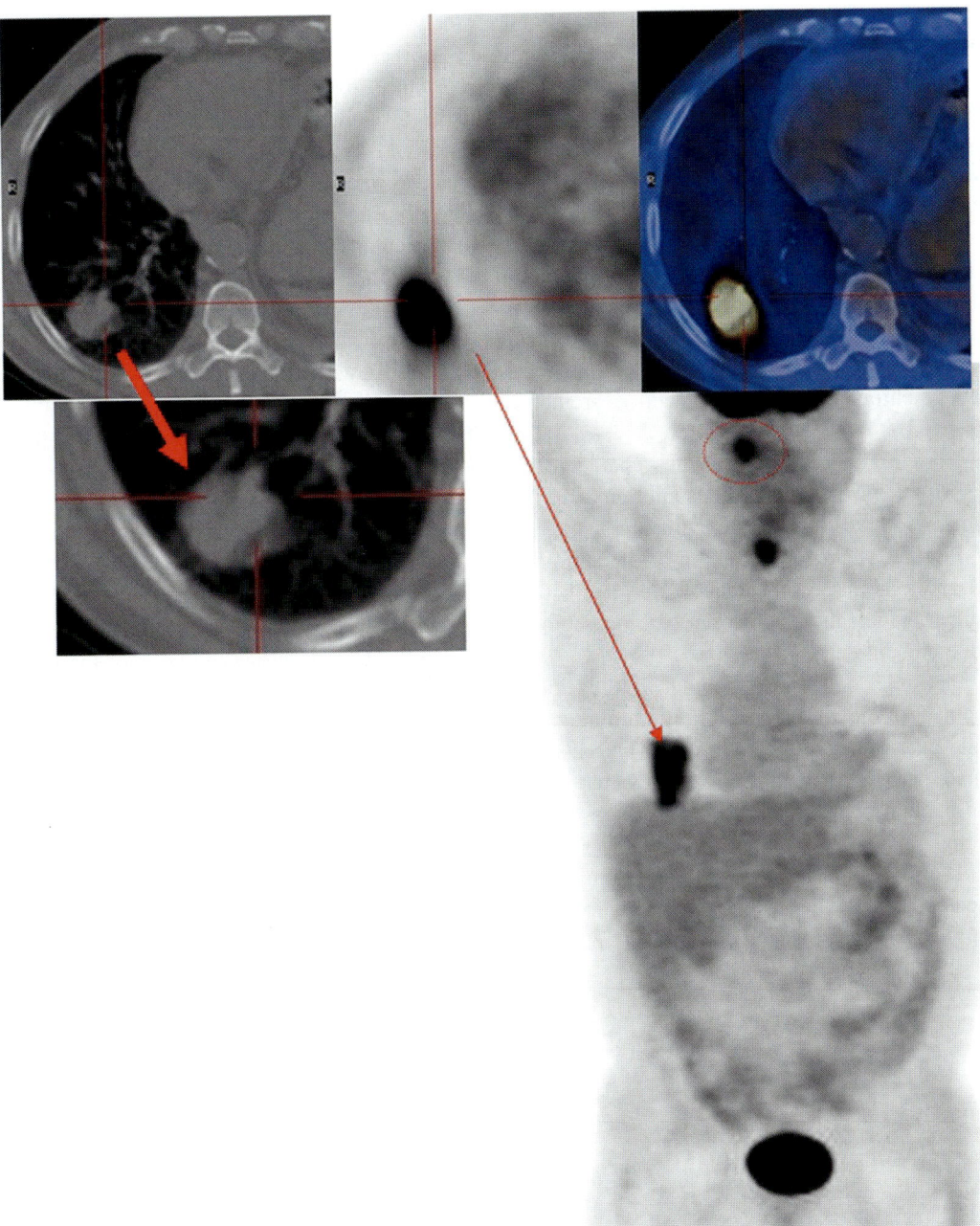

Fig. 8.3 Synchronous squamous cell carcinoma

Increased deposition of FDG to the larynx correlates to chronic inflammation, already reported in the bronchoscopic examination in medical history, SUV max 6.

On CT scans, there is a diffuse thickening of the laryngeal mucosa which shows no solid focal nodular lesions (Figs. 8.1, 8.2).

The PET scan shows widespread and increased concentration of FDG that does not resemble the typical features of nodular malignant processes.

8.4   Conclusions

The PET scan shows the right pulmonary neoplasm with a high metabolism and a skin lesion in the ipsilateral zygomatic region, which is also metabolically active, consistent with a diagnosis of synchronous squamous cell carcinoma (Fig. 8.3).

Absence of metastatic lesions characterized by high carbohydrate consumption in the remaining body segments examined.

PET-CT: marked thickening of the sub-orbital and zygomatic subcutaneous tissues, with a high metabolism of glucose. No locoregional bone erosion detected.

PET-CT: pulmonary nodule in the dorsal segment of the lower lobe of the right lung. This solid mass is uneven, with irregular margins and small peripheral dendritic branches that reach the parietal pleura. The glucose consumption is high.

The MIP image demonstrates the intense metabolism of the lesion, which is seen as elliptical rather than nodular. This effect is produced by respiratory motion artifacts that can be observed in all types of reconstructions, especially in CT-PET images. At least part of these artifacts are determined from different times and by different modes of acquisition of the two methods, the relative reconstruction algorithms, processing and re-alignment of data. In particular, while the CT scan takes only a few seconds, the PET takes 10–20 min.

8.5   Key Points

It is not always possible to determine whether:
• the patient is affected by two synchronous neoplasms,
• skin cancer is primitive while the lung is secondary,
• it is unlikely that the lung cancer produced skin metastases.

The acute and chronic diseases of the larynx frequently lead to high metabolic activity secondary to nonspecific inflammatory phenomena. In these cases, you must
• obtain a detailed medical history,
• correlate with CT images to exclude morphological lesions,
• send the patient to an ENT specialist for a laryngoscopy.

Bone-Destroying Metastases in Thyroid Undifferentiated Carcinoma

9

9.1   Clinical History

A 71-year-old man with increasing pain in the right jaw for 2 months.

- Thyroid Ultrasound: inhomogeneous glandular structure, presence of some iso-hypoechoic nodules, the most evident at the isthmus measuring 47 × 35 mm, at the middle third of the left lobe measuring 29 × 25 mm; another one measuring 20 × 10 mm is at the base of the right lobe. Subcentimetric lateral cervical lymph reactive nodes on both sides.
- Facial bones CT: large structural lithic alteration in the right body of the mandible extended to the rising branch. Osteolysis of the right basisphenoid with erosion of the clivus. Osteolytic alterations of the body of C2 with involvement of the epistropheum and the body of C3.
- Chest X-ray: morphostructural bone alteration with swollen appearance of the posterior portion of the ninth right rib.
- Bone scan: (See Fig. 9.1).

9.2   Diagnostic Question

Search for occult malignancy in patients with bone metastases: definition of glucose metabolism.

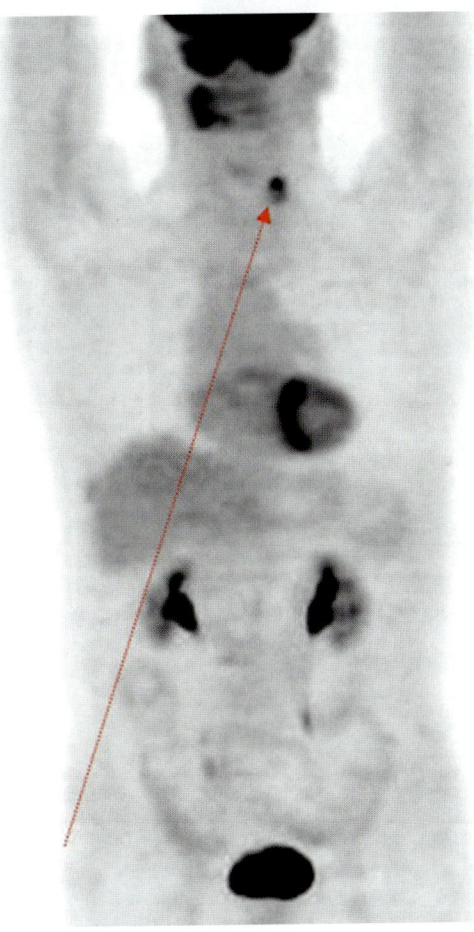

Fig. 9.1 Pathological accumulation of radiocompound on the right in the jaw and the ipsilateral ninth costal arch

P. F. Rambaldi, *Whole-Body FDG PET Imaging in Oncology*,
DOI: 10.1007/978-88-470-5295-6_9, © Springer-Verlag Italia 2014

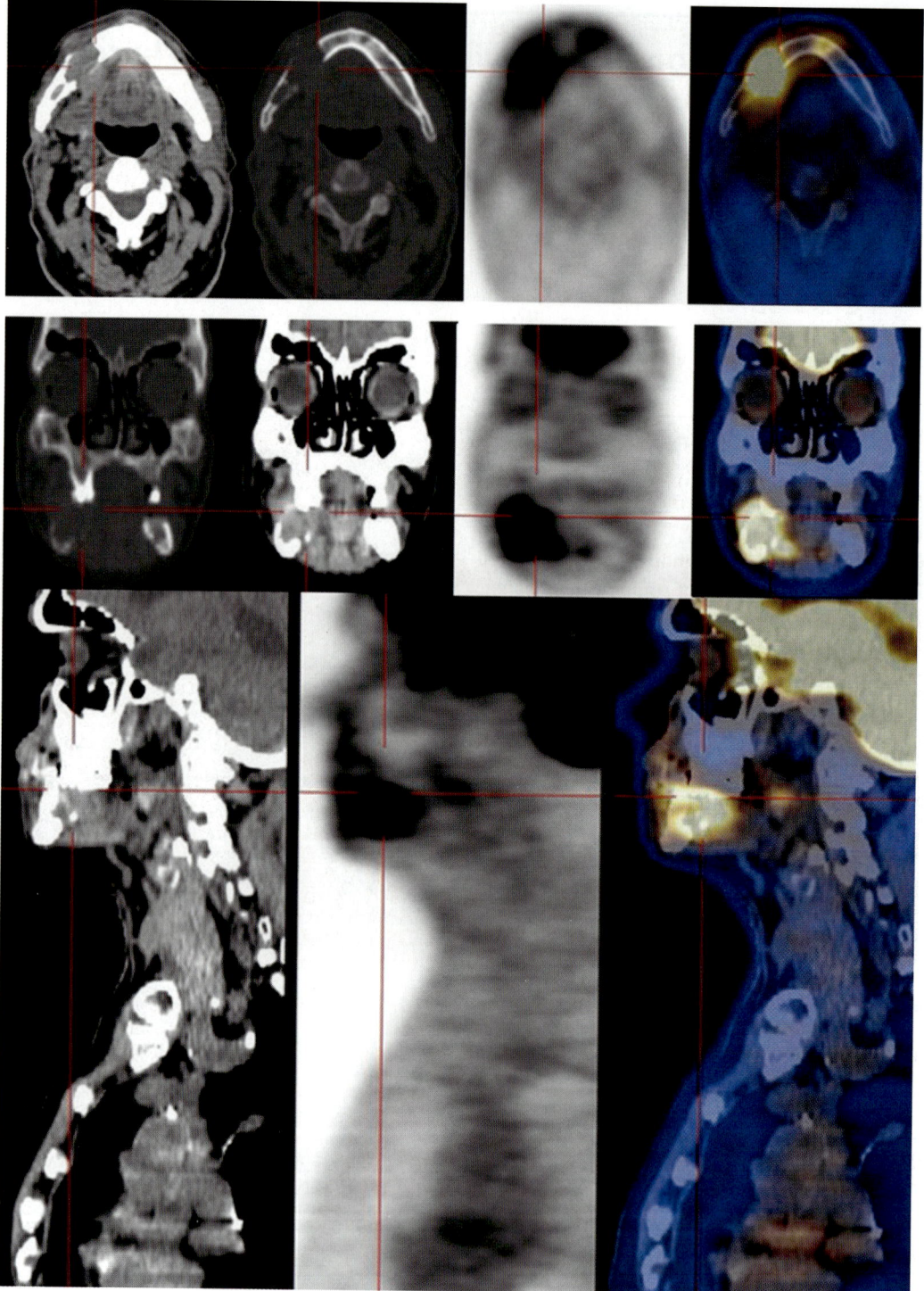

Fig. 9.2 At CT-PET, there is an evident structural alteration of the right jaw with extended osteolysis and cortical interruption; presence of newly formed solid replacement tissue invades surrounding tissues. The lesional glucose metabolism is high

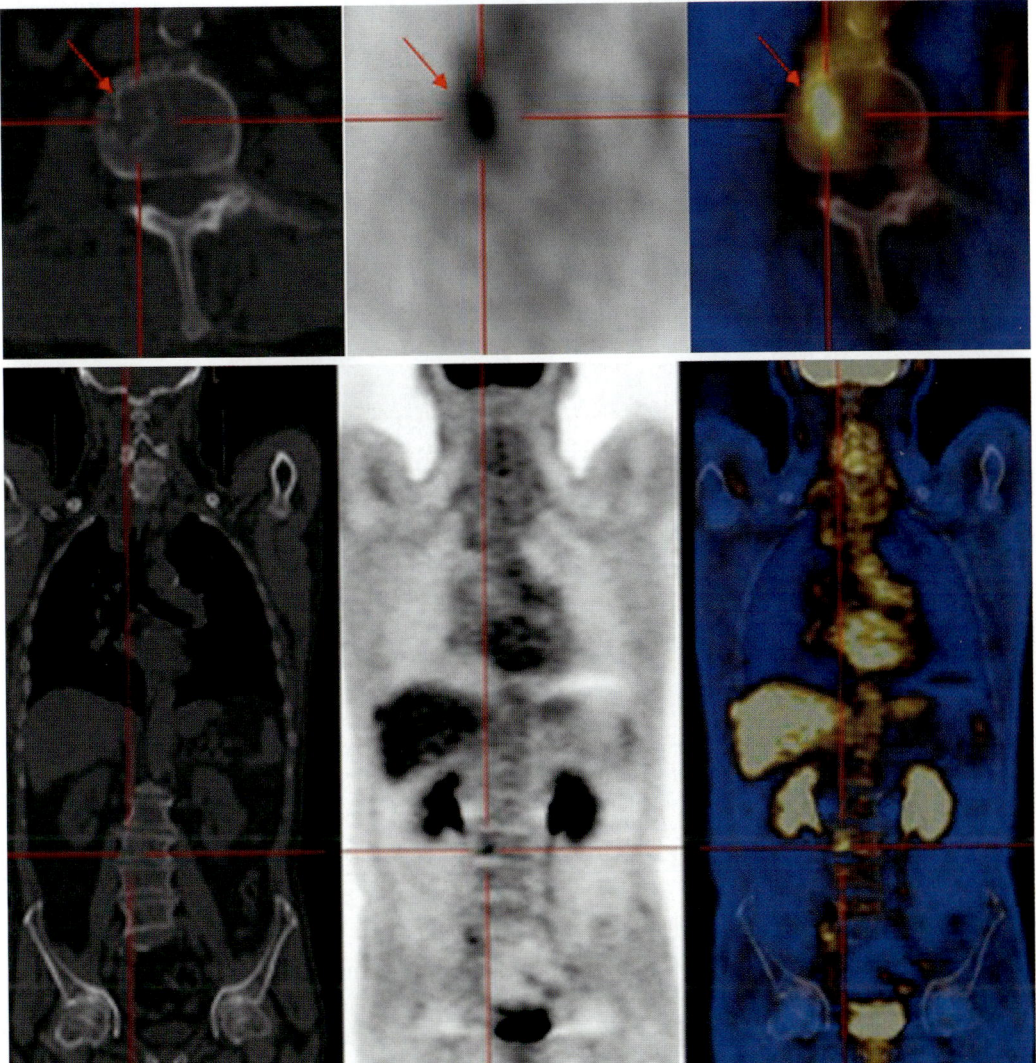

Fig. 9.3 At CT-PET, the right emisoma of L3 shows a focal morphostructural alteration which seems lytic, but there is no interruption of the cortex, the lesional margins are sclerotic and lesional metabolism is low. These elements suggest a benign, slow-growing condition, due to arthritic resorption phenomena of trabecular type

9.3   Report

Bone lesions reported in history at the right jaw and the ninth ipsilateral costal arch, have intense glucose consumption, SUV max 11 (Fig. 9.1).

Presence of left thyroid nodule with a high metabolism, SUV max 8, of doubtful meaning, to be studied by FNAB.

Slight increase in the consumption of FDG of the basisphenoid to the right, in some of the cervical (C2, C3) and a lumbar vertebrae (L3) due to degenerative involutive remodeling of osteoblastic benign type, SUV max 1.5.

No areas of pathological glucose deposition in the remaining body segments examined.

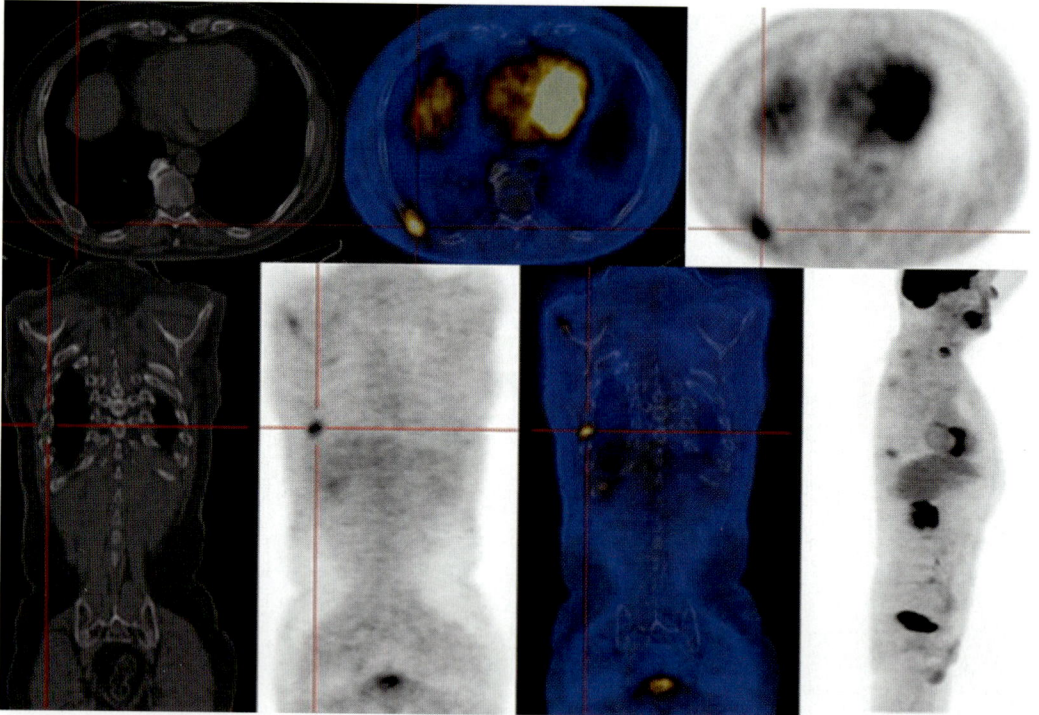

Fig. 9.4 CT-PET shows a morphostructural alteration of lytic type of the ninth posterior right costal arch that is swollen, with widespread cortical thinning. The metabolism of FDG of the lesion is high

9.4   Conclusions

The PET shows alteration of glucose consumption in the mandible and the ninth right costal arch due to metastatic disease (Fig. 9.1).

Presence of thyroid nodule with a high metabolism to evaluate cyto-histologically.

Note: the following FNAB of the thyroid nodule showed a left undifferentiated carcinoma. (See also Figs. 9.2, 9.3, 9.4, 9.5).

9.5   Key Points

In Italy, the nodular thyroid disease is widespread, and it is generally benign in nature.

On PET scans, it is the frequent occasional finding of nodular thyroid spots with high metabolic activity. This element itself is not pathognomonic of malignancy; indeed, it is totally nonspecific and is compatible with:

• toxic adenoma in functional autonomy;

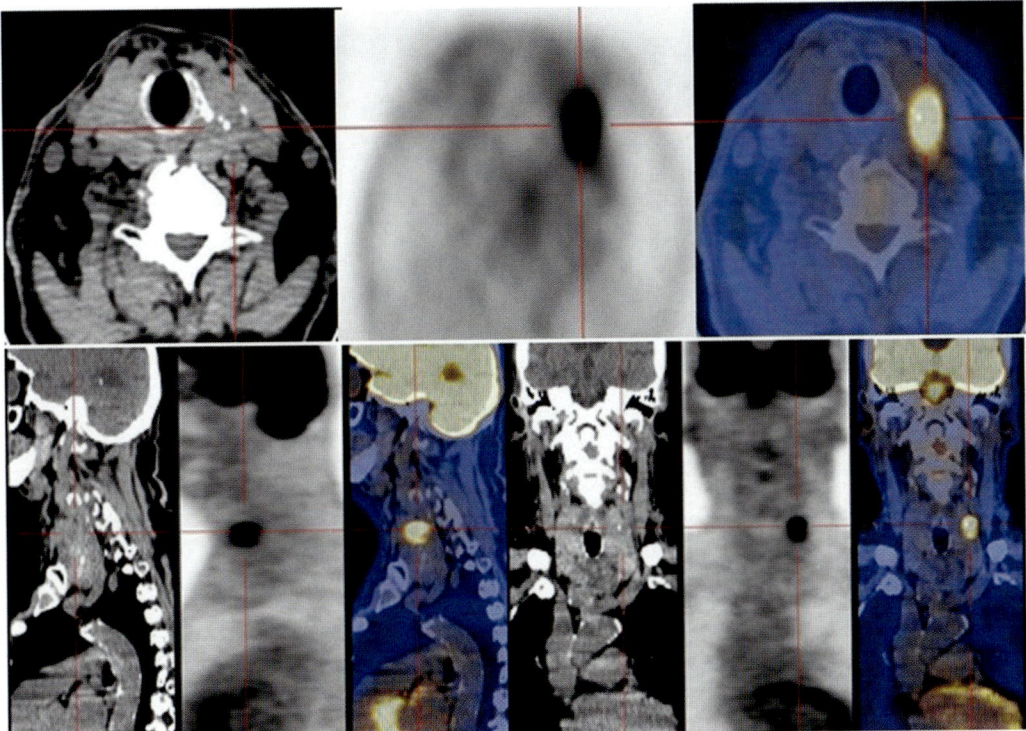

Fig. 9.5 CT-PET: multinodular goiter that exceeds the jugular region with evidence in the middle third of the left lobe of a solid, uneven nodule, with calcifications, characterized by intense focal consumption of glucose

- benign non-active nodule with high cellularity, cold on a thyroid scintigraphy;
- primary or secondary malignant disease.

In any event, the occasional finding of a thyroid hot spot to PET is a doubtful element and should be reported.

It is useful to obtain endocrinological advice, the determination of the hormonal profile, morphofunctional condition of the gland, and possibly a FNAB.

In a patient with bone metastases and occult primary tumor, the incidental finding at FDG-PET of a hot spot requires a thyroid FNAB.

- Adenocarcinomas and undifferentiated carcinomas of the thyroid have high consumption of glucose.
- The differentiated carcinomas generally have a limited metabolism of FDG.

10.1 Clinical History

58-year-old man with nasopharyngeal radio-chemotreated cancer, in remission for 18 years, with recent onset of increasing pain in the jaw.

- CT: median and left paramedian rhino-sphenoidal morphostructural alteration. Multiple areas of rarefaction of the ipsilateral maxillary and mandibular branches. Ipsilateral lymph node swellings, measuring about 15 mm in the submandibular.

Oncological report: patient with mandibular osteomyelitis seen at CT scan, that shows abnormalities related to bone suffering from radiation therapy in the ethmoido-sphenoidal region. Biopsy: chronic inflammation. The clinical and fiberoptic endoscopic evaluation of the district is oncologically negative. The oral cavity shows a thoroughly necrotic diastase, very sore at the level of the retromolar pad.

10.2 Diagnostic Question

Pathological fracture of the left mandible: search for focal lesions with a high metabolism of glucose.

10.3 Report

Abnormal glucose consumption to the mandibular left image shows a clear fracture, SUV max 6.5.

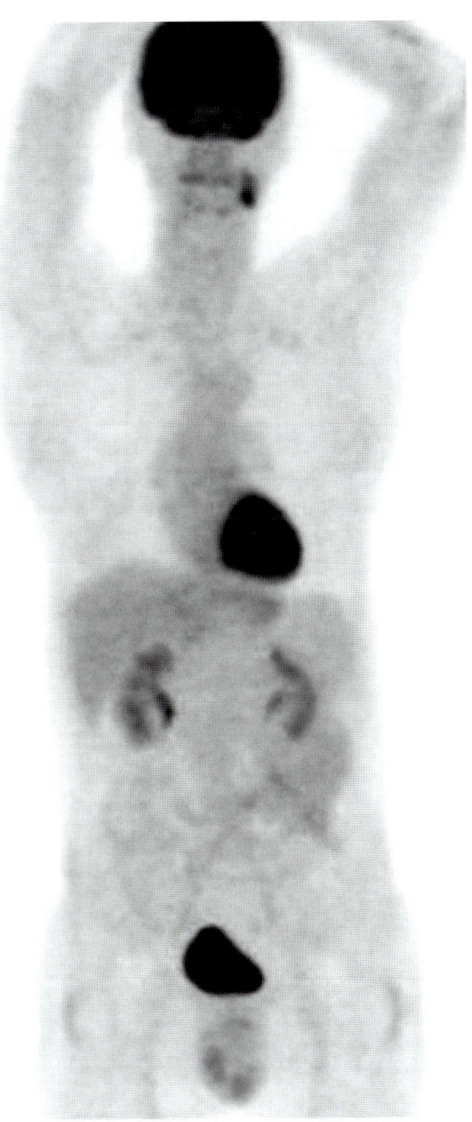

Fig. 10.1 MIP image: pathological glucose consumption in the left mandible. Absence of focal lesions with a high metabolism in other parts of the body indicating a recurrence of disease

P. F. Rambaldi, *Whole-Body FDG PET Imaging in Oncology*, DOI: 10.1007/978-88-470-5295-6_10, © Springer-Verlag Italia 2014

No areas of abnormal metabolism in the remaining parts of the body examined.

10.4 Conclusions

The PET scan shows significant increase in glucose consumption at the left mandibular region due to secondary late post-actinic fracture with metabolic activation. (See Figs. 10.1, 10.2).

10.5 Key Points

- In fractures, secondary to primary or metastatic tumors, bone appears swollen and dysmorphic for the presence of newly formed tissue with secondary disruption of cortical bone.
- In this patient, CT does not show the presence of newly formed tissue in the fracture, and the increase in glucose metabolism is determined

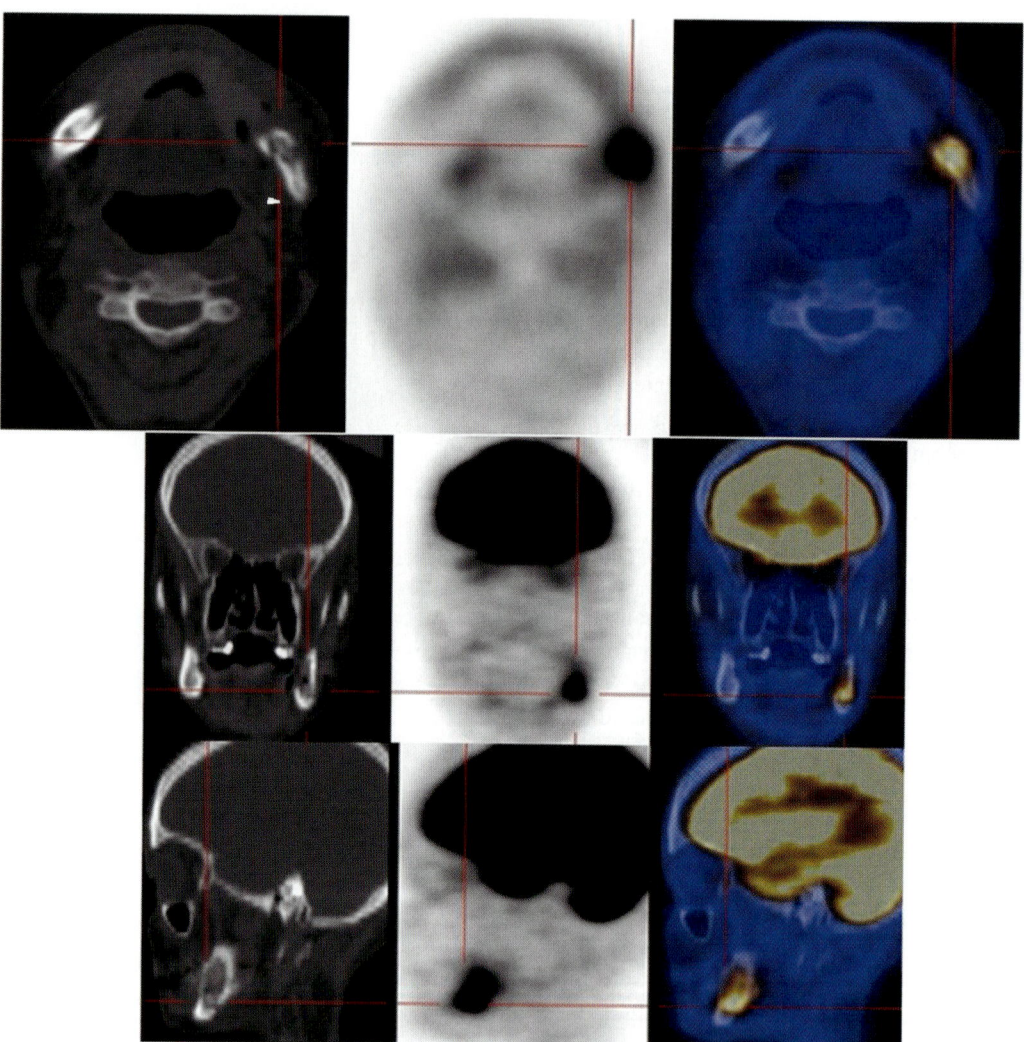

Fig. 10.2 CT-PET: gross structural alteration of the left mandibular bone trabeculae extended to the vertical branch, irregular thinning of the bone cortex, interrupted at intervals, due to dystrophic—degenerative phenomena and post-actinic late fracture. The high metabolism is determined by medullary reparative reactive activation

by the reaction and the osteoblastic bone marrow reactive reparative activation.

- A locoregional recurrence of nasopharyngeal carcinoma is generally associated with lymphadenopathy characterized by pathological metabolism.

- A carcinoma of the nasopharynx in remission for 20 years rarely results in a solitary metastatic bone lesion.

- There are not primary or secondary malignancies in any other parts of the body.

Nodal Metastases in Nasal Squamous Carcinoma

11

11.1 Clinical History

67-year-old man.

Excision of skin lesion of the lateral canthus of the right eye. Histopathologic diagnosis: "Basal cell epithelioma with areas of squamous metaplasia." Radiotherapy was performed.

11 years after, excision of a lesion at the left nasal pyramid and subsequent histological diagnosis of invasive squamous cell carcinoma with, moderately differentiated clear cell appearance.

After 4 years, onset of left lateral cervical lymphadenopathy.

- Ultrasound: in the left lateral cervical region, coarse solid, fused, inhomogeneous mass, with involvement of the submandibular and supraclavicular lymph nodes in the posterior triangle.
- CT: Large left submandibular lesion (5 × 5 cm), inseparable from the parotid gland, exceeds the angle of the jaw, arriving at the skin. This lesion has a solid, irregular structure, with central area of reduced enhancement after contrast medium injection, due to colliquative necrosis. Massive deep ipsilateral laterocervical lymphadenopathy.
- Microscopic diagnosis: sample consisting of fragments excised from the lateral cervical region: the morphological image shows diffuse infiltrating undifferentiated, small cell carcinoma.
- Chest CT: in the left apical region, fibrotic striae can be seen, with related bronchiectasis and mediastinal-para-aortic area of low density tissue thickening; ipsilateral mediastinal attraction. Parenchymal consolidation stria in the apical right region with no enhancement after contrast medium.

11.2 Diagnostic Question

Search for focal lesions with high glucose metabolism in patient with submandibular lymph node metastasis, and retroclavicular left lateral cervical infiltrating small cell carcinoma.

11.3 Report

Intense focal pathological consumption of glucose in multiple coarse lymph nodes, in the submandibular and laterocervical left retroclavear regions, SUV max 9.8.

Modest increase in glucose deposition to the nasopharynx by nonspecific inflammation SUV max 3.5.

Non-pathological metabolism mediastinal mass seen on CT.

Absence of pathological areas of concentration of FDG in the remaining parts of the body examined.

11.4   Conclusions

The PET scan showed nodal metastasis in the submandibular and laterocervical left retroclavear with high FDG metabolism, probably secondary to the previously excised ipsilateral squamous cell carcinoma of the nasal pyramid (Fig. 11.1).

No other focal lesions. Histological re-evaluation needed.

CT: massive submandibular solid, patchy lymph node swelling with irregular margins, inseparable from the adjacent tissues. It is associated in the ipsilateral deep lateral cervical region with adenopathy with similar densitometric characteristics.

The MIP image:

- allows you to appreciate the extent of the massive lymph node involvement and the intensity of FDG consumption;
- excluded abnormal metabolism of the mediastinal mass on CT reported in medical history;
- does not detect nodules characterized by abnormal glucose consumption in other parts

Fig. 11.1 The PET demonstrates the high carbohydrate metabolism of both masses (*arrows*)

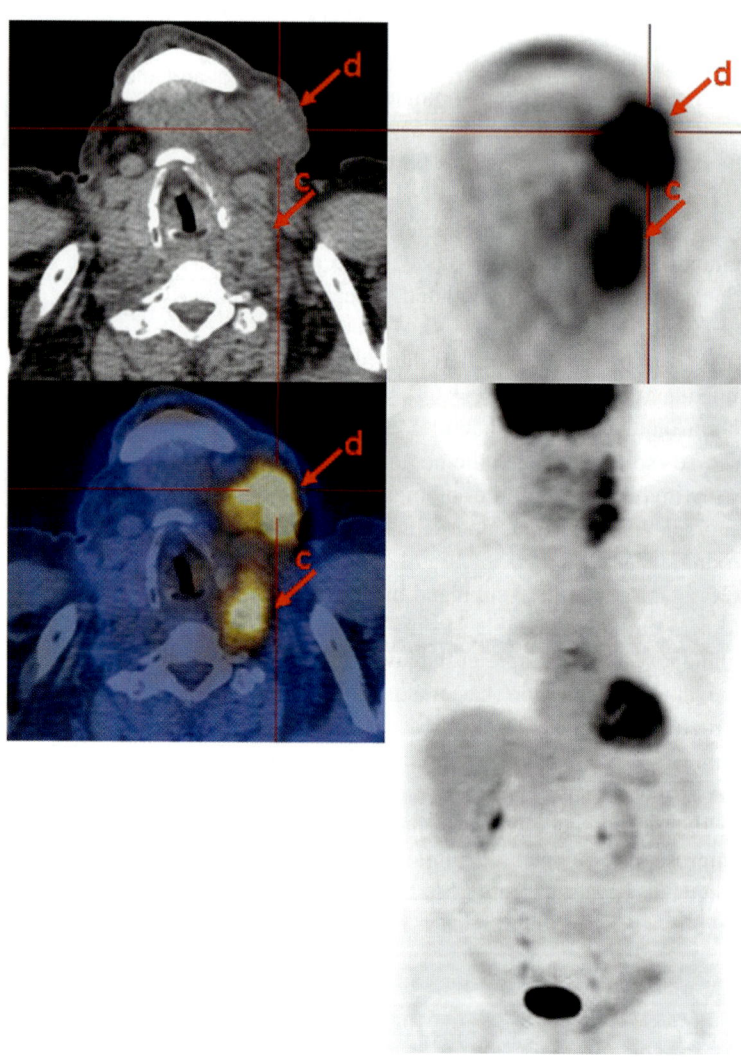

Fig. 11.2 The CT-PET shows a metastatic lymph node increased in size, hypodense, characterized by pathological metabolism, in the left sub-mandibular region (a). In the same axial section there is widespread modest increase in glucose deposition to the nasopharynx, but CT shows no nodular morphological alterations, therefore this can be attributed to non-specific inflammation (b), this element is evident in the MIP reconstruction

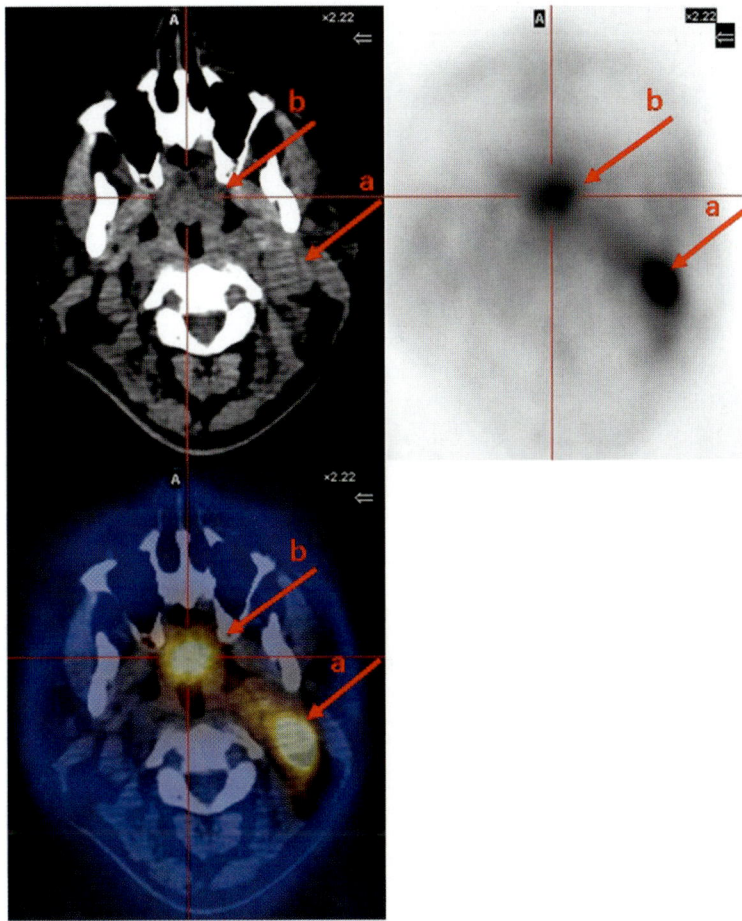

of the body due to unknown neoplastic conditions.

In these cases it is useful to re-evaluate all PET scans, CT and fusion images, reconstructed according to different axes, to rule out an occult malignancy. (See Fig. 11.2).

11.5 Key Points

PET is not always able to identify occult malignancy. In some patients, the primary lesions are very small, below the resolving power of the technique and have poor glucose metabolism.

When the PET-CT scan shows a focal consumption of glucose for suspected occult pathology, it is necessary to suggest any diagnostics additions in the report.

The nodal lesions are ipsilateral to the previously excised lesion of the nasal pyramid. A review of histological preparations would be helpful.

Final Diagnosis: undifferentiated metastases from squamous cell carcinoma.

Jugular Ulcerated Cutaneous Spinalioma

12

12.1 Clinical History

72-year-old man suffering from myelodysplastic syndrome, shows an ulcerated skin lesion of nature yet to be determined at the jugular region.

LDH = 1.290 mu/ml (NV 230-460).

12.2 Diagnostic Question

Search for focal lesions with high glucose metabolism in patient with an alleged skin spinalioma of the jugular region.

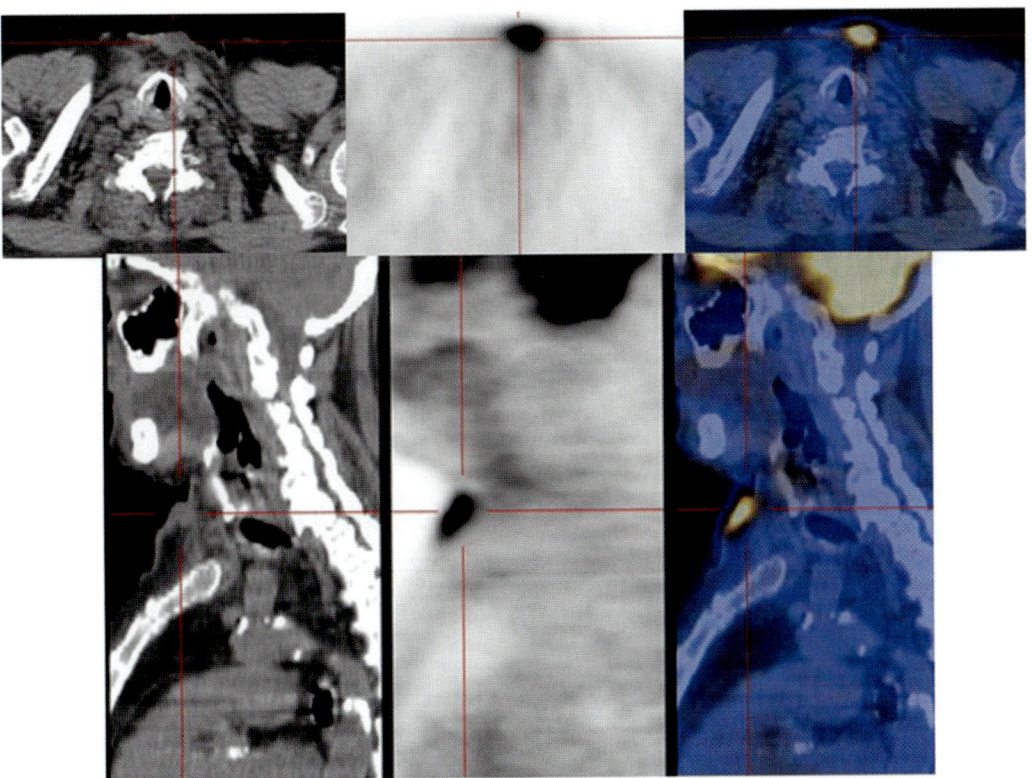

Fig. 12.1 CT shows a heterogeneously hypodense nodular thickening of the subcutaneous tissues at the jugular region, that the PET shows to have a high metabolism of glucose

P. F. Rambaldi, *Whole-Body FDG PET Imaging in Oncology*,
DOI: 10.1007/978-88-470-5295-6_12, © Springer-Verlag Italia 2014

12.3   Report

The clinically appreciable ulcerated jugular mass shows a high increase in the consumption of glucose, SUV max 8.5.

No areas of abnormal metabolism in the remaining parts of the body.

12.4   Conclusions

The PET scan shows high carbohydrate metabolism of the skin lesion at the jugular, probably a spinalioma, to be confirmed histologically (Fig. 12.1).

12.5   Key Points

- Data in the literature reported a high local aggressiveness of squamous cell carcinomas and the rate of distant metastases up to 7 %.
- In these tumors, the PET is not only useful to define the staging and grading lesion, but also to exclude synchronous diseases.

13.1 Clinical History

62-year-old woman with rectal cancer:

- CT scan performed during staging: multiple hypodense cystic hepatic nodules, the greater being at the sixth segment, measuring 25 × 20 mm. Wall thickening of the rectum-sigma due to a neoplasm, with inhomogeneity of the perirectal fat tissue. Outcomes of hysterectomy.

- Cancer markers: CEA = 5.1 ng/ml (nv = 0–5).

  Anterior resection with total mesorectal excision for mucinous adenocarcinoma, infiltrating the perivisceral fat.

  Pathological stage: pT3, pN1, PMX, G2. Adjuvant chemotherapy.

- CT scan performed after one year: multiple hypodense hepatic cystic nodules, the greater being at the sixth segment, measuring

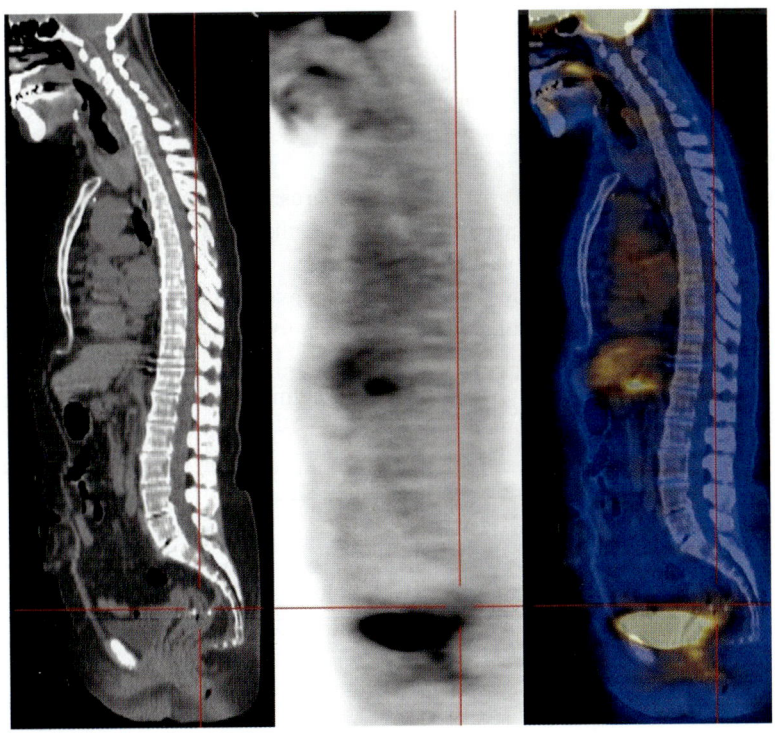

Fig. 13.1 Sagittal CT-PET reconstruction: in correspondence of the rectal anastomosis, at the level of the metal clips, solid, inhomogeneous tissue which has no pathological glucose consumption can be seen. This element is attributable to post-surgical scarring

P. F. Rambaldi, *Whole-Body FDG PET Imaging in Oncology*,
DOI: 10.1007/978-88-470-5295-6_13, © Springer-Verlag Italia 2014

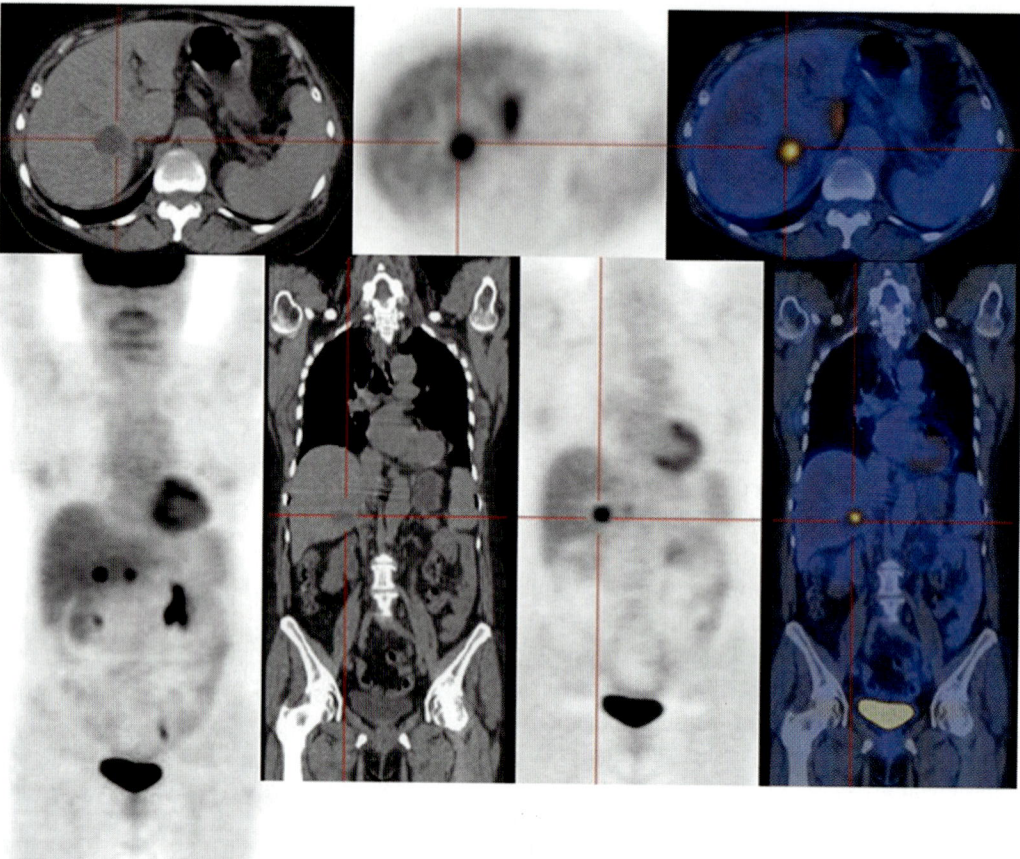

Fig. 13.2 PET scan shows two hepatic nodules, respectively at the VI and II segment that have high consumption of glucose. CT scan identifies only that the sixth segment

29 × 27 mm. Fair left hydroureteronephrosis with a calculus wedged in the ureter at the pelvic segment. Outcomes of hysterectomy.
- Colonoscopy: ulceration of the colon above the anastomosis; histology was negative for malignant cells.
- Cancer markers: CEA = 12.2 ng/ml (nv = 0–5).

13.2 Diagnostic Question

Search for focal lesions with high glucose metabolism in patient with surgically treated rectal cancer: recent increase in the value of the CEA.

13.3 Report

Presence of two hepatic nodules characterized by high carbohydrate consumption, respectively, at the VI and II segment, SUV max 10. No pathological metabolism at the other subcentimetric hepatic nodules reported at CT, probably due to the resolving limits of the technique.

The recto-colonic anastomosis shows mild consumption of FDG, that is no similar to that of focal nodular lesions and therefore is attributable to non-specific inflammation, SUV max 2.6. (See Figs. 13.1, 13.2).

13.4 Conclusions

The PET scan today shows two metastatic liver nodules with high carbohydrate metabolism, showing recurrence of disease.

13.5 Key Points

PET has a decisive diagnostic role when observing a gradual increase over time in the values of the cancer markers, and the contrast-enhanced CT is negative or doubtful.

The two CT scans reported in history show multiple hepatic nodules as cystic. The biggest one at the sixth segment measured 25 × 20 mm presurgery, while at follow-up performed after one year, it measured 29 × 27 mm, so we can say that

- PET has high accuracy in the metabolic characterization of liver nodules measuring more than a centimeter.

- a lump showing volumetric progression over time is suspected.
- a lump that after adjuvant chemotherapy shows volumetric progression did not respond to treatment.
- the persistence of high metabolism after chemotherapy defines a category of patients with a worse prognosis.
- not always the PET allows the characterization of subcentimetric hepatic nodules.

In this patient, it should be remembered that the subcentimetric liver nodules described by TC reported in history are metastatic, but a PET does not show pathological lesional metabolism due to resolving limits.

In fact, in the conclusions of our report, we should state: "presence of multiple liver metastases characterized by cystic appearance, two of which show high glucose metabolism as demonstrated by PET scans. Abnormal FDG consumption of other lesions can't be seen due to the resolving and biological limits of technique."

14.1 Clinical History

35-year-old woman with cancer of the posterior hemi-circumference of the anal canal, a centimetric lump at the base of a hemorrhoidal varicose vein: "carcinoma of the transitional colo-anal epithelium in mixed non-keratinizing cells large cell and basaloid morphological variant".

- Chemo-radiotherapy and subsequent intraluminal rectal brachytherapy in HDR mode. Follow-up at three months.
- PET: negative for focal lesions.

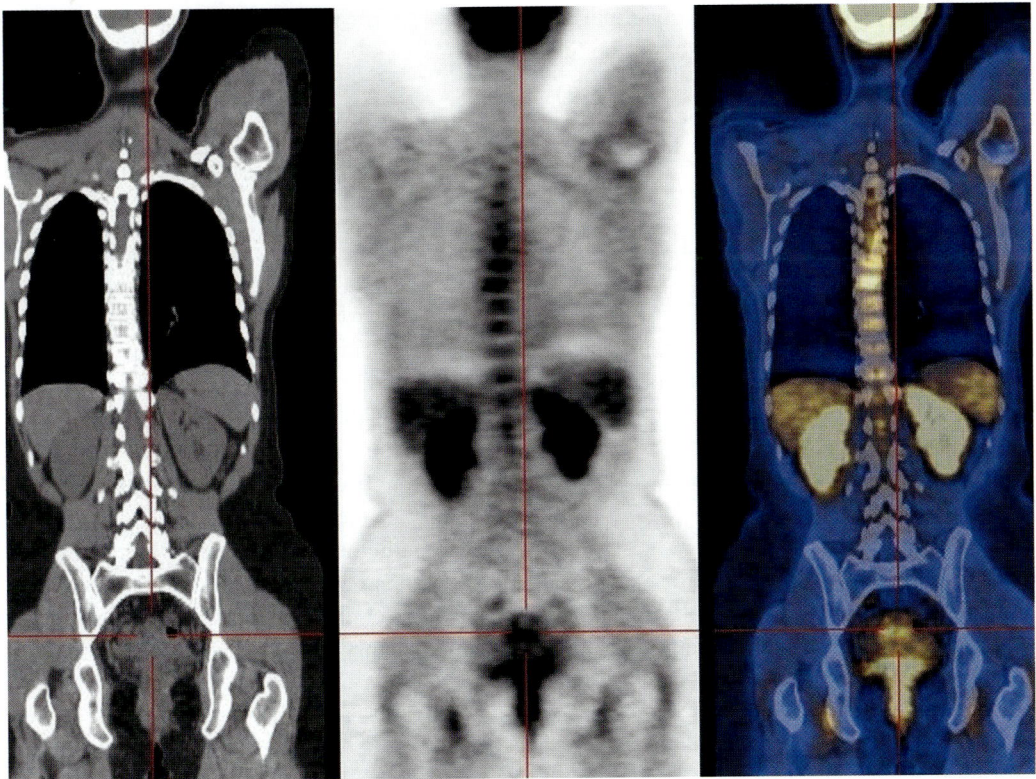

Fig. 14.1 MIP image: presence of slight and widespread increase in the glucose consumption of the axial skeleton, typical of bone marrow rebound

P. F. Rambaldi, *Whole-Body FDG PET Imaging in Oncology*,
DOI: 10.1007/978-88-470-5295-6_14, © Springer-Verlag Italia 2014

- Abdomen, pelvis MRI: hyperintensity of the cancellous bone of the sacrum, due to brachytherapy. After radio-chemotherapy, the lesion in the proximal portion previously described at 3 cm from the anal sphincter and the thickening of the mucosal surface are not seen. The solution of continuity in the posterior anal wall is not seen anymore.
- Rectal-sigmoidoscopy: ano-rectal cancer in remission, light macroscopic actinic proctopathy.

14.2   Diagnostic Question

Search for focal lesions with high glucose metabolism in patient with chemo-radiotreated carcinoma of the anus. Follow-up at six months.

14.3   Report

The PET scan shows no areas of abnormal glucose consumption in body areas examined (Fig. 14.1).

Modest increase in metabolism in the lower rectum-anus due to post-actinic fibrosis, SUV max 2.3.

14.4   Conclusions

The PET scan is negative for recurrence of disease with high glucose metabolism. (See Figs. 14.2, 14.3).

14.5   Key Points

- Compared with other diagnostic techniques, including MRI and transrectal ultrasound, CT-PET allows a precise and accurate restaging of

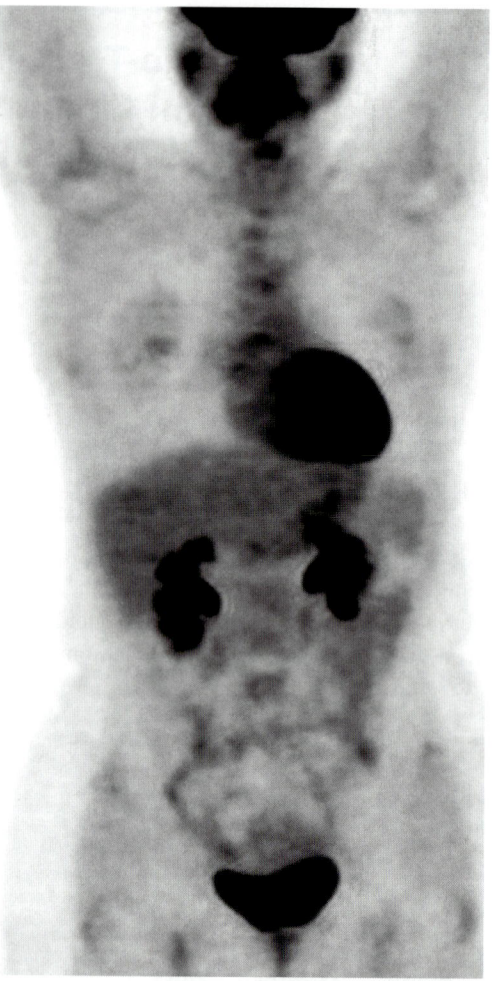

Fig. 14.2 Absence of lytic bone lesions on CT and focal areas with high metabolism at PET, excludes progression of skeletal disease

patients with cancer of the colon-rectum and anus after radiochemotherapy, with high accuracy because it defines the biological vitality of the tumor.
- After radiotherapy, there is a slight increase in metabolism due to post-actinic inflammation. Then, after three months, the activity of the inflammatory lesion reduces; the presence of

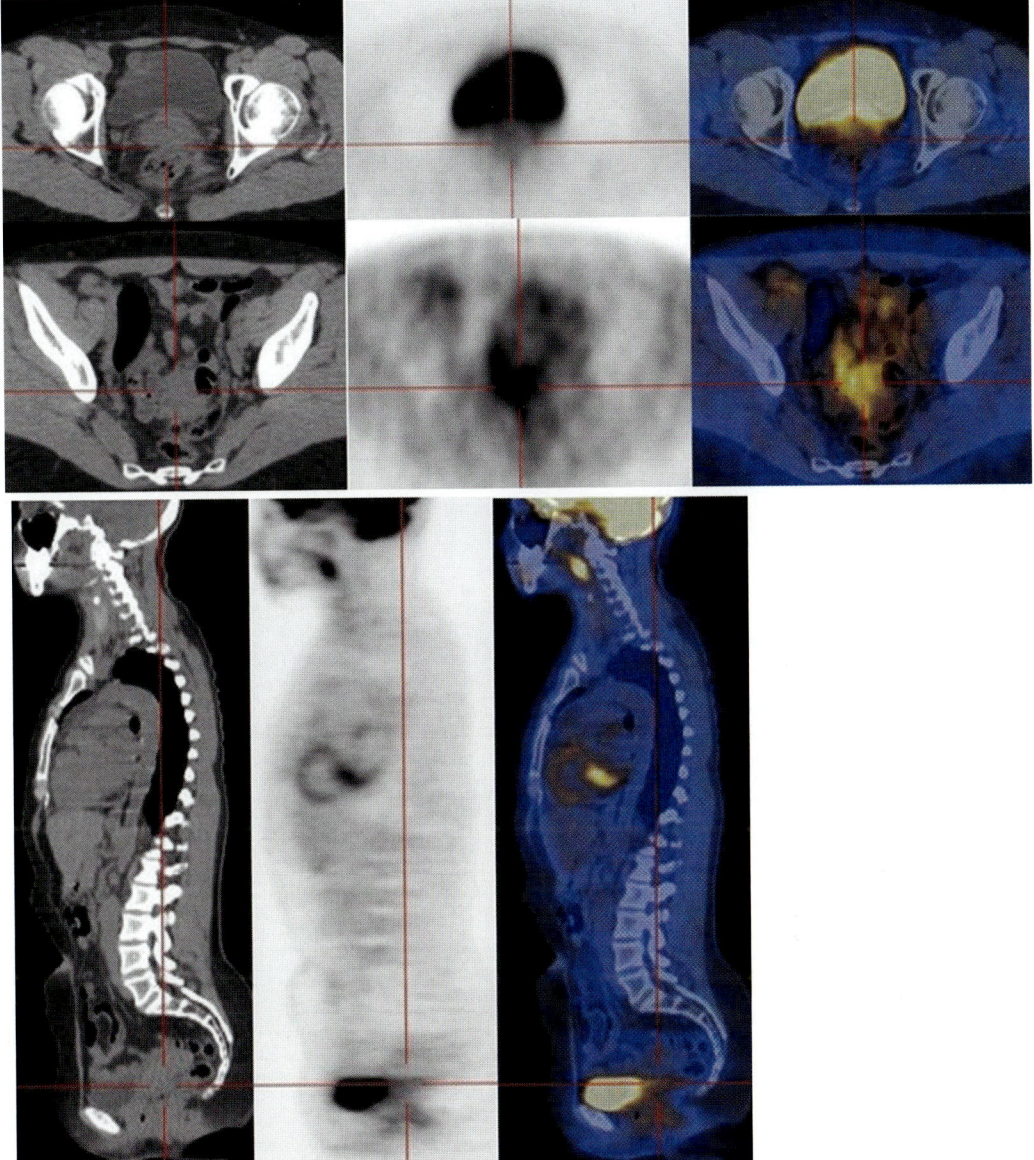

Fig. 14.3 On CT-PET, the rectal carbohydrate consumption is low due to radiation proctitis. There are no focal solid nodules with a high metabolism indicating a recurrence of disease

fibrosis will then reduce the local glucose consumption dramatically.

- The radiation proctitis is characterized by a glucose consumption higher than that of the liver, while the fibrosis has a lower activity.

- In some cases, there is still a modest increase in glucose consumption even several months after the end of the radiotherapy, and this element suggests chronicity of the inflammatory process (chronic proctitis).

Liver Metastases in Mucinous Adenocarcinoma of the Colon: Low Metabolism of FDG

15

15.1 Clinical History

73-year-old man undergoes surgery for mucinous adenocarcinoma of the colon, G2 pT3, pN0, PM0, and adjuvant chemotherapy.

Follow-up at three months.
- CT: negative for focal lesions.
- Cancer markers: normal.

Follow-up at six months.
- CT: negative for focal lesions.
- Cancer markers: CA50 = 46.1 U/ml (nv 0–25), CA19-9 73.7 U/ml = (nv 0–37); CEA 47.3 ng/ml = (nv 0–5).
- Colonoscopy: negative for recurrence of disease.

Follow-up to eight months.
- Cancer markers: CA50 = 354.0 U/ml (nv 0–25), CA19-9 = 102.9 U/ml (0–37 nv); CEA = 55.3 ng/ml (nv 0–5).
- Ascites.

15.2 Diagnostic Question

Search for focal lesions with high glucose metabolism in patient with surgically and chemo-treated colorectal cancer, with progressive increase of the cancer markers.

15.3 Report

Presence of multiple subcentimetric hepatic and splenic nodules which do not show focal consumption of glucose, SUV max 2.1 (Fig. 15.1).

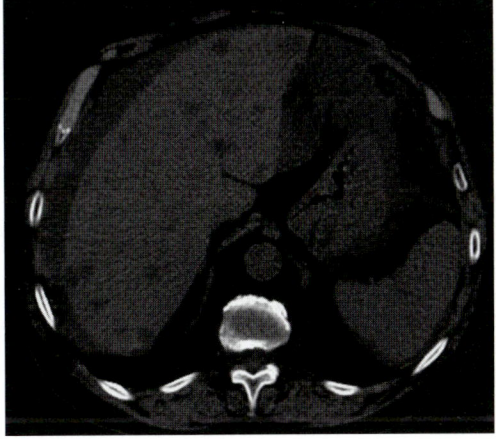

Fig. 15.1 Multiple subcentimetric hepatic nodules

Major ascites.

Subcentimetric pulmonary nodule in the left anterior basal segment, with low metabolism, SUV max 0.8 (Fig. 15.2).

15.4 Conclusions

The PET-CT scan showed multiple subcentimetric secondary lesions of the liver and spleen characterized by restricted carbohydrate consumption. It is associated with a pulmonary nodule also be referred to metastatic disease. (See Fig. 15.3).

NB: mucinous carcinomas may have little carbohydrate consumption.

15.5 Key Points

- The limited consumption of glucose by the liver and spleen subcentimetric metastases is

P. F. Rambaldi, *Whole-Body FDG PET Imaging in Oncology*,
DOI: 10.1007/978-88-470-5295-6_15, © Springer-Verlag Italia 2014

Fig. 15.2 Subcentimetric pulmonary nodule in the left anterior basal segment, with low metabolism, SUV max 0.8

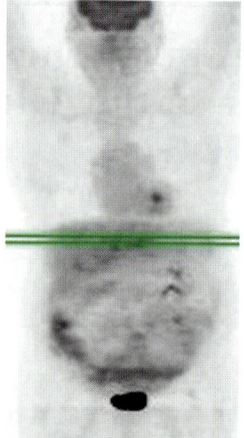

determined by the biological and resolving limits of the technique.

- Pharmacological interference caused by previous chemotherapy treatments must always be excluded.
- Liver metastases from carcinoid tumors and those of some histological types such as mucinous carcinomas may express a low metabolism of glucose.

- The demonstration of low metabolic activity of the lesion should not be considered simply a "false negative" of PET-FDG, but in fact this information suggests a different metabolic and biological behavior of the tumor, from which to extrapolate useful prognostic considerations.
- Some possible "false negatives" determined by a limited metabolism of glucose in a PET scan can be identified and indicated by a careful study of CT images, and later integrated with other imaging techniques (MRI, US, contrast-enhanced CT).
- PET-FDG is not the method of choice in restaging after chemotherapy in patients whose baseline scan had neoplastic lesions characterized by low consumption of glucose.
  N.B.
- In patients with recent-onset of ascites, a primary or secondary neoplastic condition should always be suspected.
- The presence of liver and spleen metastases or peritoneal carcinomatosis can determine this condition.
- In these cases, the advanced stage of the disease suggests a poor prognosis.

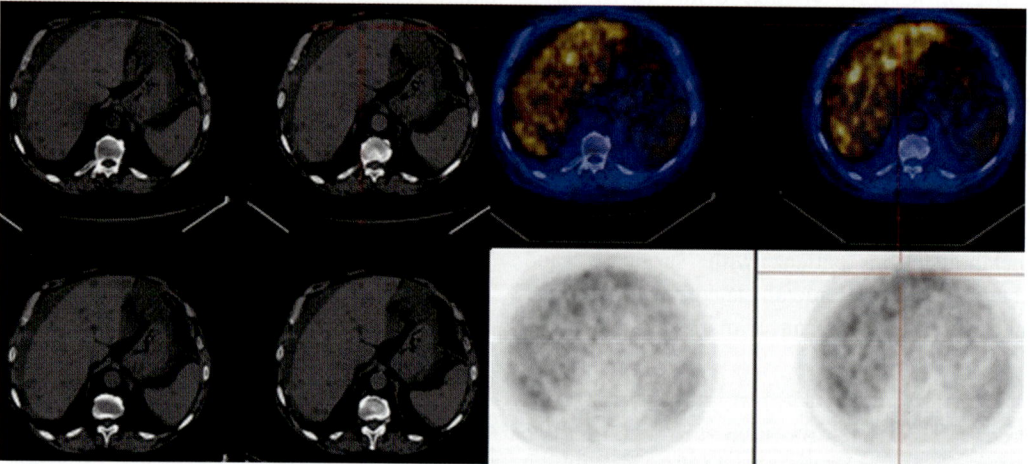

Fig. 15.3 At the liver and spleen, CT demonstrates multiple subcentimetric hypodense nodules that do not show any glucose metabolism due to the biological and resolving limits of the technique. Conspicuous ascites can be seen

Hepatic Metastases from Carcinoma of the Transverse Colon: Persistent Disease After Thermal Ablation

16

16.1 Clinical History

56-year-old man who underwent colectomy for adenocarcinoma of the transverse colon (pT4, pN0, PMX), but not radio-adjuvant chemotherapy.

Follow-up after one year:
- Abdomen CT: subcapsular, hypodense nodule in liver segment V, measuring 22 × 17 mm, doubtful for repetitive injury.
- Ultrasound: hypoechoic, probably metastatic nodule in the V hepatic segment measuring 35 × 31 mm.
- Cancer Markers: CEA = 8.3 ng/ml (nv 0–5).
- needle aspiration of hepatic injury: positive secondary lesion from adenocarcinoma.

Thermal ablation of metastatic liver lesion.

16.2 Diagnostic Question

Patient with liver metastasis from adenocarcinoma of the colon: restaging after ablation.

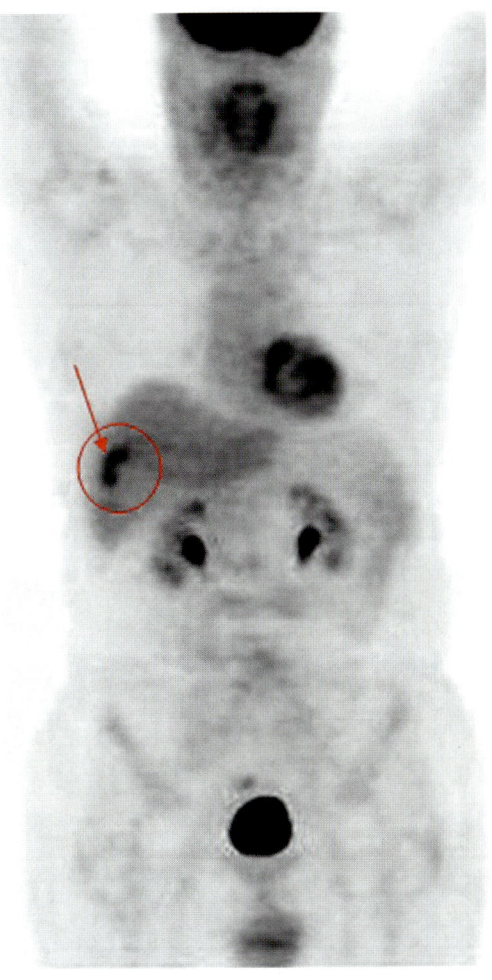

Fig. 16.1 MIP image demonstrates the persistence of high metabolism of the hepatic lesion in the fifth segment. The other two secondary nodules do not appear in MIP reconstruction because they are subcentimetric and also have only a limited increase in carbohydrate consumption, and their activity is masked by the background activity of the liver and the physiological renal excretion

P. F. Rambaldi, *Whole-Body FDG PET Imaging in Oncology*,
DOI: 10.1007/978-88-470-5295-6_16, © Springer-Verlag Italia 2014

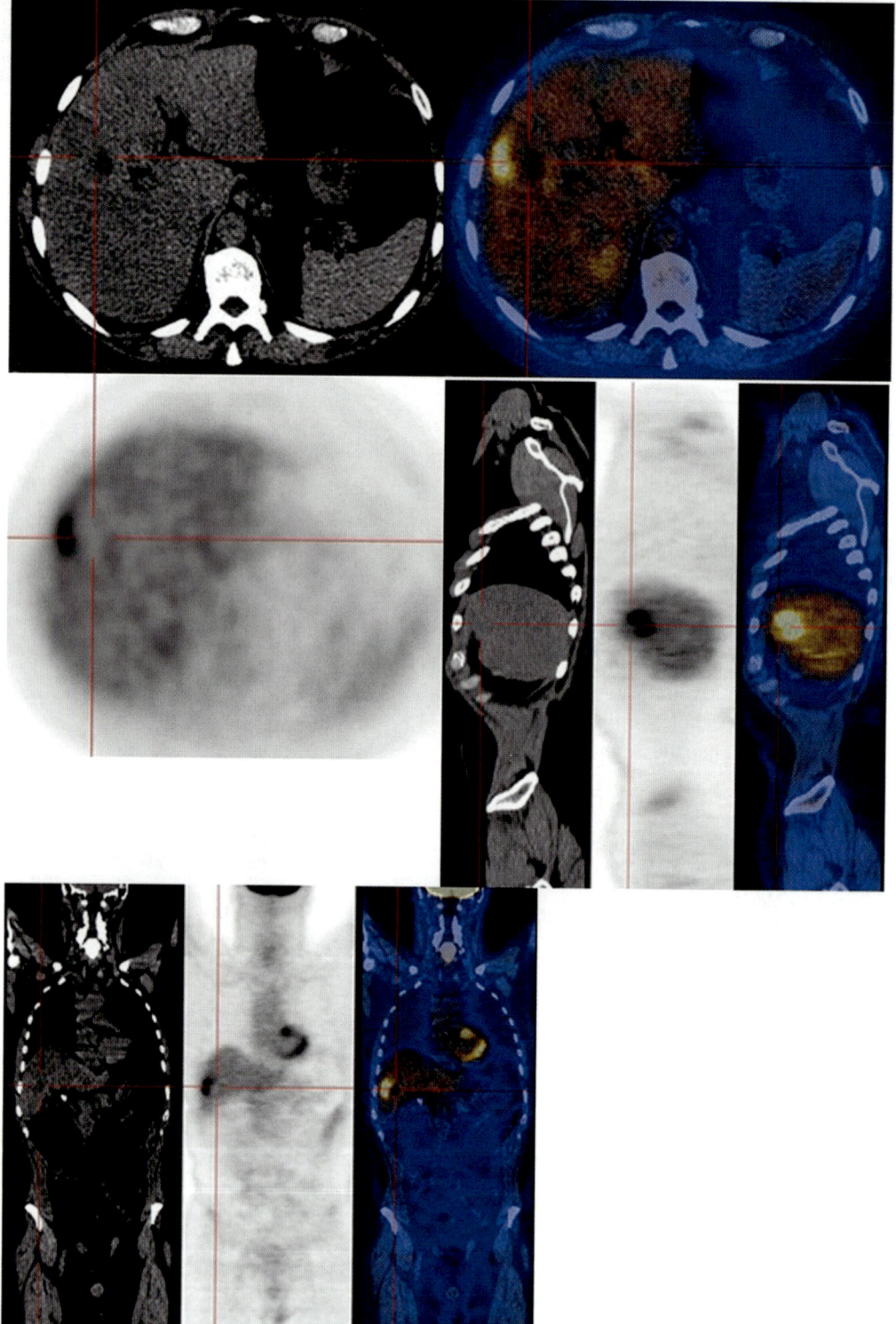

Fig. 16.2 The CT scan shows a subcapsular, uneven mass in the hepatic V segment, with markedly hypodense internal component due to colliquation

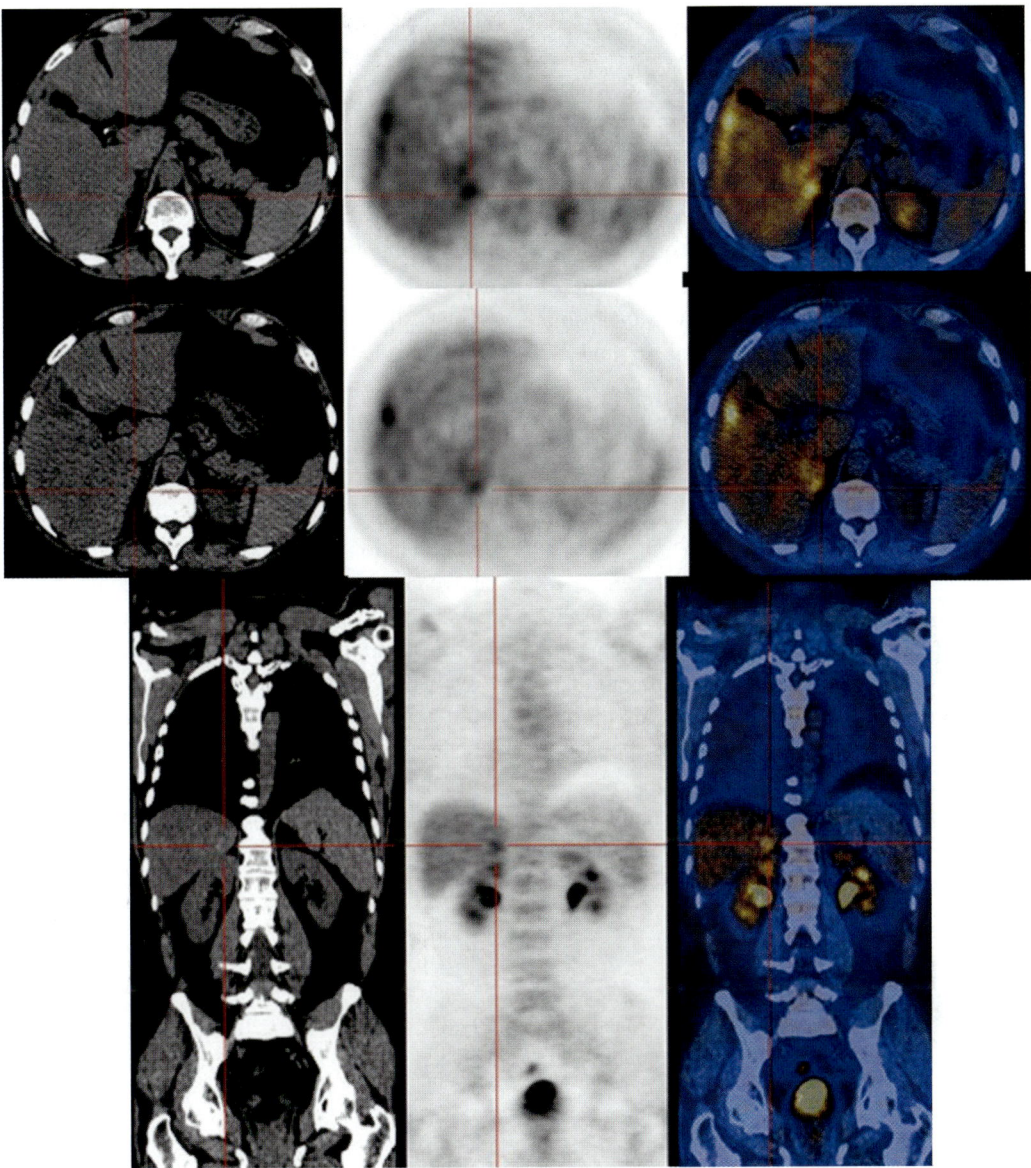

Fig. 16.3 CT-PET: Small paracaval, metabolically active lump in the VI hepatic segment, not detected on CT

16.3 Report

The PET shows pathological glucose consumption of a subcapsular hepatic mass in segment V, SUV max 6, with an internal low-metabolism section, due to colliquation secondary to thermal ablation.

Two subcentimetric nodules characterized by altered glucose metabolism in liver segment VI, respectively in the paracaval and subcapsular regions are seen, with SUV max of 3.3 and 2.2, respectively.

No areas of abnormal FDG consumption in the remaining parts of the body examined.

16.4 Conclusions

The PET scan suggests progression of disease for the presence of three repetitive hepatic lesions with a high carbohydrate metabolism, the most evident, already treated with thermal ablation, shows only a partial response to treatment.

This mass is mostly cold on PET and only on the lateral subglissonian side metabolic activity corresponding to the vitality of the residual tumor can be seen. The success of the ablation can be considered incomplete. (See Figs. 16.1-16.3).

16.5 Key Points

Colorectal cancer frequently causes liver metastases.

- Generally, this involves multiple secondary lesions.
- Sometimes during follow-up solitary hepatic repetitive nodules are diagnosed, but this is still a poor prognostic sign because it shows the high potential of the tumor to determine metastasis.
- The ablation of a solitary liver lesion does not have any influence on the outcome of the disease, having just a palliative function.
- The questionable lesions should always be evaluated in much more targeted techniques: ultrasonography, MRI, contrast-enhanced CT, or biopsy.
- In the presence of multiple hepatic metastases, systemic chemotherapy is suggested.

Surgically Treated Adenocarcinoma of the Rectum: Locoregional Recurrence with Lymph Node Metastases

17

17.1 Clinical History

Low anterior resection of the rectum due to stenosing moderately differentiated adenocarcinoma (G2, pT3, pN1, PMX) in a 62 year old patient.

Follow-up after one year.

- CT: intercavo-aortic lymphadenopathy (10–12 mm) originating below the hilum of the kidney.
- PET: small nodular areas of hyperaccumulation in the paraortic region.

The patient undergoes chemotherapy.

17.2 Diagnostic Question

Restaging three months after chemotherapy: search for focal lesions with a high metabolism of glucose.

17.3 Report

Pathological glucose consumption of three lymph nodes in the paraortic region, below the renal arteries, SUV max 14, with extension up to the aorto-iliac bifurcation, SUV max 7.

Modest increase in FDG deposition of the colo-rectal stoma, SUV max 5.6, due to possible recurrence of locoregional disease, to be confirmed histologically.

Modest right hydroureteronephrosis.

17.4 Conclusions

The PET scan (Fig. 17.1) shows recurrence of disease for lymphadenopathy with high glucose metabolism. It is associated with locoregional recurrence, to be confirmed by colonoscopy (Fig. 17.2).

17.5 Key Points

The metabolic data must be critically evaluated in relation to adjuvant chemotherapy, especially intensity of the metabolic activity at the PET-FDG.

P. F. Rambaldi, *Whole-Body FDG PET Imaging in Oncology*,
DOI: 10.1007/978-88-470-5295-6_17, © Springer-Verlag Italia 2014

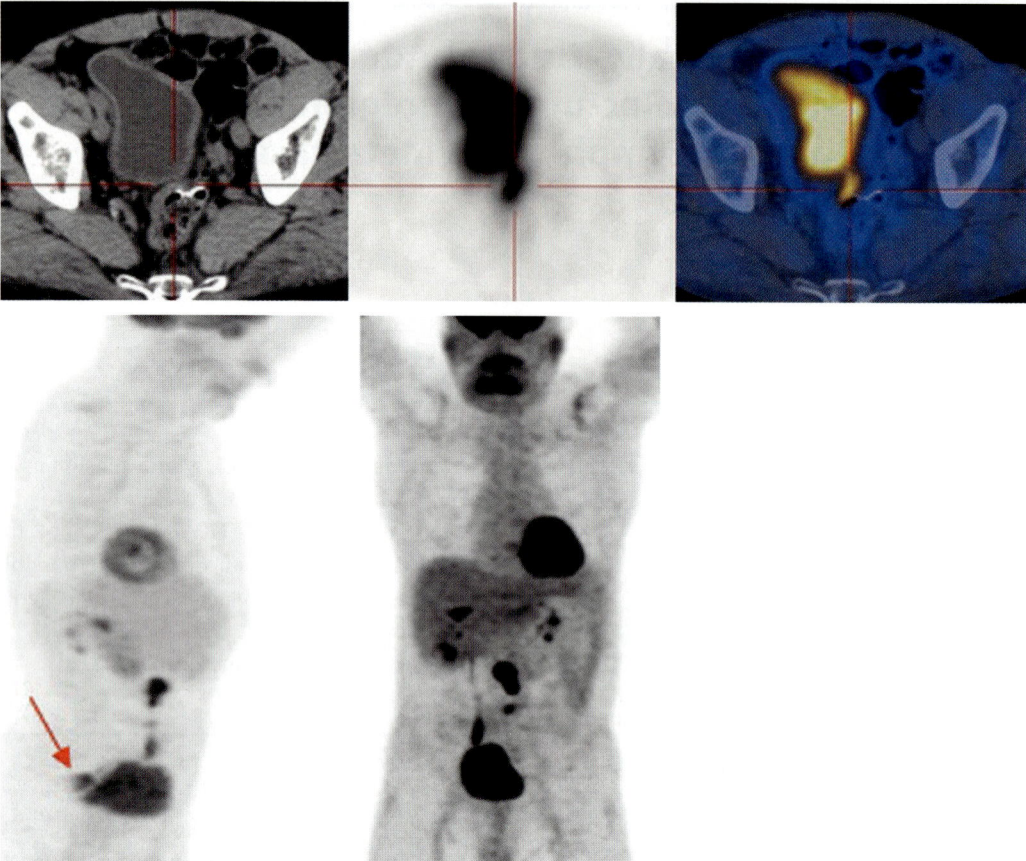

Fig. 17.1 The PET-CT examination demonstrates modest thickening tissue with high carbohydrate metabolism in correspondence of the rectal anastomosis adjacent to the metal clips, in contiguity with the posterior wall of the bladder

Therefore, in this patient, we can say that metastatic disease has not responded to treatment and is in progress for the following reasons:
- the consumption of glucose of the nodal lesions is very high.

- CT shows volumetric progression of metastatic lymph nodes compared with the scan performed before chemotherapy.
- there is locoregional recurrence.

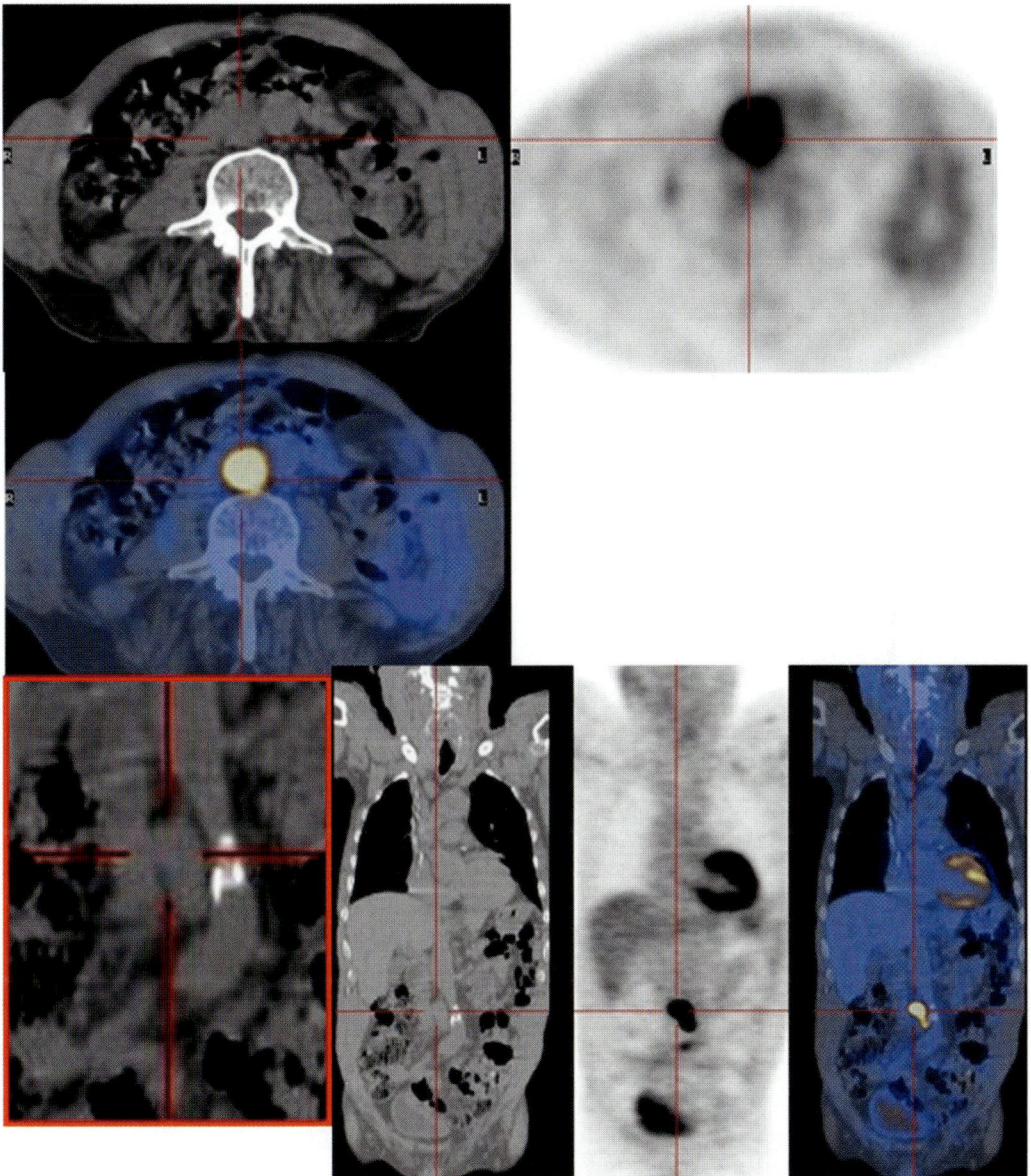

Fig. 17.2 The PET-CT scan shows a conglomerate of lymph nodes measuring 22 x 25 mm in the axial plane and characterized by high metabolism. This mass extends from the intercavo-aortic region, through a plane passing over the renal arteries, reaching the aorto-iliac bifurcation

NB: The lumbo-aortic and intercavo-aortic lymph nodes are frequent site of metastasis, so the PET and CT images must always be carefully considered.

Rectal Adenocarcinoma and Hepatic Metastases: Partial Response to Chemotherapy

18

18.1 Clinical History

Anterior rectal resection in a 59-year-old male with moderately differentiated adenocarcinoma, G2, pT3, pN0 (node 0/12), PMX.

Radio-adjuvant chemotherapy was not performed.

Post-surgical revaluation.

- CT: Negative for focal lesions.

- cancer markers: CEA = 3.3 ng/ml (0–5). Follow-up at six months.
- Chest XR: right parieto-basal pleuritic remnants. Not parenchymal lesions.
- CT: the presence of two small lung nodules in postero-basal segments of the lower lobes bilaterally and two centimetric subglissonian, hypodense hepatic nodules, respectively at I–II and VI segment.

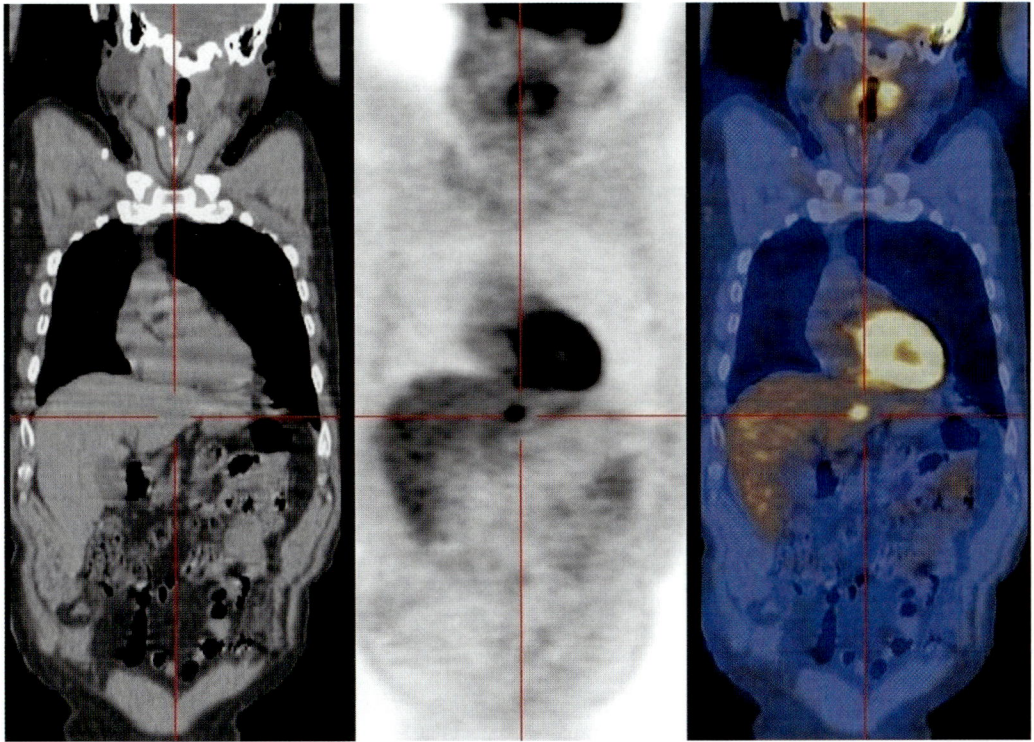

Fig. 18.1 PET scan before chemotherapy

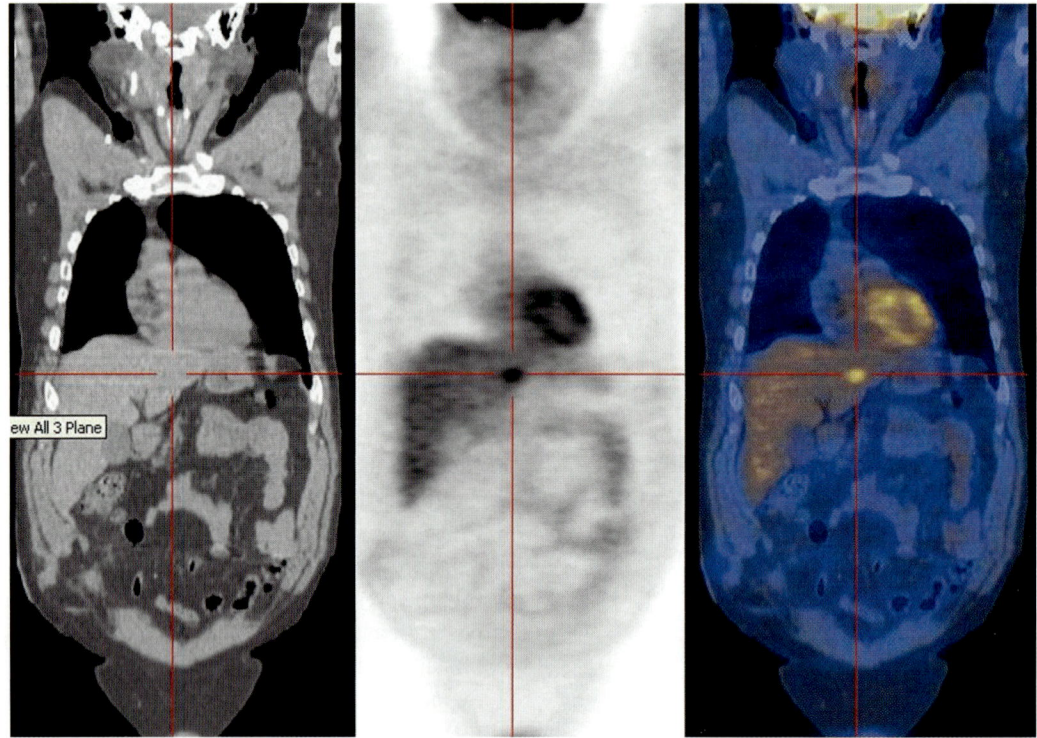

Fig. 18.2 PET scan after chemotherapy shows partial response to treatment

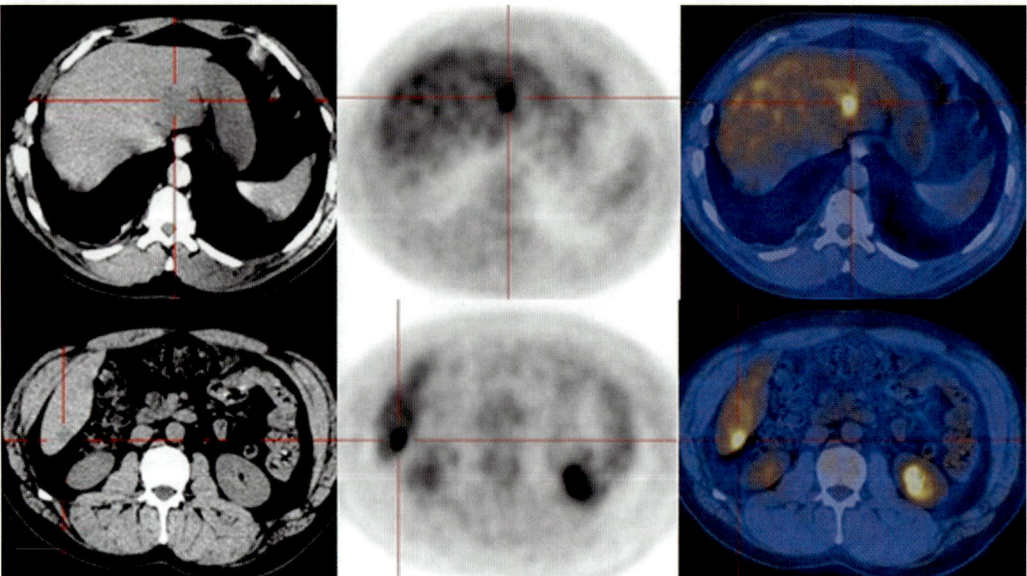

Fig. 18.3 CT-PET performed before chemotherapy: evidence of two centimetric, hypodense subglissonian metastatic nodules, characterized by high metabolism, respectively at I–II and VI hepatic segment

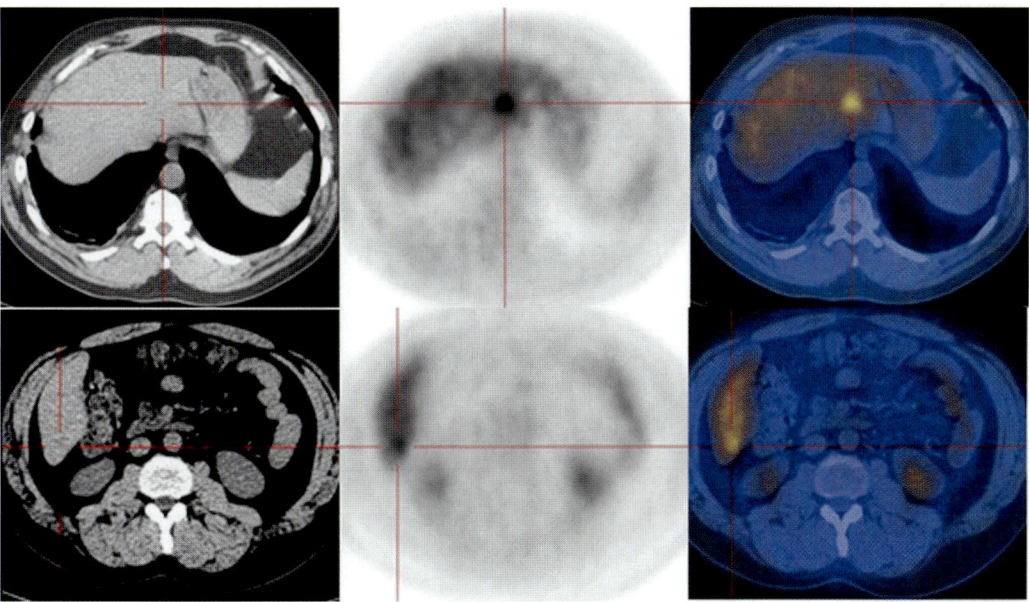

Fig. 18.4 Follow-up after chemotherapy: reduction in volume and metabolic activity of the two secondary liver nodules

- PET: pathological glucose consumption of two secondary liver nodules respectively to the I–II and VI segment.
- Cancer markers: CEA = 11.3 ng/ml (0–5). Follow-up after chemotherapy.
- CT: The small pulmonary nodules seen in the postero-basal segments bilaterally do not appear modified. Centimetric subglissonian hypodense metastatic lump in the VI hepatic segment.

18.2   Diagnostic Question

Evaluation of the response after chemotherapy in patient with liver metastases from rectal adenocarcinoma: study of glucose metabolism.

18.3   Report

The PET scan shows two hepatic nodules characterized by modest increase in carbohydrate consumption, respectively, at I–II, SUV max 2.7, and sixth segment, SUV max 2.1 (Fig. 18.1).

Absence of pathological metabolism in other body segments examined.

18.4   Conclusions

The PET scan shows partial response to treatment, due to persistence of mild metabolic activity of the two metastatic liver nodules (Fig. 18.2).

The response to treatment can be considered incomplete. (See Figs. 18.3, 18.4, 18.5, 18.6, 18.7).

18.5   Key Points

- The liver lesions detected with a high metabolism baseline PET image do not disappear completely at the follow-up after

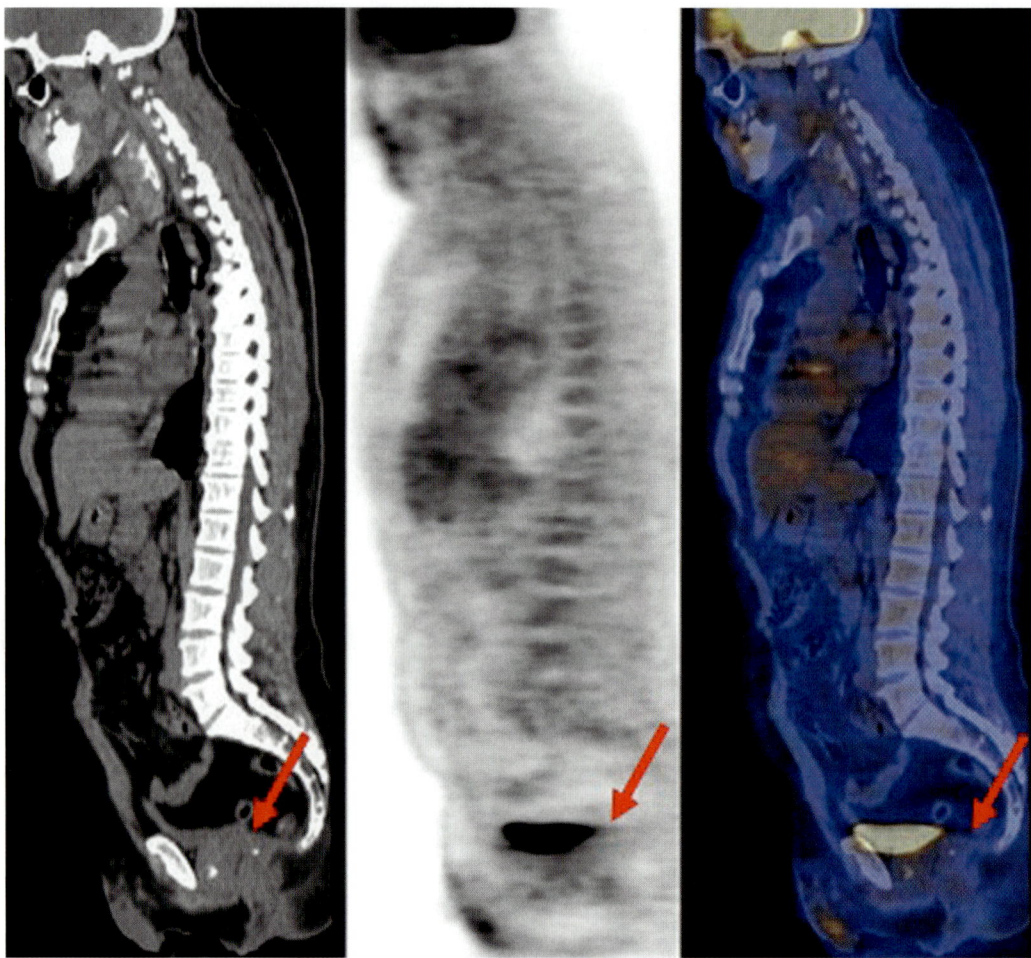

Fig. 18.5 The sagittal CT reconstruction allows identification of the metal clips at the site of the previous resection of the rectum. PET does not show pathological glucose consumption here, therefore the examination excludes loco-regional recurrence

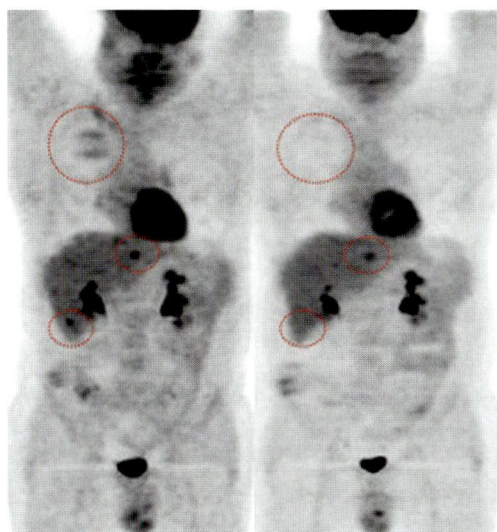

chemotherapy, so the response to treatment is incomplete (MIP image, Fig. 18.6).

- The persistence of metabolic activity is a negative prognostic index and suggests a different approach to chemotherapy.

Fig. 18.6 MIP Images before (left) and after (right) chemotherapy, show partial response to treatment

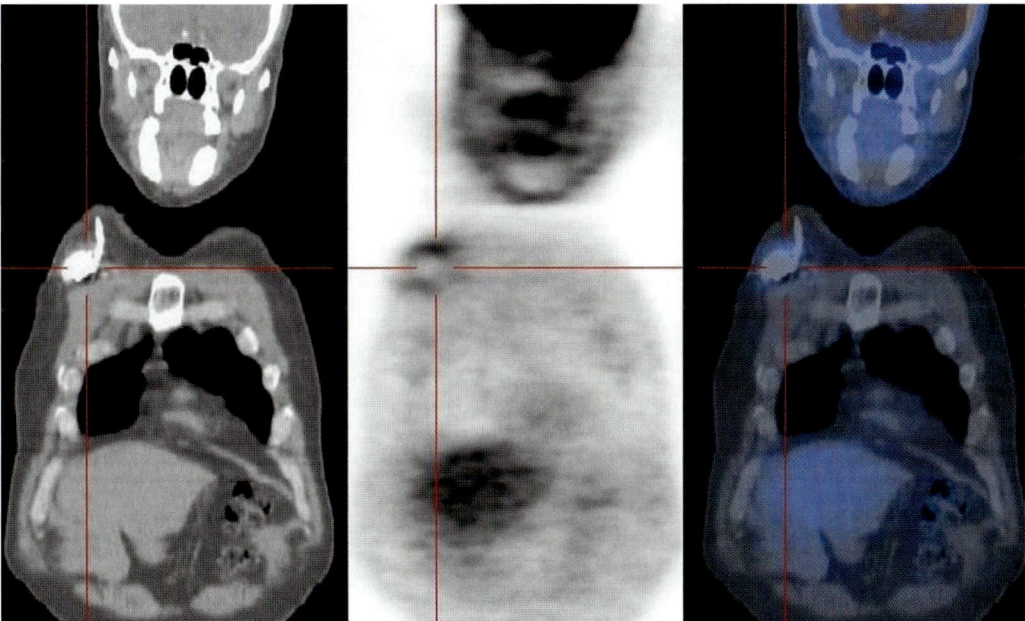

Fig. 18.7 Inflammation of the soft tissues of the anterior chest wall determined by the installation of port-a-cath, that is not seen at the successive PET scan

Sigmoid Adenocarcinoma: Post-Actinic Tardive Sacral Fracture

19.1 Clinical History

Left hemicolectomy in a 48-year-old woman with stenosing sigmoid adenocarcinoma, pT2, pN1, PM0. Chemo-radiotherapy.

Clinical control after 18 years: worsening low back pain.

- Abdomen US: absence of focal lesions.
- MRI of the abdomen and lumbosacral spine: alteration of signal at the soma of L4, compatible with angioma. Presence of two biliary cysts at hepatic segment V and VI, respectively measuring 10 and 8 mm.
- Cancer Markers: CEA = 6.8 ng/ml (0–4.5).

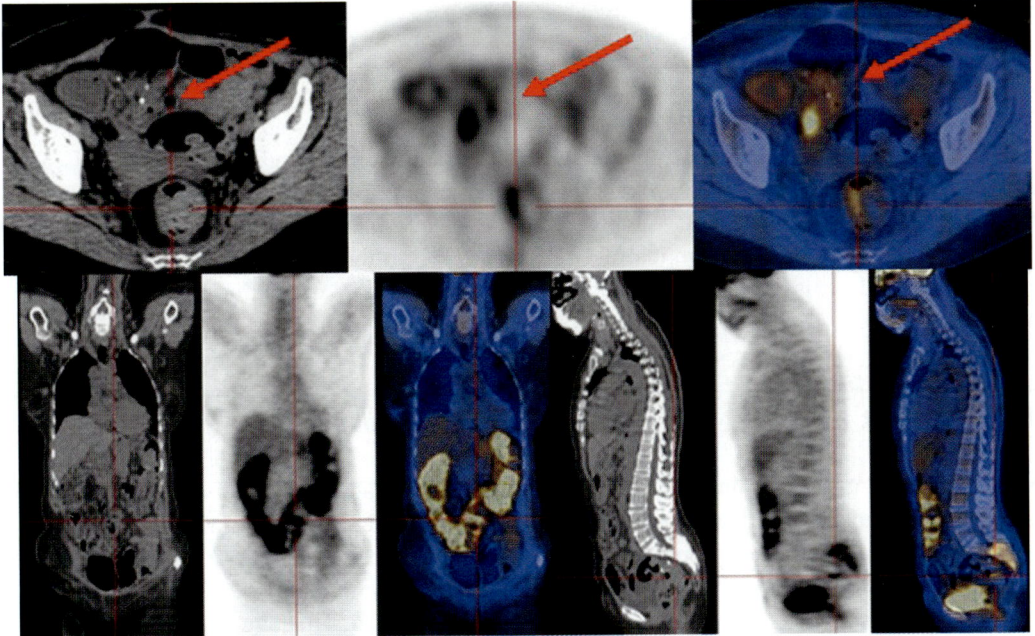

Fig. 19.1 At the peri-anastomotic bowel loops, adjacent to the metal clips, CT-PET shows a heterogeneously hypodense portion of tissue, which has negligible carbohydrate consumption. It is associated with intense and widespread increase in metabolism of the large intestine. This finding is nonspecific and must be related to the clinical signs and symptoms, in particular to nonspecific inflammatory conditions or IBD

P. F. Rambaldi, *Whole-Body FDG PET Imaging in Oncology*,
DOI: 10.1007/978-88-470-5295-6_19, © Springer-Verlag Italia 2014

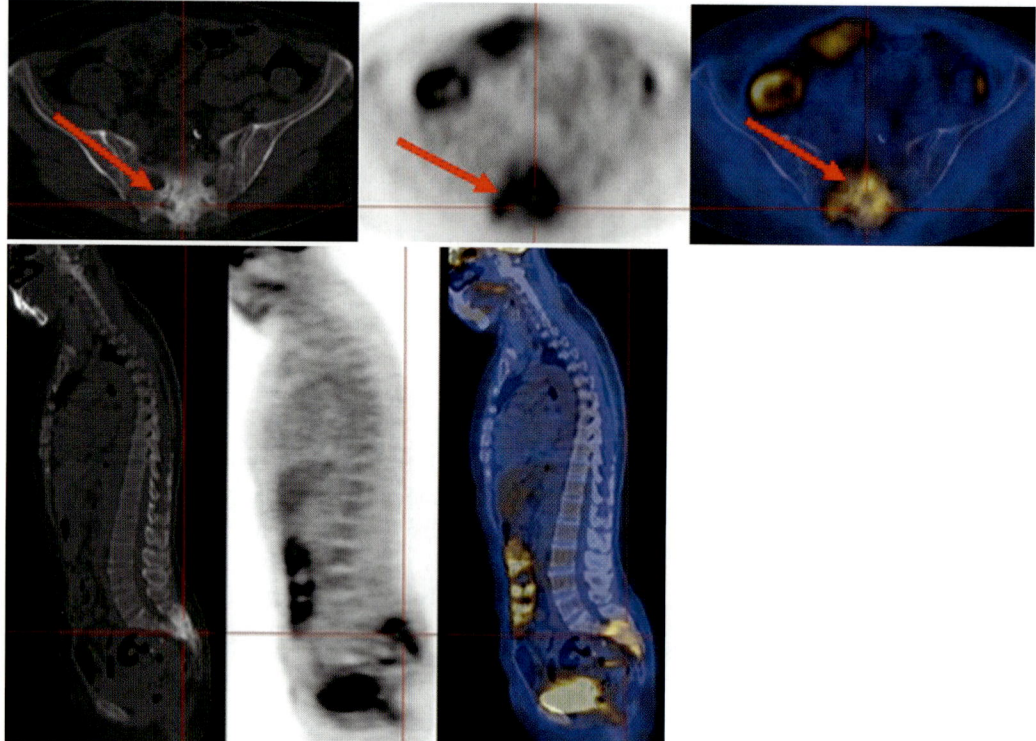

Fig. 19.2 On CT-PET there is presence of morphostructural alteration of the sacrum and coccyx, that appear diffusely thickened due to late outcomes of radiation therapy

19.2 Diagnostic Question

Patient with a history of surgically treated sigmoid cancer, morpho—structural lumbosacral spine alterations and modest elevation of CEA: search for focal lesions with a high metabolism of glucose.

The alteration described at the MRI scan at the soma of L4 has no significant deposition of FDG and therefore indicates a benign disease.

Marked increase in the metabolism of the large intestine for nonspecific activation, to correlate to the clinical signs. Absence of pathological glucose deposition in other parts of the body examined.

19.3 Report

Modest increase in the consumption of glucose at the sacrum and coccyx, due to bone marrow activation caused by fracture, morphologically evident at CT, SUV max 3.1 (Fig. 19.1).

19.4 Conclusions

The PET scan shows no focal lesions characterized by high metabolism indicating a recurrence of disease.

Modest consumption of glucose at the sacrum, due to a fracture. (See Fig. 19.2).

Axial images show a small fracture of the sacrum with modest increase in the consumption of glucose due to reparative bone marrow activation.

19.5 Key Points

- When it a high nonspecific intestinal activity is seen, a locoregional recurrence of disease can be reasonably excluded only after a thorough study of all the PET-CT images.
- In the presence of extensive inflammatory bowel disease, increase in the CEA values is a nonspecific indicator of disease.
- This patient is in complete remission for 18 years; therefore, a recurrence is unlikely. A limited bone metabolism (SUV max <3) does not bode well for a metastatic disease secondary fracture.

Radiation therapy performed in the pelvic region causes the destruction of a share of vital cellular bone marrow with subsequent fibrotic evolution and structural bone thickening. In this way, the irradiated segment loses its physiological elasticity and is more sensitive to fractures.

The stress fractures are characterized by a modest glucose consumption determined by an inflammatory reaction and osteomedullary reparative activation.

Clinical control over time through a bone scan, the determination of phosphatase and parathyroid hormones, may be useful to help determine the risk of fracture of other skeletal sites.

Locoregional Recurrence of Mucinous Adenocarcinoma of the Transverse Colon

20

20.1 Clinical History

65-year-old man who underwent colectomy for mucinous neoplasm of the transverse colon.

Follow-up performed after three years:

- presence of abdominal distension associated with light pain,
- tumor markers are normal,
- CT scan shows an abdominal mass, suspicious for recurrence.

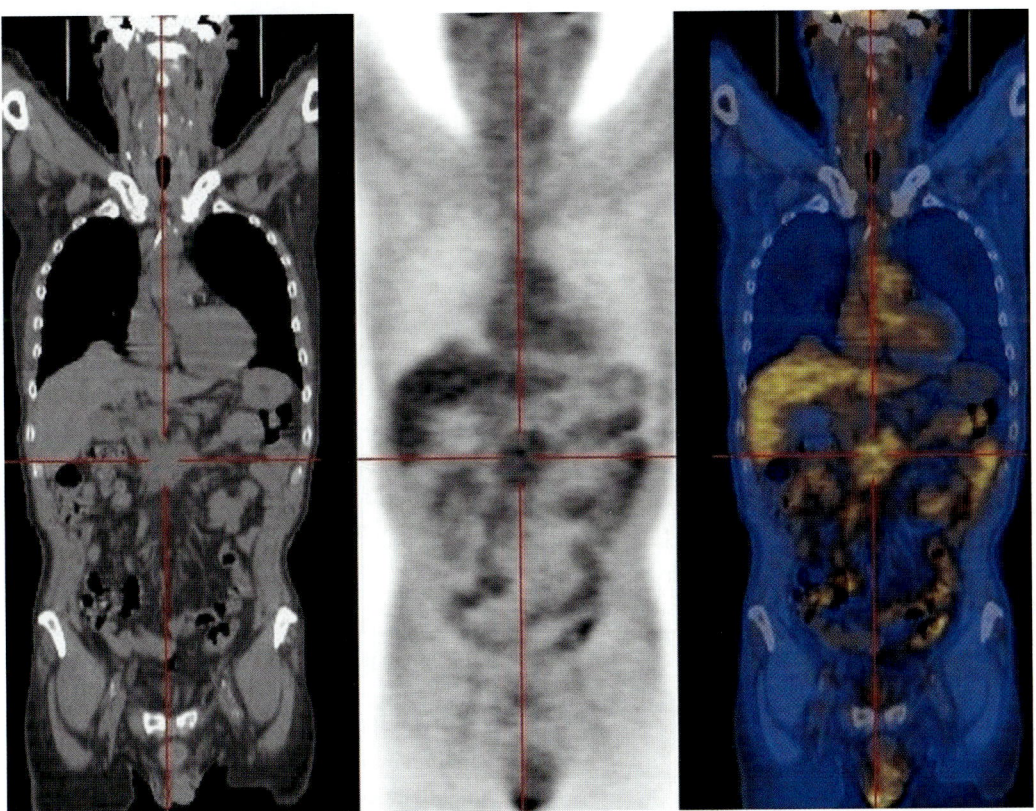

Fig. 20.1 In the celiac-mesenteric intercavo-aortic region, CT-PET demonstrates a solid mass with parenchymal density, uneven with irregular margins, not separable from the surrounding structures and characterized by limited concentration of FDG

P. F. Rambaldi, *Whole-Body FDG PET Imaging in Oncology*,
DOI: 10.1007/978-88-470-5295-6_20, © Springer-Verlag Italia 2014

Fig. 20.2 The MIP image demonstrates the limited metabolism of the abdominal mass which has a carbohydrate consumption comparable to that of the liver

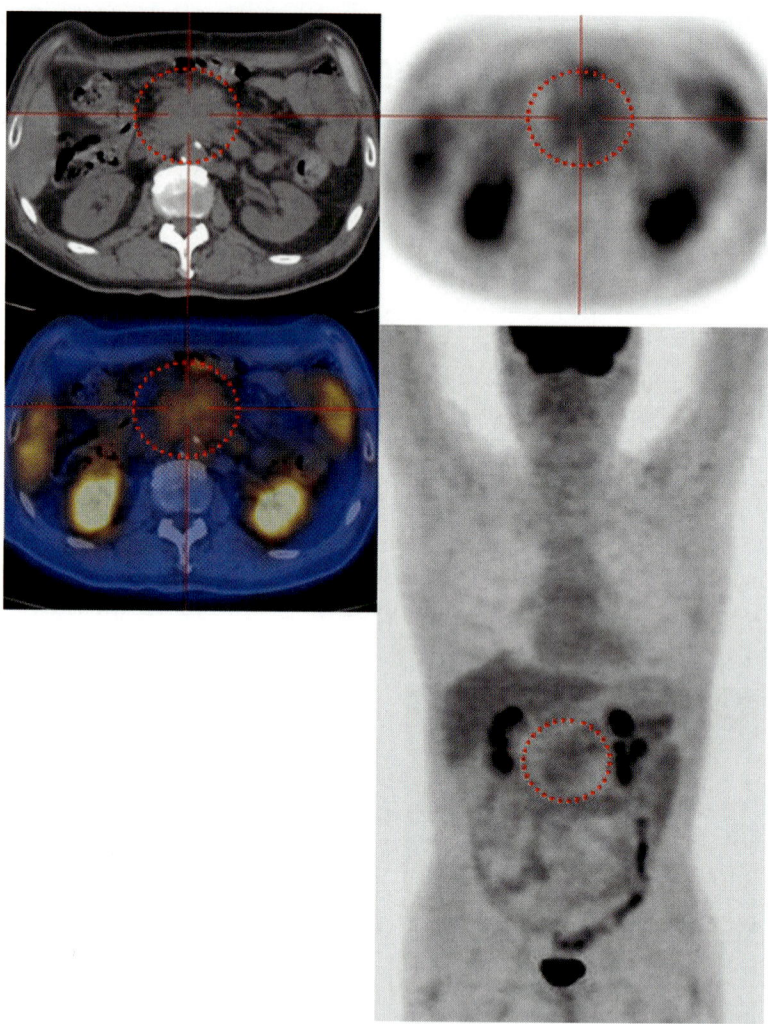

20.2 Diagnostic Question

Search for focal lesions with high glucose metabolism in patient with suspect of recurrent mucinous adenocarcinoma of the colon.

20.3 Report

The PET scan shows slight increase in glucose consumption at the mass indicated by the CT, in the celiac-mesenteric-paracaval region, SUV max 2.9 (Fig. 20.1).

Absence of significant focal areas of abnormal metabolism in the remaining body segments examined.

20.4 Conclusions

The PET scan suggests recurrence of mucinous adenocarcinoma of the colon with limited metabolism of glucose. (See Fig. 20.2).

20.5 **Key Points**

- The concentration of FDG must always be critically assessed in mucinous neoplasms which may have limited metabolism of this tracer.

- The PET-FDG is not the technique of choice in the follow-up of these tumors due to the high incidence of false negatives.
- CT allows us to determine the precise anatomic site of recurrence, even when lesional glucose metabolism is low.

Esophageal Cancer in Patient with Ulcerative Colitis

21

21.1 Clinical History

46-year-old man, underwent surgery and radio-adjuvant chemotherapy for liposarcoma of the right chest wall. Reoperation and adjuvant radiotherapy for loco-regional recurrence 5 years after.

Follow-up after eight years.

- PET-FDG: small nodular areas of hyper accumulation of doubtful meaning in the retrocarenal area.

21.2 Comorbidity

- Ulcerative colitis.

Fig. 21.1 MIP images in anterior and oblique scans show the diffuse high metabolism of the rectum and transverse, descending and sigmoid colon. Caecum and ascending colon show lesser metabolic activity

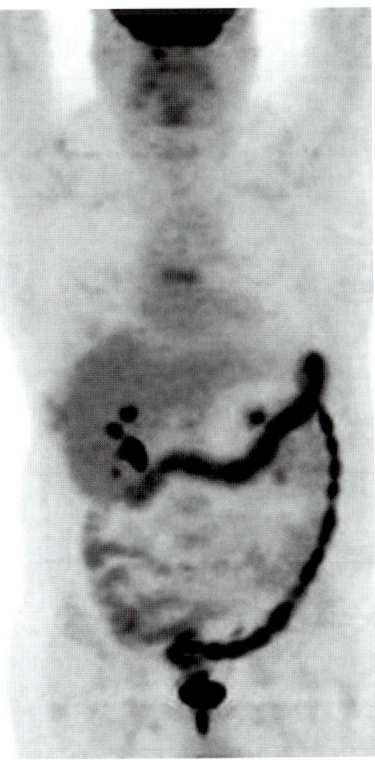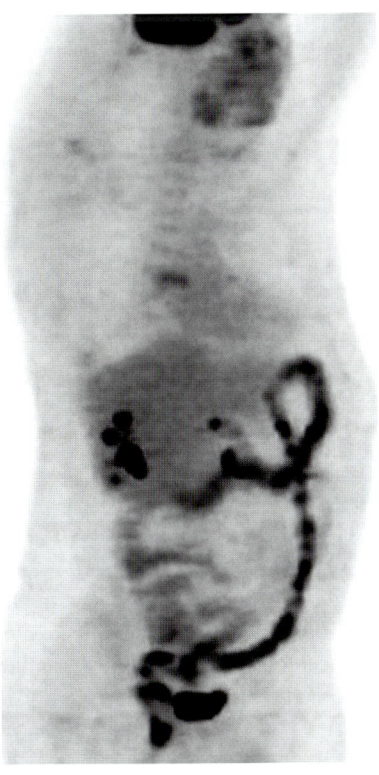

Fig. 21.2 CT-PET shows the presence of solid, inhomogeneous tissue in the posterior mediastinum, inseparable from the wall of the esophagus and showing pathological metabolism

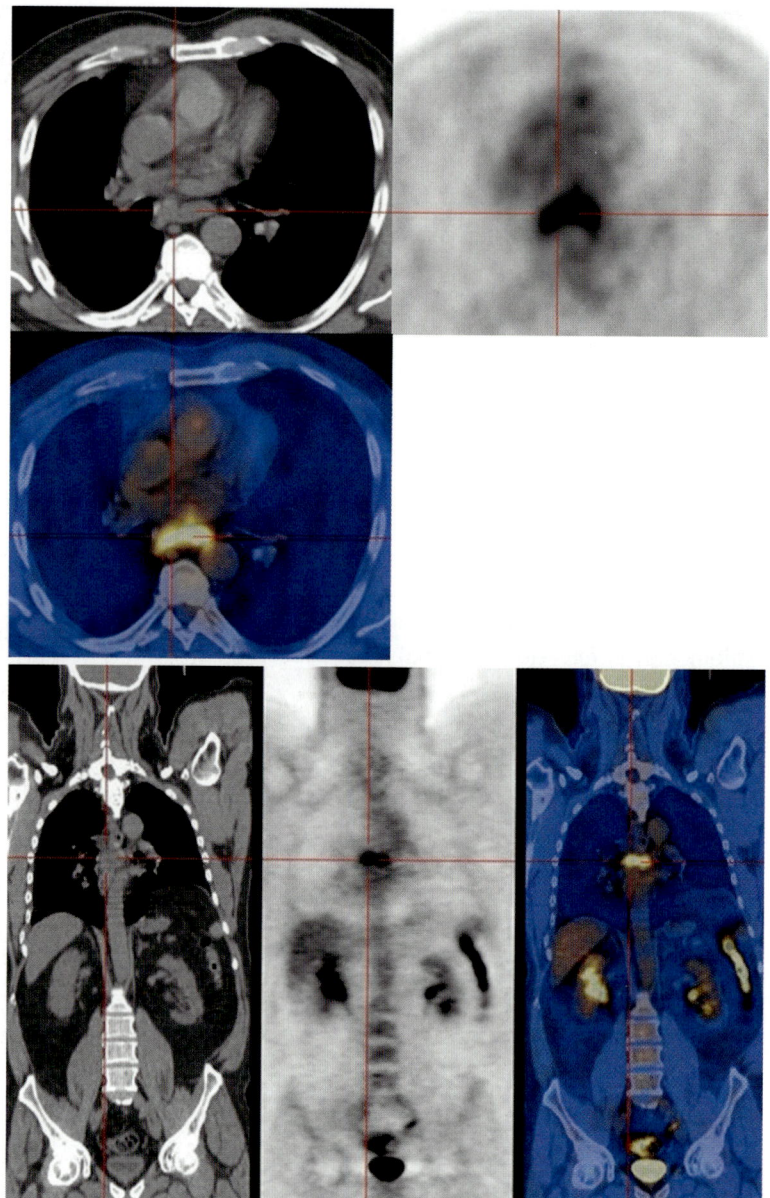

21.3   Diagnostic Question

Search for focal lesions with high glucose metabolism in patient with liposarcoma and with retrocarenal lesion of dubious nature, in follow-up.

21.4   Report

Pathological glucose consumption within the retrocarenal-paraesophageal area, SUV max 5.7 incremented in intensity and extent when compared to the previous scan.

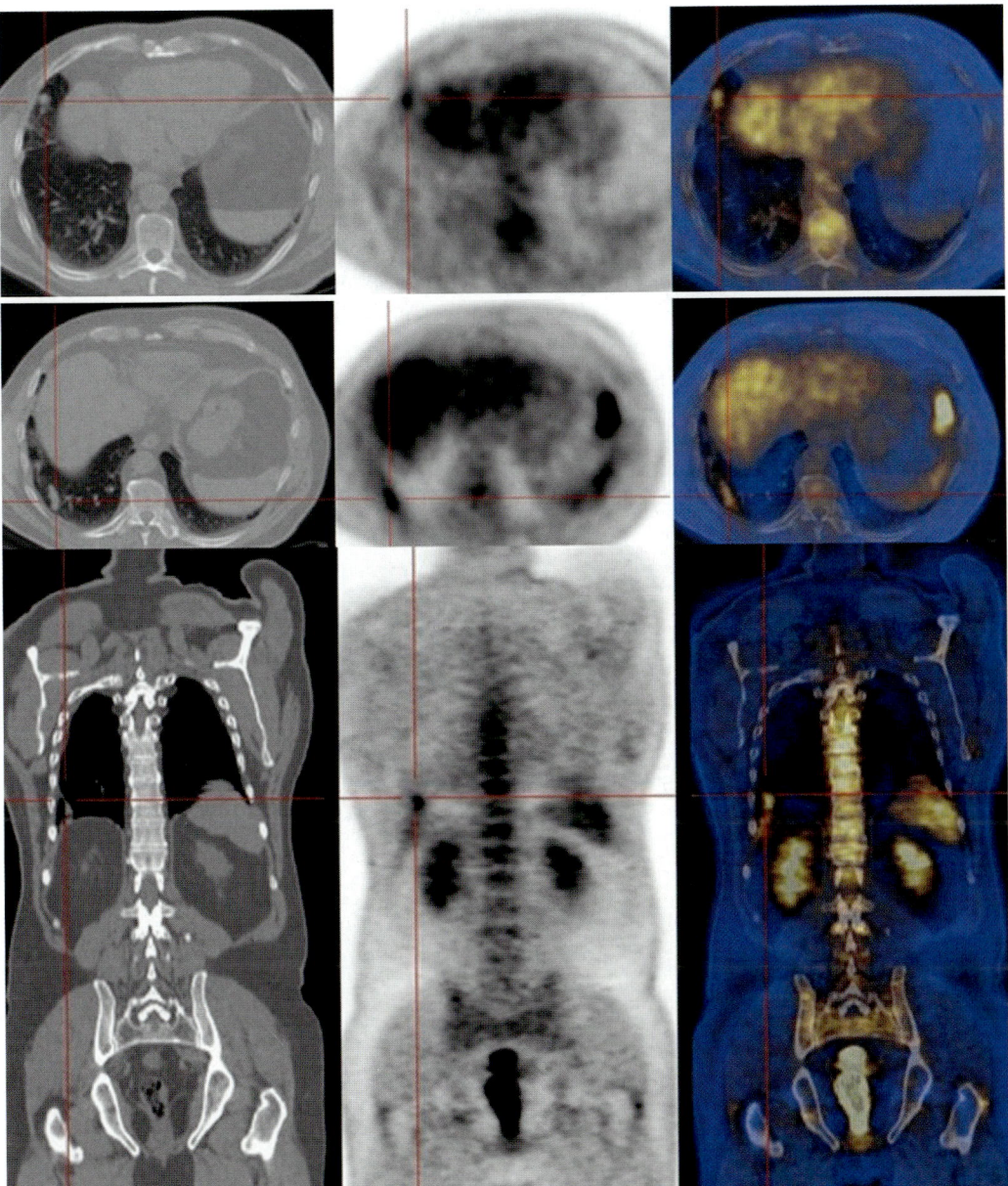

Fig. 21.3 On CT-PET a small pulmonary right anterior basal nodule and an infero-posterior ipsilateral disventilatory streak are observed. These elements are characterized by low consumption of glucose and are attributable to disventilatory-fibrotic lung damage due to chronic actinic injury, determined by the previous radiotherapy treatment, performed after the excision of the sarcoma of the chest wall

Slight increase in metabolism in an anterior basal right lung nodule, measuring one centimeter, and in an inferior—posterior ipsilateral streak SUV max 1.5, both to relate to late outcomes of radiotherapy (actinic fibrosis).

Deposition of FDG to the large intestine is more intense in the transverse, the descending and the sigmoid colon and rectum, to be referred to the previously diagnosed IBD, of discrete inflammatory activity in the current scan (Fig. 21.1).

21.5   Conclusions

The scan shows pathological glucose consumption in the esophagus, to be confirmed by endoscopy. (see Figs. 21.1–21.3).

21.6   Key Points

A primary tumor of the esophagus should always be suspected when CT-PET shows focal high metabolism lesions at the posterior mediastinum. Disventilatory phenomena frequently cause a slight increase in glucose consumption related to nonspecific inflammation. This phenomenon is more common in patients receiving radiation therapy that induces reactive actinic fibrosis.

Esophageal Cancer and Secondary Nodal Metastases

22

22.1 Clinical History

67-year-old patient with dyspepsia, heartburn and gastro-oesophageal reflux.

- EGD: ulcerated lesion in the middle third of the esophagus.
- TC: The presence of lymph node swelling in the lodge of Barety in the aortopulmonary window, in the subcarinal and right hilar areas. Lymphnodes measuring less than a centimeter and found in the porto-caval and interaorto-caval areas are not of pathologic interest.

22.2 Diagnostic Question

Staging of esophageal carcinoma: search for lesions with a high metabolism.

22.3 Report

Abnormal glucose consumption in the middle third of the esophagus, SUV max 8.9.

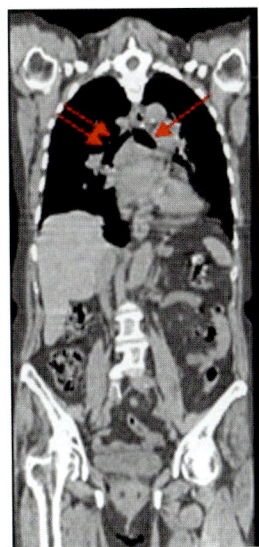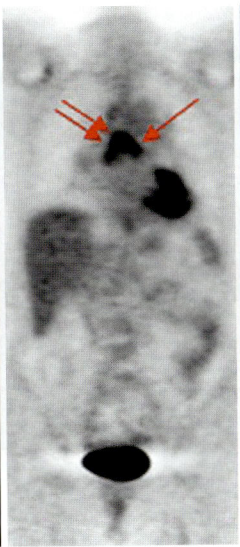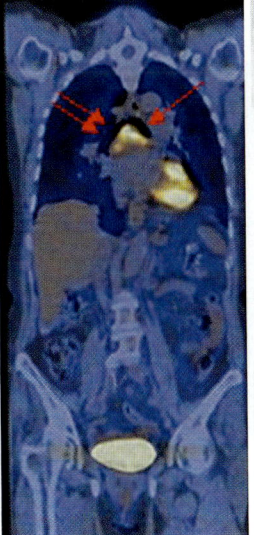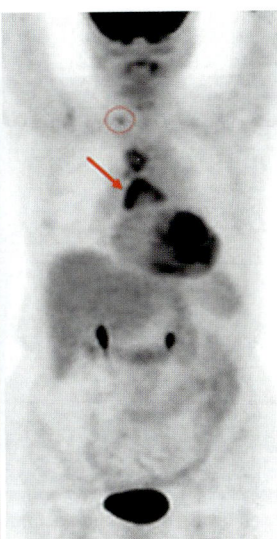

Fig. 22.1 The MIP image shows intense FDG deposition in an esophageal coarse lesion with mediastinal involvement. The use of PET-CT coronal reconstruction allows the definition of the precise location of lymph node metastases in the subcarinal area (*arrows*)

P. F. Rambaldi, *Whole-Body FDG PET Imaging in Oncology*,
DOI: 10.1007/978-88-470-5295-6_22, © Springer-Verlag Italia 2014

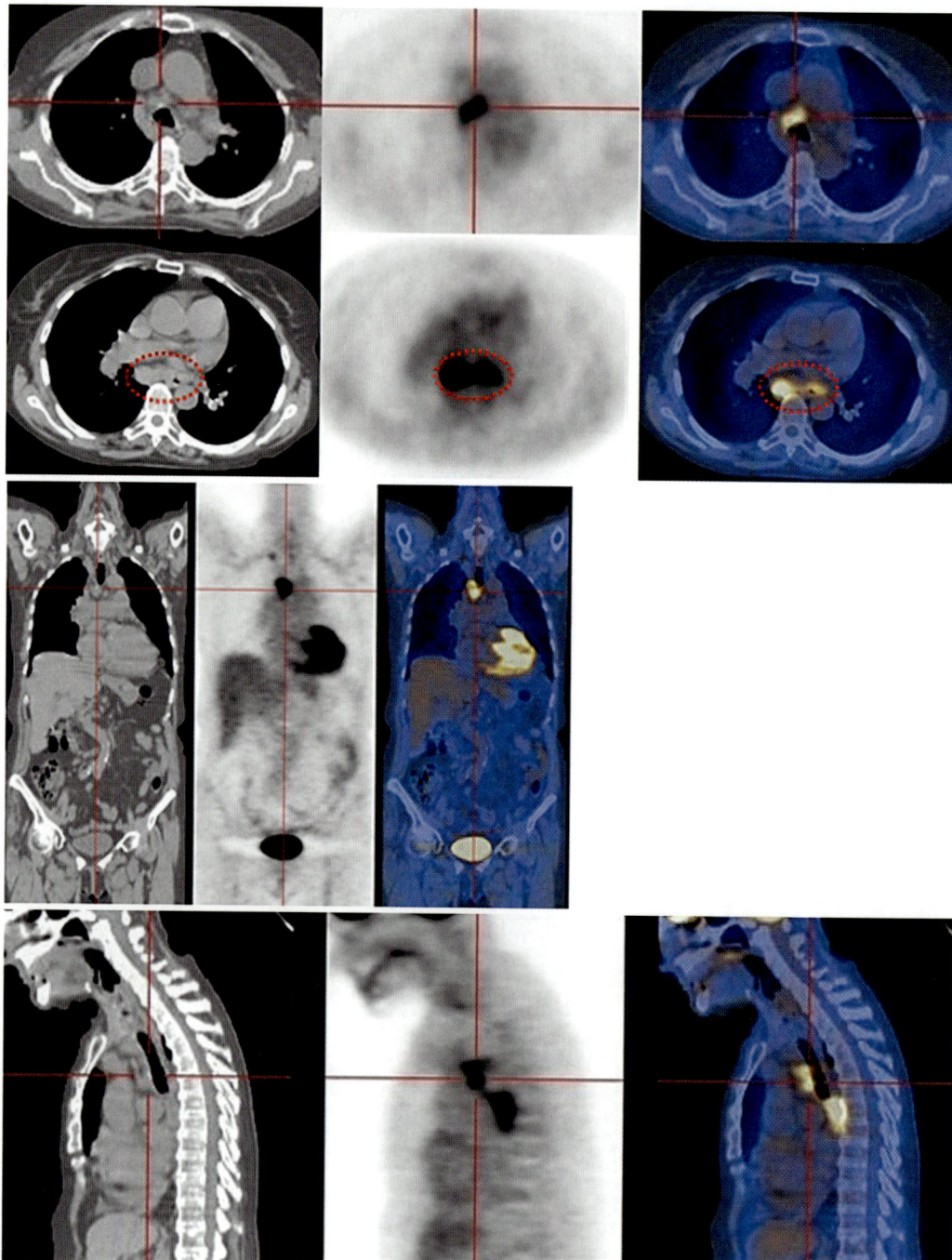

Fig. 22.2 PET-CT demonstrates abnormal glucose metabolism in the middle third of the esophagus and subcarinal lymph nodes that appear enlarged (sagittal reconstruction). Cranially, the lumen of the organ is enlarged due to the neoplastic stenosis and concomitant compression determined by the neoplasm

Presence of multiple adenopathies with intense glucose metabolism in Barety's space, the aortopulmonary window, in the pre- and subcarinal and the right pulmonary hilum, SUV max 11, and to a lesser extent in the ipsilateral clavicular fossa, SUV max 2.4. Lymph nodes measuring less than a centimeter and identified by the TC, as reported in the clinical history in the porto-caval and interaorto-caval do not have pathological carbohydrate consumption.

No significant areas of abnormal FDG metabolism in the remaining body segments examined.

22.4   Conclusions

The PET shows esophageal cancer and multiple lymph node metastases with a high metabolism (Fig. 22.1). (See also Fig. 22.2).

22.5   Key Points

- There are no precise strategies in the initial staging of esophageal cancer.
- In cases of lymph node involvement and/or the presence of distant metastases already documented by CT, nuclear medicine defines the metabolic activity of the tumor and cell vitality and grading.
- This information is preliminary to the treatment and neoadjuvant radio-chemotherapy is needed to verify the subsequent metabolic response to restaging.

Locoregional Recurrence of Carcinoma of the Uterus with Lymph Node Metastasis that Determines Lymphedema and Obstructive Hydronephrosis

23.1 Clinical History

Radical hysterectomy with bilateral salpingo-oophorectomy preceded by neoadjuvant chemo-radiotherapy for adenocarcinoma of the uterine cervix in a 65-year-old woman.

Restaging after surgery:
- PET-FDG: accumulation (SUV max 3.2) of the tracer at the level of the lesser pelvis between the rectum and bladder in the right paramedian region, adjacent to the metal clips. On the right there is a small absorbing area (SUV max 2.8), due to the external iliac lymphadenopathy. On the left there are some weak uptakes corresponding to small sub-centimetric lymph nodes located in the para-aortic region, beside the renal lodge. This finding is not conclusive: tumor recurrence versus post-surgical inflammation.

Check after adjuvant chemotherapy:
- Recent onset of unilateral lymphedema of the lower right limb.
- CT: para-aortic left (25 × 20 mm) and right iliac-obturator lymphadenopathy (36 × 35 mm). Irregular solid tissue swelling in the posterior pelvis 47 × 30 mm, due to

locoregional recurrence. Presence of right hydroureteronephrosis.

23.2 Diagnostic Question

Search for focal lesions with high glucose metabolism in patient with a history of carcinoma of the uterine cervix that currently shows right lower limb lymphedema associated with pain and paresthesias.

23.3 Report

Coarse mass characterized by abnormal glucose consumption at the level of the lesser pelvis, that extends posteriorly from the vaginal vault to the bladder, with underactive area due to colliquation areas contained within, SUV max 8.

Presence of multiple lymph nodes with intense glucose metabolism in the left para-aortic, SUV max 5, iliac-obturator right, SUV max 6.5, and presacral ipsilateral regions, SUV max 4.4. This latter formation determines ipsilateral obstructive hydroureteronephrosis (Fig. 23.1).

P. F. Rambaldi, *Whole-Body FDG PET Imaging in Oncology*,
DOI: 10.1007/978-88-470-5295-6_23, © Springer-Verlag Italia 2014

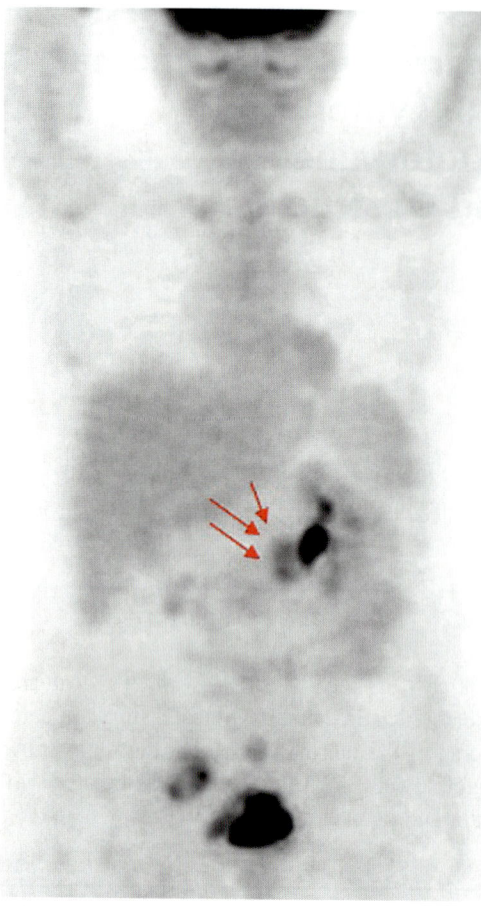

23.4   Conclusions

The PET scan shows extended locoregional recurrence associated with nodal satellite involvement that is responsible for right lower limb plexopathy and ipsilateral obstructive uropathy.

The sequence of images (Figs. 23.2–23.6) shows the morpho-functional dissociation: at the CT, the right kidney is increased in size but has slight parenchymal function. Cortical thickness is slightly thinned (Fig. 23.2, *red arrows*), the pelvis is severely dilated and has a predominantly exophytic development. We observe the presence of contrast administered during a CT scan performed a few days before (Fig. 23.2, *yellow arrows*), for the same reason contrast can be seen in the bowel (Fig. 23.2, *blue arrows*). The PET shows weak deposition of glucose in the right renal cortex (Fig. 23.2, *red arrows*), while there is absent activity in the excretory cavity (Fig. 23.2, *yellow arrows*). This item indicates the limited function of the parenchyma and poor filtration caused by the tumoral obstructive ureteral infiltration. The parenchymal concentration of glucose is not predictive of recovery of renal function, after the obstruction was removed with a stent implantation.

Fig. 23.1 Presence of some lymph nodes in the left para-aortic region that compress the pyeloureteral junction without causing obstruction (MIP image)

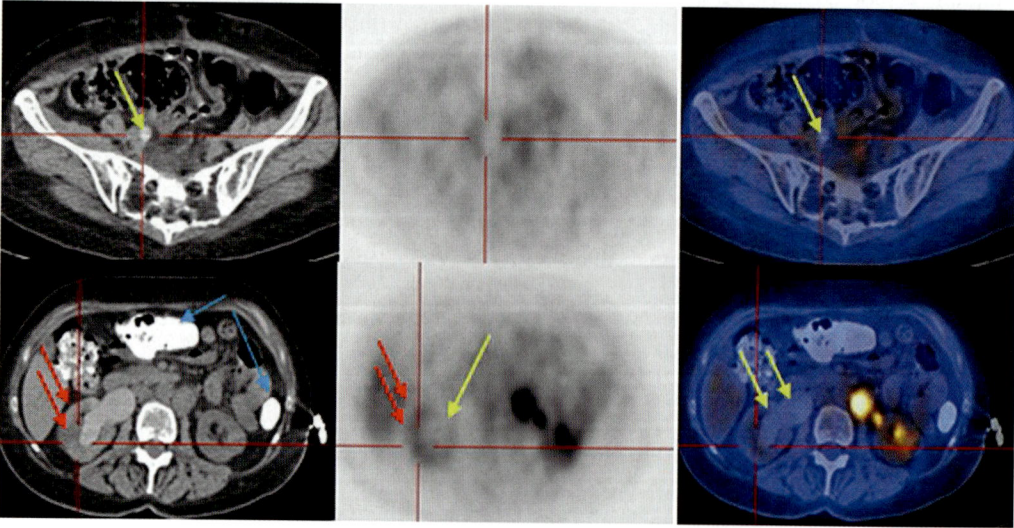

Fig. 23.2 MIP image 1

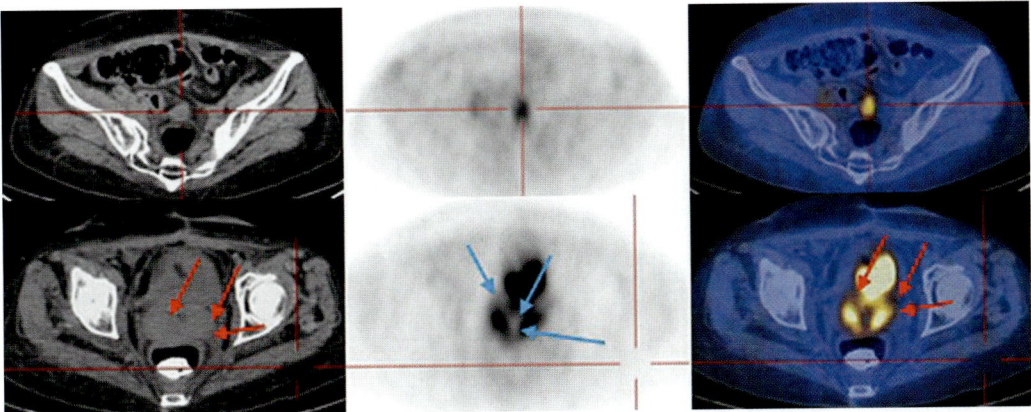

Fig. 23.3 At the CT there is a solid, irregular mass, not dissociable from the bladder anteriorly and posteriorly from the rectum (*red arrows*). At PET scan this lesion presents a cold core compatible with fibrosis determined by previous radiotherapy and / or from the colliquative component (*blue arrows*). The high metabolic activity of peripheral areas documents the vitality of the tumor, and recurrence

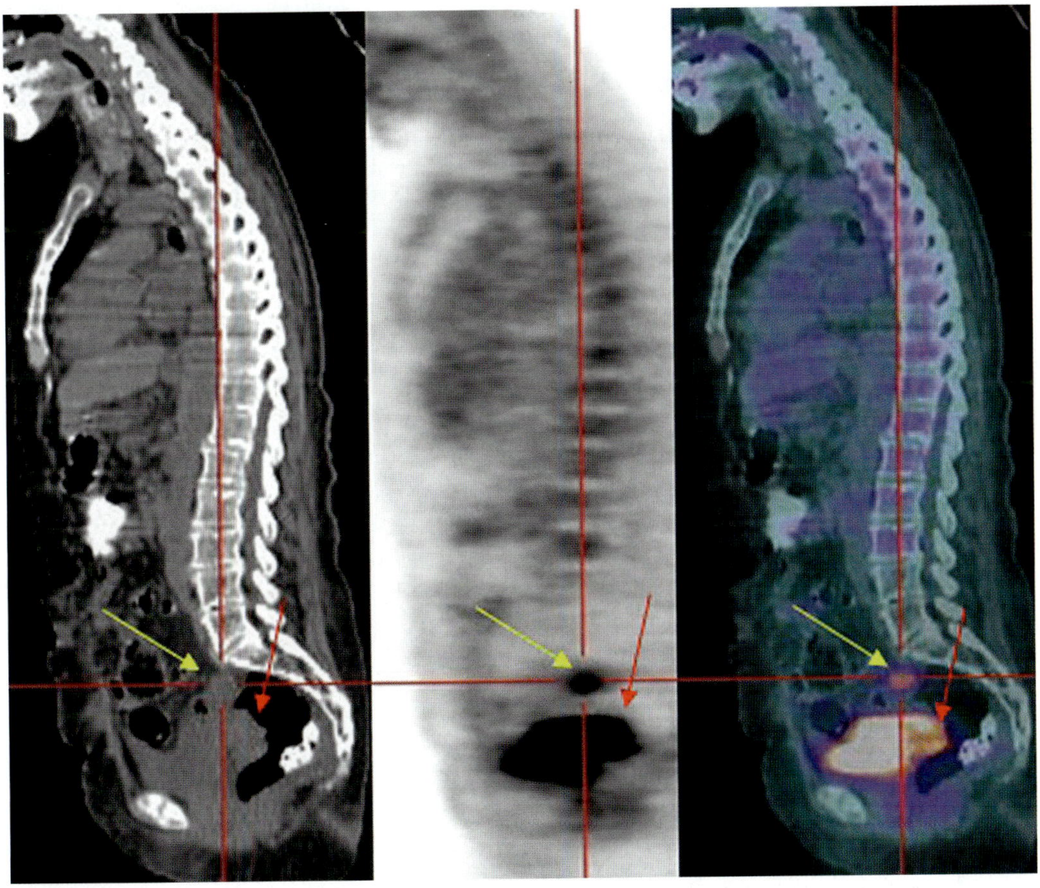

Fig. 23.4 In the sagittal reconstructions presacral adenopathy is seen (*yellow arrows*), with a high metabolism. Bone marrow activation is associated with post-chemotherapy rebound

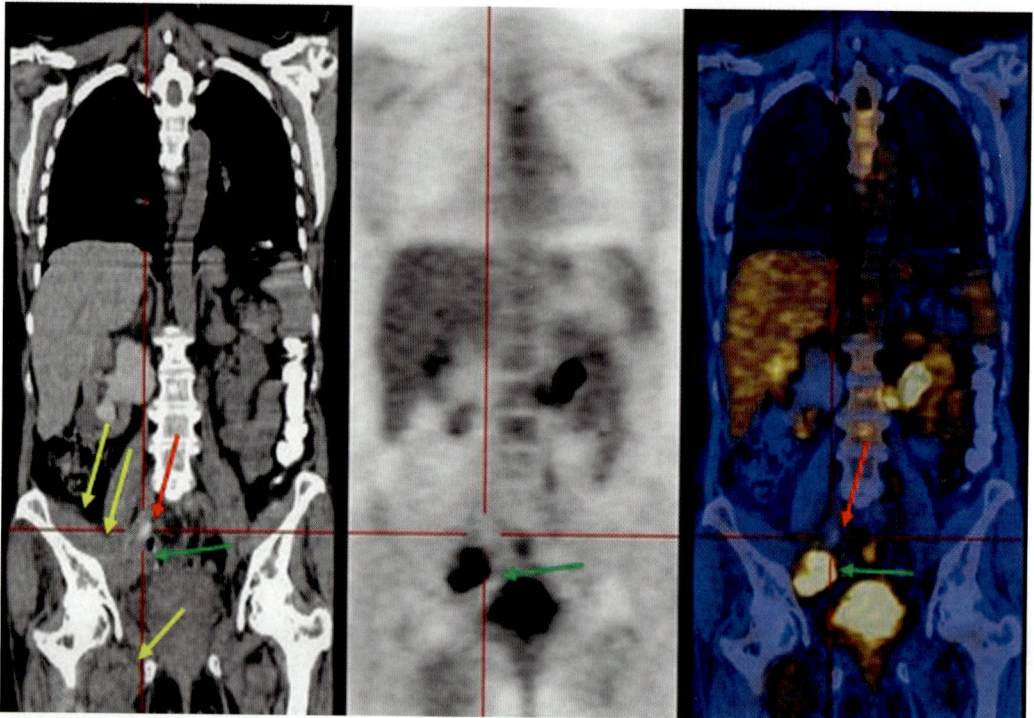

Fig. 23.5 The CT-PET shows high metabolism in a right obturatory nodal mass (*green arrows*) that determines thickening of the iliopsoas muscle and soft tissues of the ipsilateral lower limb (*yellow arrows*) with altered drainage (lymphedema). This nodal conglomerate infiltrates and blocks the ipsilateral ureter, which is dilated upstream. In the lumen of the ureter there is contrast administered in a previous CT examination (*red arrows*)

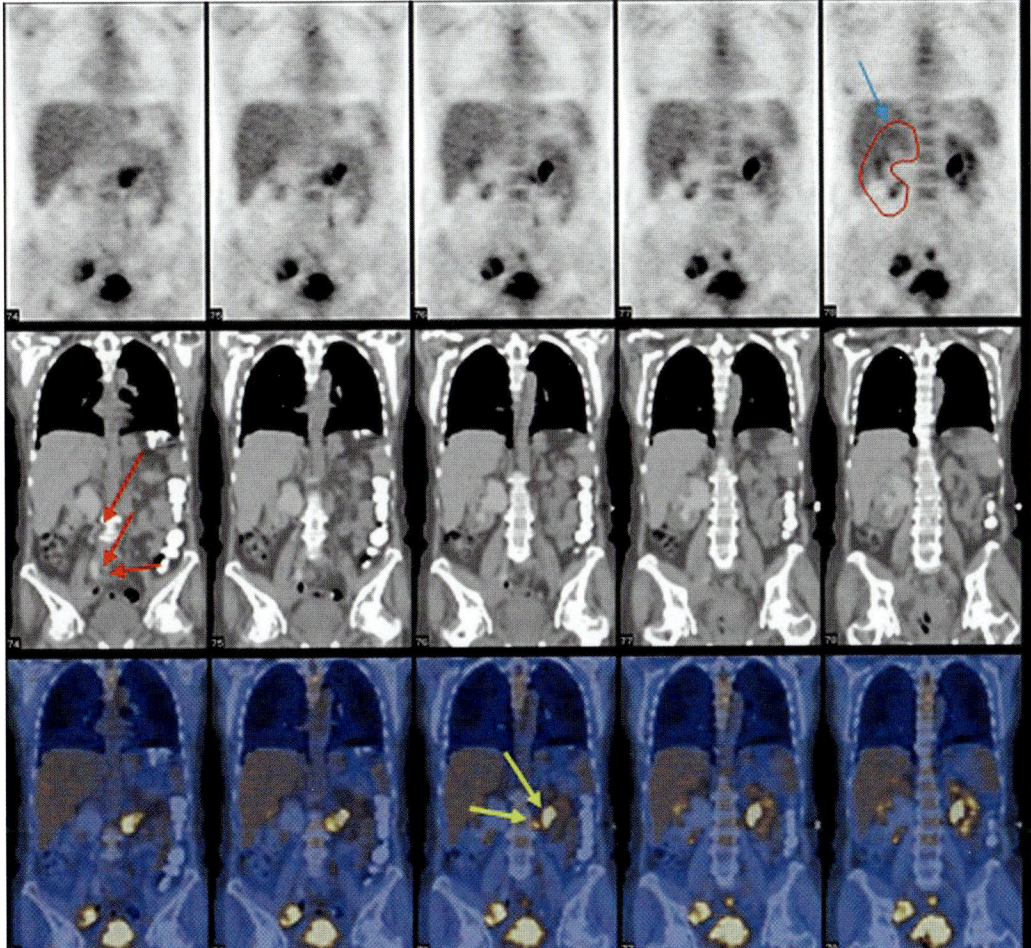

Fig. 23.6 At PET-CT in the right urinary system there is the presence of contrast medium administered during a CT scan performed a few days before (*red arrows*). This, however, is not predictive of functional recovery of the parenchyma (*blue arrow*) in the case of stent implantation. The left kidney (*yellow arrows*) is not blocked even if it shows moderate dilatation of the pelvis which is compressed, at the junction by a para-aortic lymph node with a high metabolism

23.5   Key Points

- The clinical progression of disease is suggested by the presence of pain associated with paresthesia of the lower right limb, which is swollen (lymphedema).
- The PET confirmed disease progression and localized critical districts.

- The intense metabolic activity demonstrates the chemoresistance of the tumor.

   In these cases, it is urgent to have a palliative approach:
- treatment of pain;
- treatment and management of lymphedema, or at least, slowing its progression,
- urological advice to enhance or preserve renal function.

Ovarian Cancer and Peritoneal Carcinosis: Follow-up After Chemotherapy

24

24.1 Clinical History

Radical hysterectomy, bilateral salpingo-oophorectomy and systematic pelvic lymphadenectomy for ovarian cancer in a woman of 55 years of age.

The follow-up performed at five years shows abdominal and pelvic recurrence:
- CT: centimetric nodes in the jugulo-digastric region bilaterally. Inhomogeneous spleen with hypodense nodule to the upper third measuring 25 mm, unchanged from the previous controls. 25 mm solid nodular swelling in the pelvic left paramedian region, also unchanged, compared with the previous CT.
- PET-FDG: presence of some areas of solid tissue with pathological glucose consumption in the pelvis, the most obvious in the left obturatory (SUV max 19), right internal iliac (SUV max 4.9) and ipsilateral pericolic stations (SUV max 10). Pathological increase in the metabolism of glucose to report to peritoneal involvement of some serous nodules adherent to the spleen (SUV max 5), the diaphragm (SUV max 4) and the liver in correspondence of the II and III segment (SUV max 8 and 6). Conclusions: The PET scan shows recurrence of disease with a high metabolism.
  Restaging after chemotherapy:
- CT: reactive centimetric lymph nodes of in the lateral cervical region bilaterally. Spleen-density is inhomogeneous due to the presence at the upper pole of a formation of reduced tissue

attenuation (4.4 cm), increased in size when compared to the previous examination. Presence of some swelling in the iliac—obturator lymph nodes bilaterally, with a maximum diameter of 2.5 cm to the left, 1 cm to the right.
- PET-FDG nodule with a high metabolism in the left obturatory region (SUV max 11), reduced in intensity and size compared to the previous control. No pathological consumption of FDG in the peritoneal, splenic and hepatic areas previously up taking, due to response to chemotherapy.

24.2 Diagnostic Question

Restaging 3 months after chemotherapy in woman with recurrent metastatic ovarian cancer: search for focal lesions with a high metabolism of glucose.

24.3 Report

The PET scan shows multiple nodules characterized by abnormal glucose consumption at the pelvis, the most evident in the obturatory, SUV max 22, left presacral, SUV max 19, right internal iliac, SUV max 5.2, and pericolic ipsilateral stations, SUV max 6.

Pathological increase of glucose metabolism due to peritoneal involvement in two subglissonian nodules in the II and III hepatic segments, SUV max 13 and 18 respectively and in

P. F. Rambaldi, *Whole-Body FDG PET Imaging in Oncology*,
DOI: 10.1007/978-88-470-5295-6_24, © Springer-Verlag Italia 2014

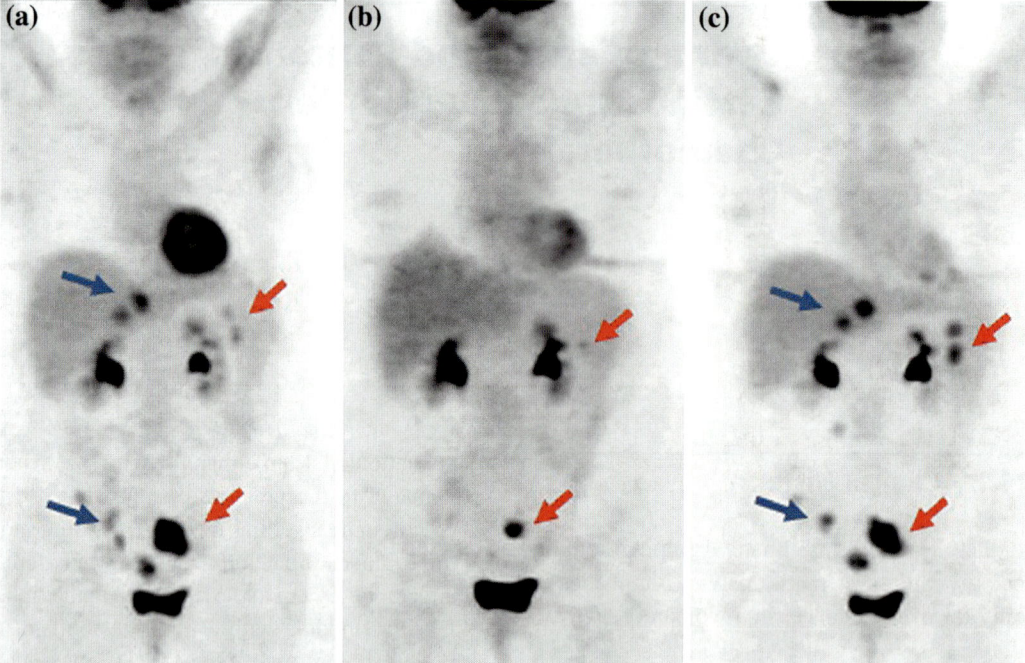

Fig. 24.1 The PET shows high basal metabolism of glucose, multiple peritoneal nodules evident in the pelvis, on the surface of the liver and spleen, due to recurrence from illness (a). Follow up after chemotherapy (b) shows the incomplete response to treatment with persistent vitality of a peritoneal malignant nodule in the left obturatory region and a small mass adherent to the medial aspect of the spleen. Three months after chemotherapy, PET-CT showed a net progression of the disease (c)

two splenic lesions on the medial side and the upper pole with SUV max of 9 and 14 respectively.

24.4   Conclusions

PET scan shows progression of the peritoneal carcinomatosis. (See Figs. 24.1–24.6).

24.5   Key Points

- The peritoneal carcinomatosis is a different WAY of tumor dissemination (vs. hematogenous and lymphatic); tissue implants of the diaphragm, liver, spleen, and other districts should be differentiated from lesions of hematogenous origin and lymph nodes because the treatment protocol is different.

- Often, the multiplanar CT and CT-PET are an aid in the differential diagnosis of secondary injuries caused by peritoneal dissemination, more than in those of hematogenous and lymphatic origin.

   Not all data in the literature report an optimal accuracy of nuclear medicine techniques in the diagnosis of peritoneal carcinomatosis secondary to advanced ovarian cancer.

- If a PET-CT examination performed during staging is positive, it shows that the tumor has biological affinity for FDG, and this technique will then be registered in the subsequent restaging.

- The persistence of carbohydrate consumption in the lesion documented by CT-PET performed at restaging suggests chemoresistance of the tumor, and a poor prognosis.

   The value of the SUV max is affected by artifacts, so we can say that:

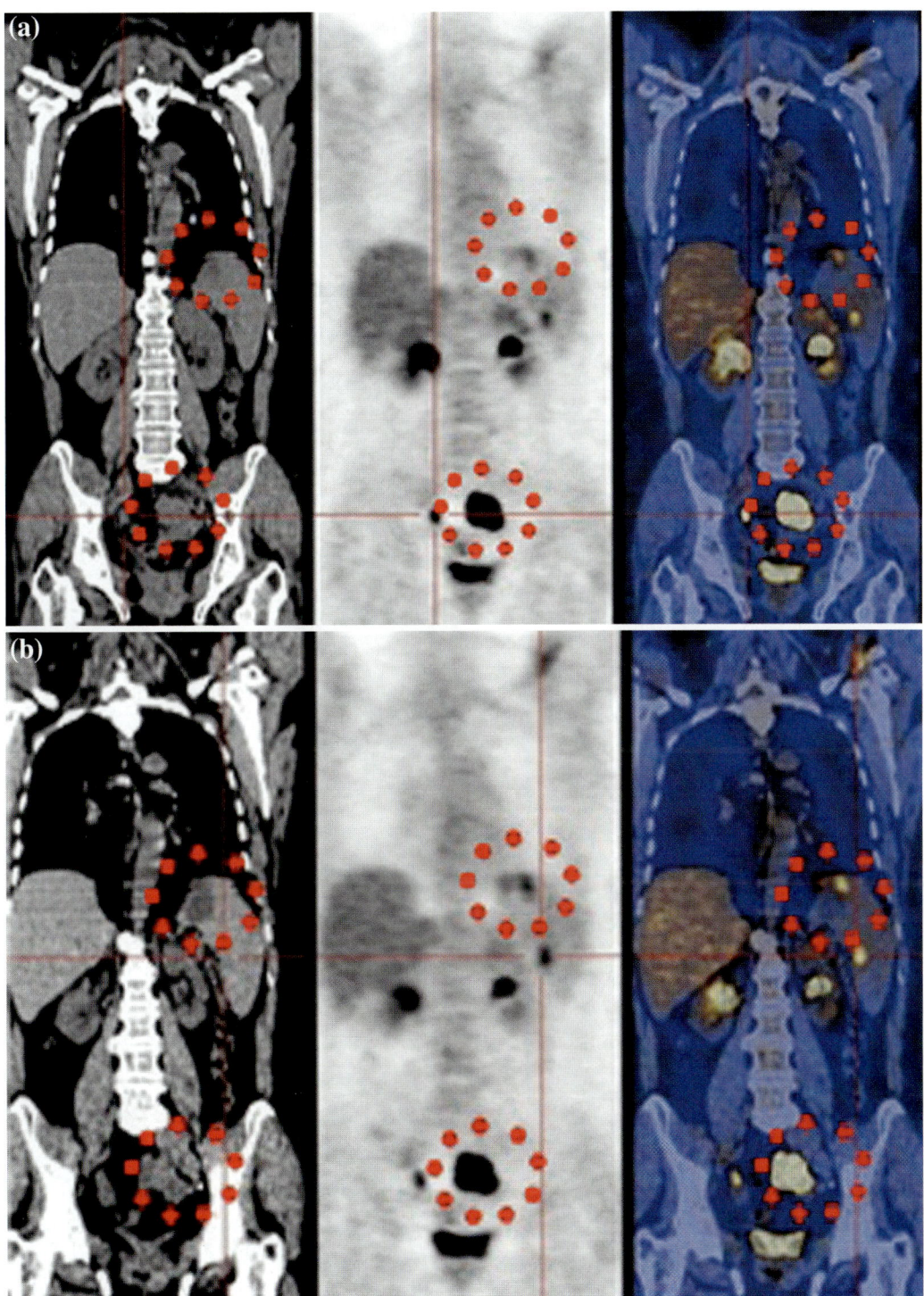

Fig. 24.2 CT-PET performed before chemotherapy (a) shows peritoneal carcinomatosis with multiple nodules with high metabolism, some pelvic, other splenic adherent to the surface. At the scan done 3 months after chemotherapy, the CT-PET (b) shows the recovery of metabolic and morphological pathology in the same districts reported on previous examination

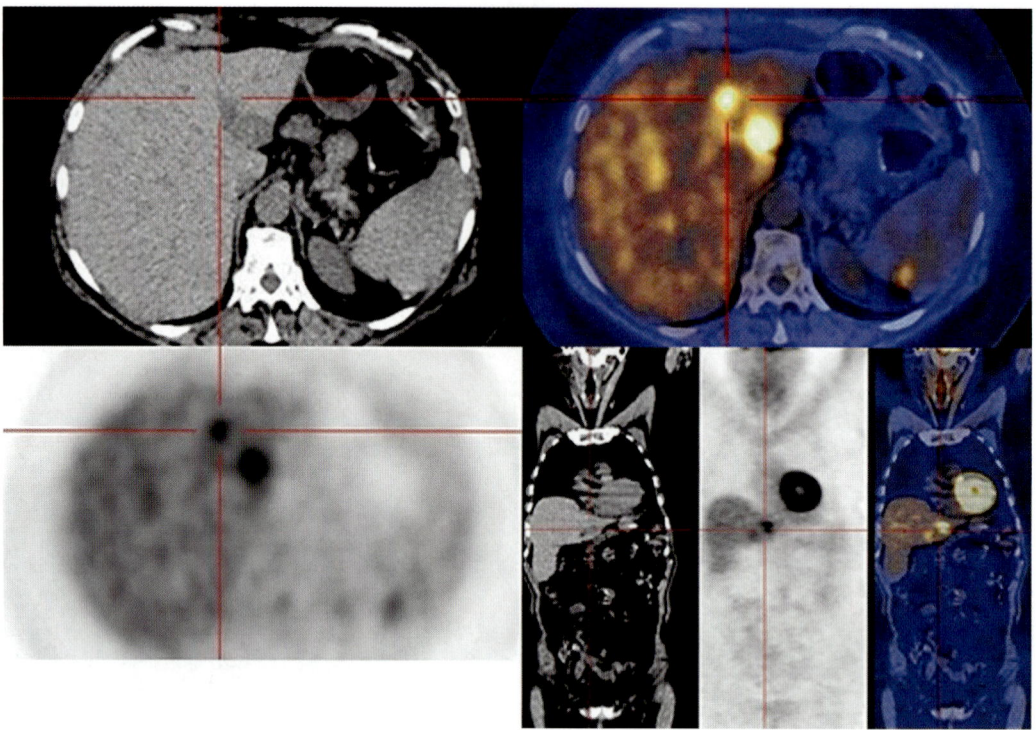

Fig. 24.3 CT before chemotherapy shows two hypodense nodules at the falciform ligament in the II–III hepatic segment, that PET shows to have elevated glucose consumption

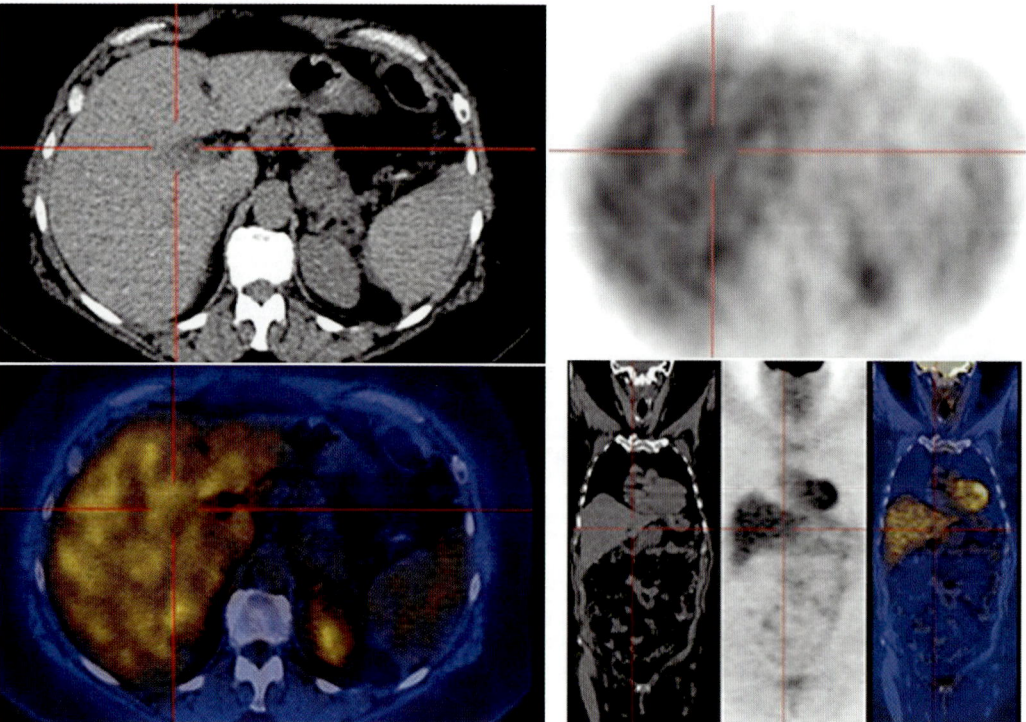

Fig. 24.4 At the scan performed after chemotherapy, both PET and CT show the morphological and metabolic disappearance of the metastatic nodules adherent to the hepatic parenchyma

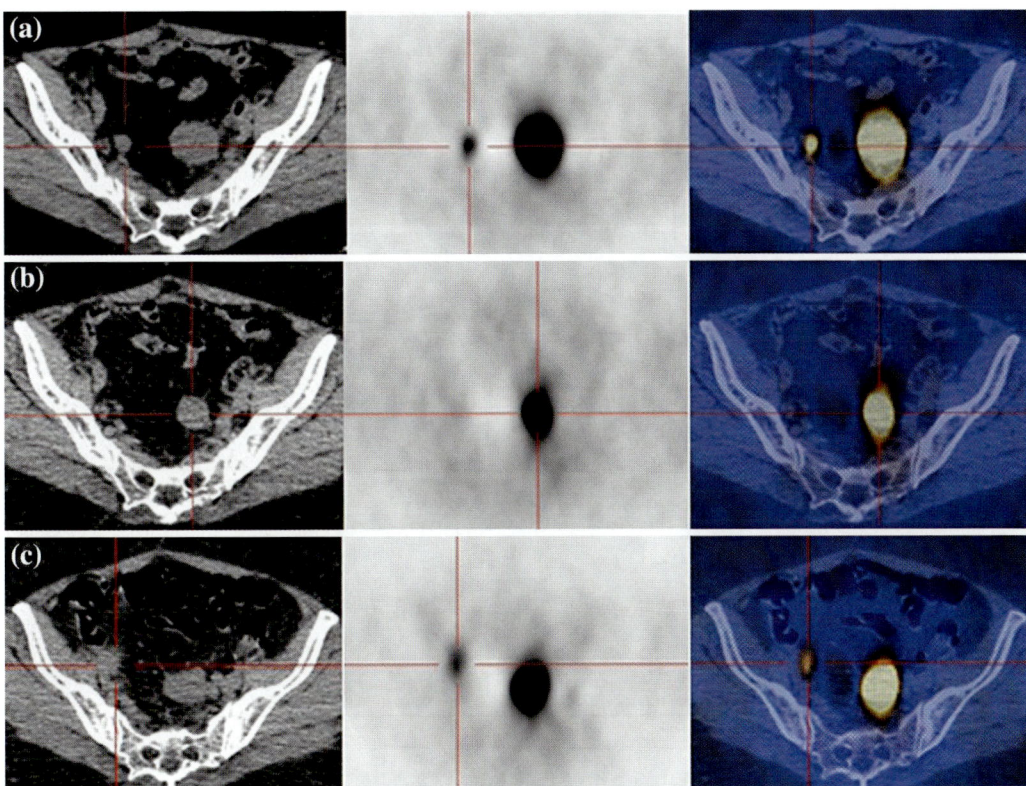

Fig. 24.5 The CT-PET performed before chemotherapy (Figs. 24.5a and 24.6a) shows multiple peritoneal solid metastases with high metabolism, some adherent to the splenic surface. The study performed at the end of treatment (Figs. 24.5b and 24.6b) shows the reducing of both the volume and the biological activity of the disease. Subsequent reassessment CT-PET performed three months after (Figs. 24.5c, 24.6c) shows the volumetric and metabolic recovery of carcinomatosis. The sequence of coronal reconstructions provides a detailed view of the spread of the abdominal and pelvic carcinomatosis (Fig. 24.6d)

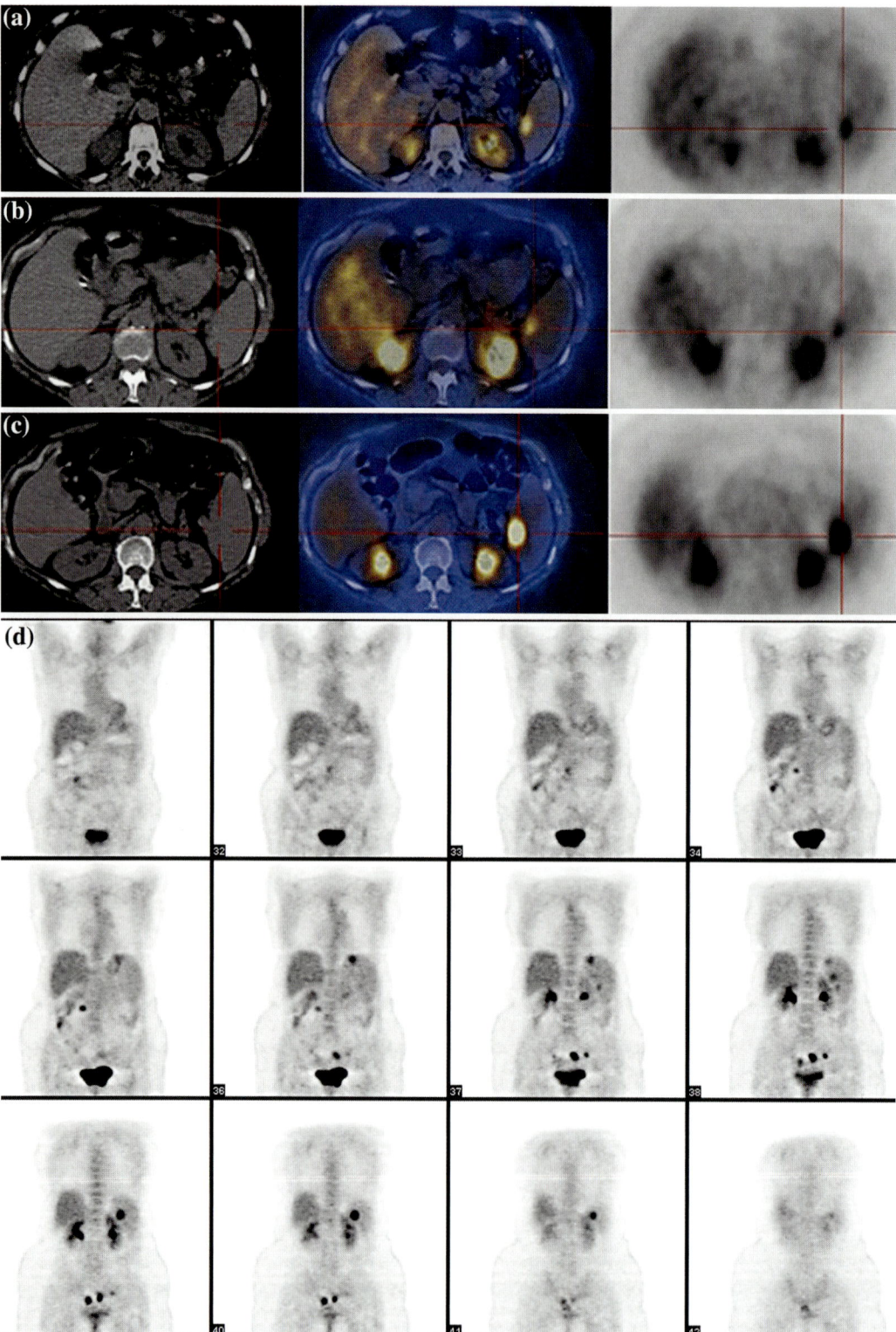

Fig. 24.6

- not always the SUV max enables the assessment of therapeutic response, especially when the examination is performed in different structures with different equipment;
- the comparison with appropriate window of the MIP images before and after chemotherapy allows a simpler assessment of the therapeutic response, especially in the definition of questionable lesions;
- CT and CT-PET images are of aid in cases of doubt.

Ovarian Cancer: Diagnosis and Progression of Disease

25.1 Clinical History

37-year-old woman who underwent laparoscopic radical hysterectomy, salpingo-right lumbar-aortic and pelvic lymphadenectomy for squamous—large cell, well-differentiated (G1) cervical carcinoma. Adjuvant chemotherapy performed.

- Follow-up at three years: negative except for a hypodense oval mass in the left iliac-obturatory region, maximum diameter of 32 mm, substantially unchanged over time.
- Follow-up at 3 years and 6 months: PET-FDG shows modest consumption of glucose (SUV max 2.8) in the mass already previously reported in the left iliac-obturatory region, probably originating from the uterine appendages.
- Follow-up at 4 years: the total body CT demonstrates a volumetric expansion of the left iliac-obturatory mass which has a maximum diameter of 73 × 65 mm, which is poly-lobed, shows internal septa, with solid inhomogeneous tissue inside. Centimetric nodes in the intercavo-aortic and inguinal regions bilaterally.
- The cancer markers are normal: CEA, CA19.9, CA125, CA15.3, TPA.

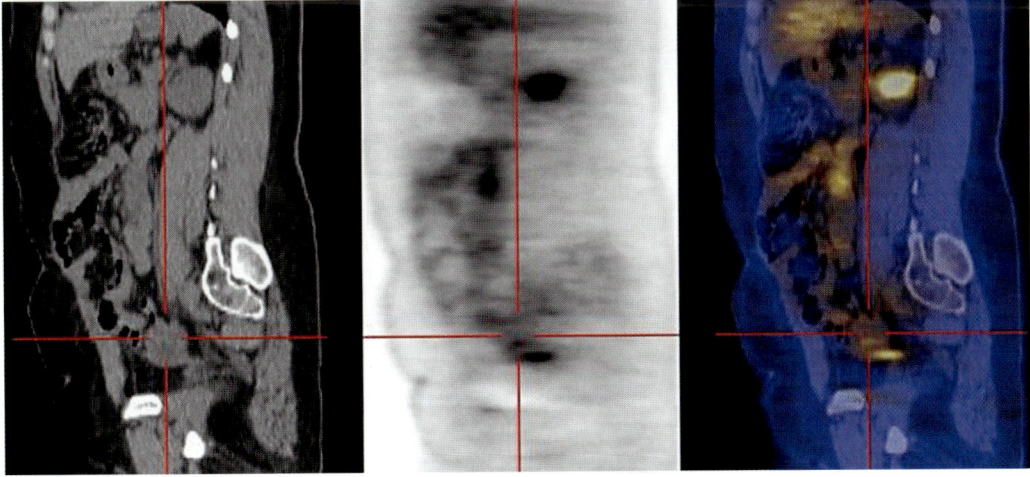

Fig. 25.1 Coarse iliac-obturatory left mass, shows modest consumption of glucose, SUV max 2.5

P. F. Rambaldi, *Whole-Body FDG PET Imaging in Oncology*,
DOI: 10.1007/978-88-470-5295-6_25, © Springer-Verlag Italia 2014

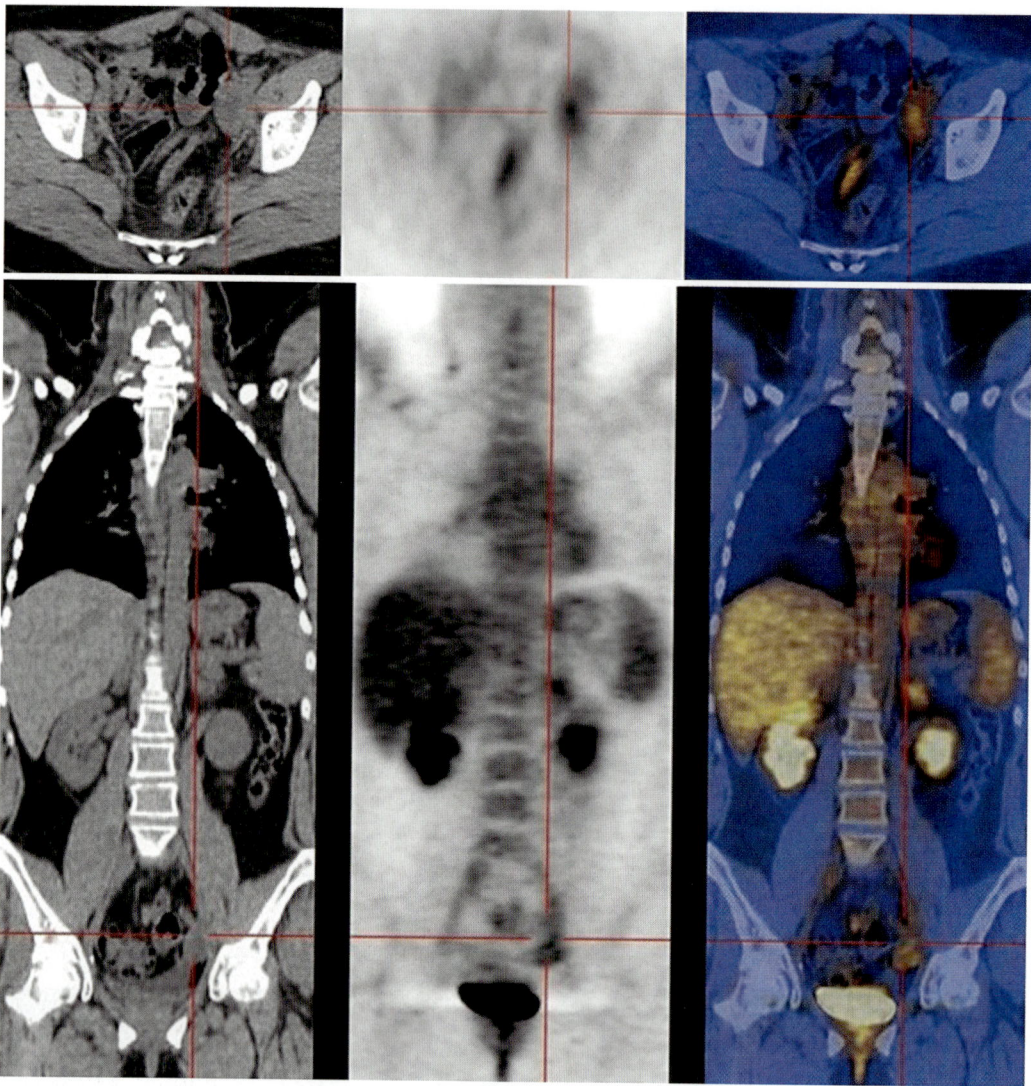

Fig. 25.2 At the CT-PET baseline study a lump in the left iliac-obturator is evident, of adnexal origin, hypodense, heterogeneous, characterized by very low levels of glucose

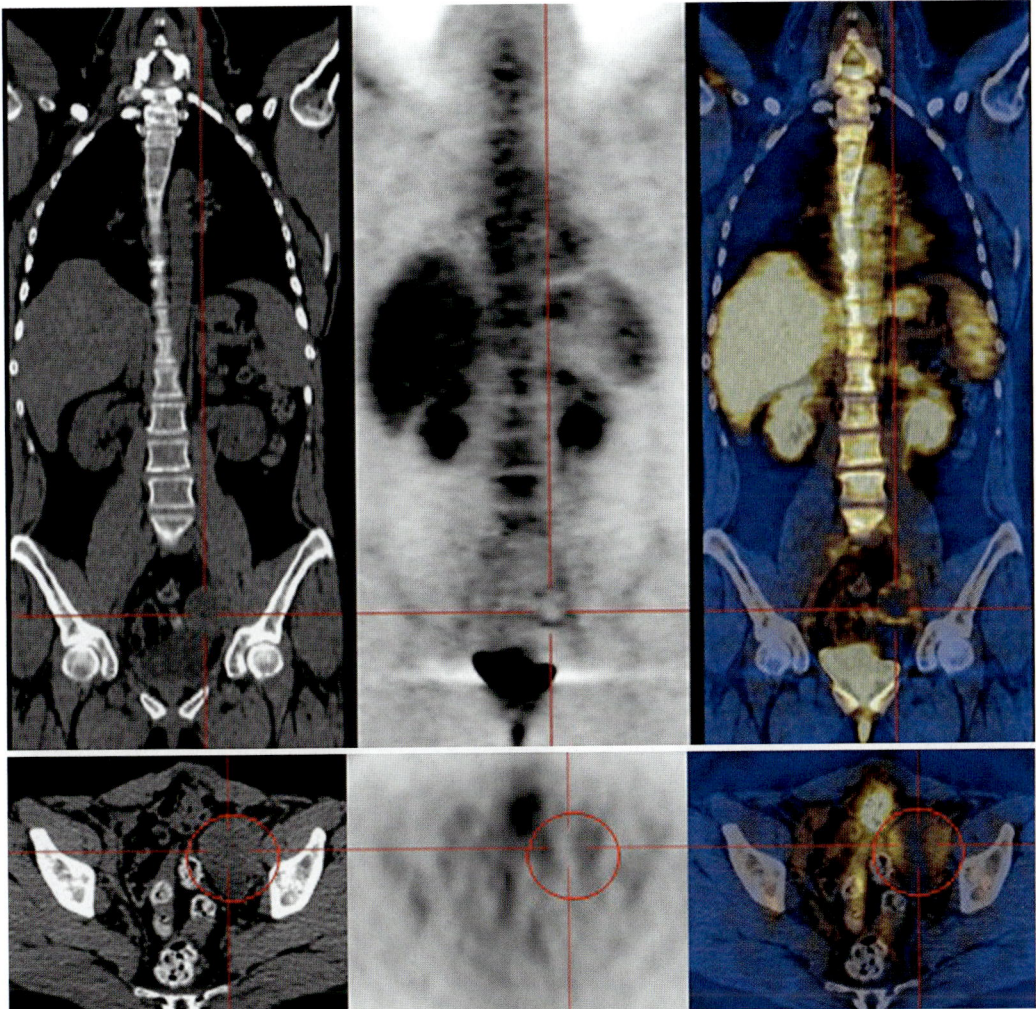

Fig. 25.3 At the CT-PET study performed after six months, compared to the previous 62 examination the nodule in the left iliac-obturatory region shows increase in volume (73 x 65 mm), and appears poly-lobed, with internal septa, heterogeneously hypodense solid tissue. The PET-FDG shows modest carbohydrate consumption only on the margins of the lesion that appears to be substantially made of large shares of colliquative or serous areas

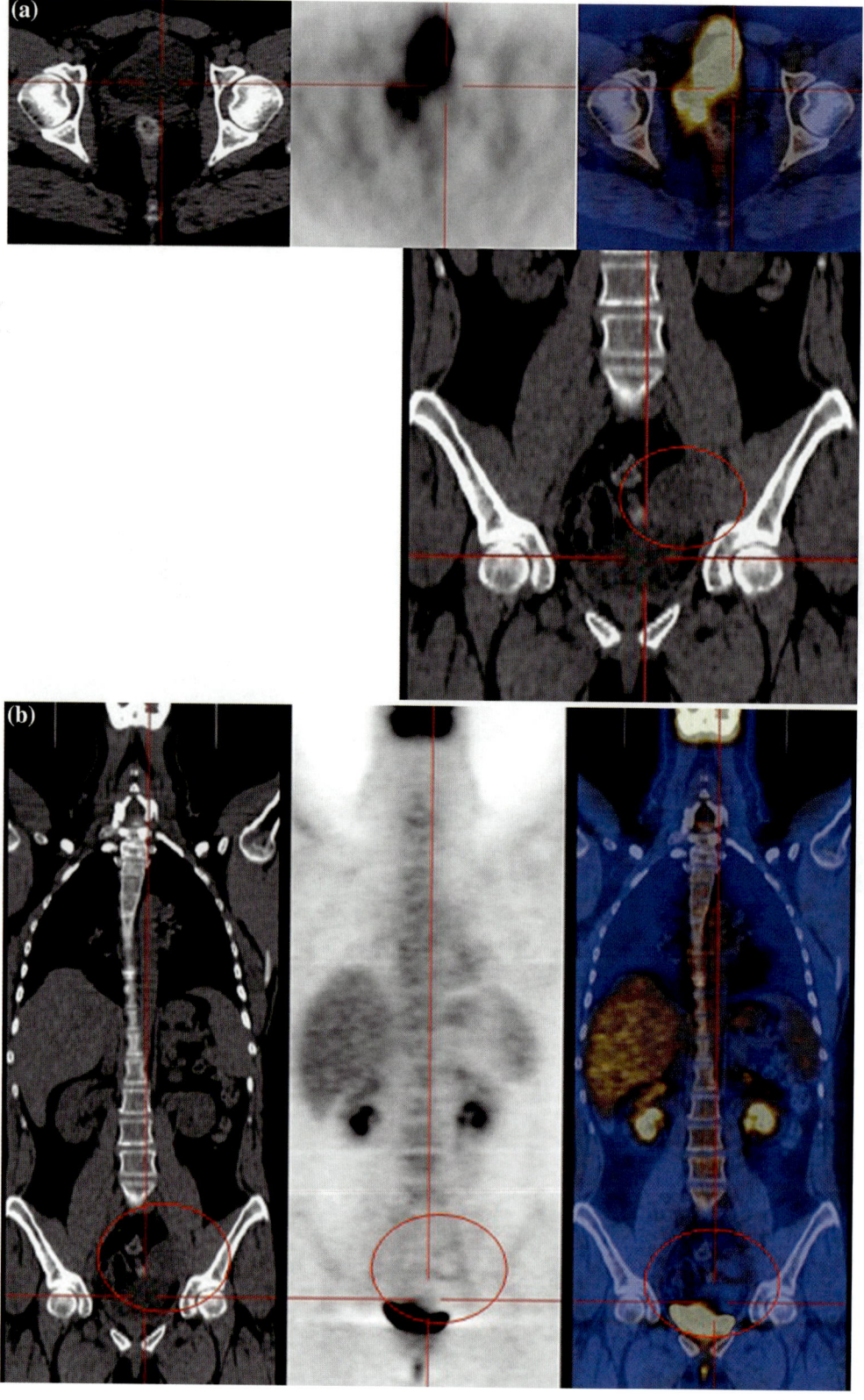

◀ **Fig. 25.4** **a** PET-CT scan after six months the axial scan shows the characteristics of the massive formation that appears hypodense, with internal septa, touching the bladder. **b** The coronal reconstructions allow a better view of the lesion that has little glucose consumption

25.2 Diagnostic Question

Search for focal lesions with high glucose metabolism in patient with a history of cervical cancer and likely adnexal mass, suspicious for pelvic recurrence.

25.3 Report

The coarse iliac-obturatory left mass, shows modest consumption of glucose, SUV max 2.5.

Non-pathological metabolism of intercavo—aortic and inguinal lymph nodes on both sides reported at CT in clinical history, SUV max 0.8 (Fig. 25.1).

No focal lesions in the remaining body segments examined.

25.4 Conclusions

The iliac-obturatory left mass, partially colliquated or serous, shows very low levels of glucose. Its volumetric increase showed at CT

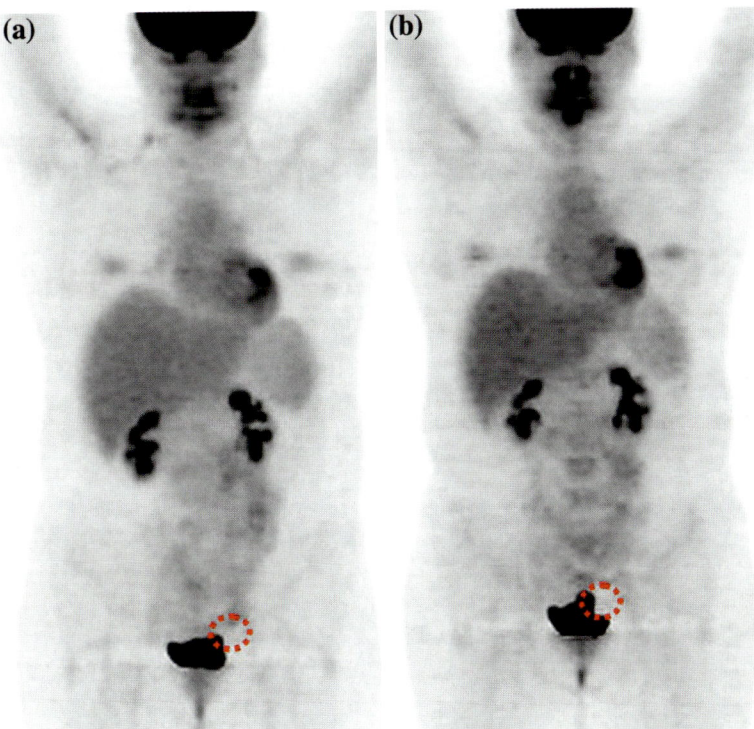

Fig. 25.5 **a** The morphology of the bladder appears to be regular at the basal control while the study performed at six months shows a clear relationship with the neoplastic adnexal mass that has sharply increased in volume.**b** The MIP images of both scans show that this tumor has a low carbohydrate consumption, an element that characterizes some histological types of ovarian cancer

suggests an evolving condition to be studied with MRI and then by typing. (See Figs. 25.2–25.5).

25.5   Key Points

- The subsequent histological examination showed a serous type of ovarian cancer at the left ovary that had not been removed in the

previous surgery, so you should remember that:

- the increase in the volume of a lesion over time should always be considered as suspect, even when the FDG-PET demonstrates restricted carbohydrate consumption, in which case a surgical option is recommended.

Staging of Metastatic Sarcoma of the Uterus

26

26.1 Clinical History

47-year-old woman with histologically typed uterine sarcoma, reported lower abdominal pain during the staging.

- CT: symmetric lungs with a 5-mm lesion in the right upper lobe, adjacent to the fissure. On the left side, two other milli-metric mantlar nodules can be found in the apical segment of the upper lobe and the dorsal aspect of the lower lobe. Morpho-structural alteration of the uterus. Right uterine appendages increased in size and patchy. Multiple swollen lymph-nodes (max = 17 mm) in the intercavo-aortic, precaval areas and iliac areas bilaterally.

26.2 Diagnostic Question

Staging of sarcoma of the uterus: search for focal lesions with a high metabolism of glucose.

26.3 Report

Pathological glucose consumption of a patchy uterine mass with areas of low metabolism on the inside, due at least in part to colliquation, SUV max 13.

Intercavo-aortic precaval and bilateral iliac lymphadenopathies, SUV max 5.

P. F. Rambaldi, *Whole-Body FDG PET Imaging in Oncology*,
DOI: 10.1007/978-88-470-5295-6_26, © Springer-Verlag Italia 2014

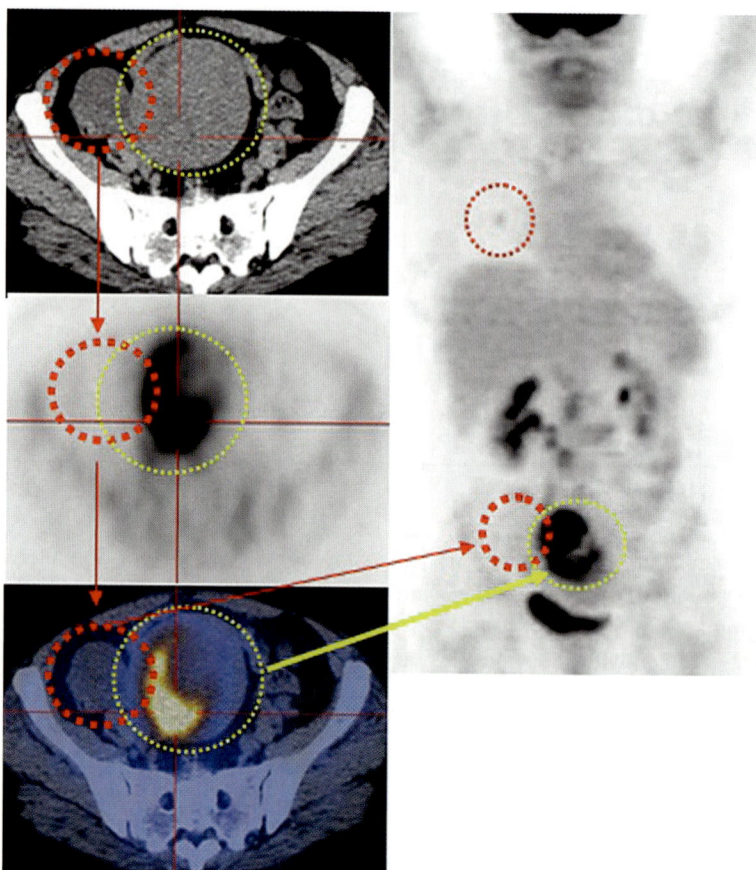

Fig. 26.1 In the MIP image a small right pulmonary nodule with restricted carbohydrate consumption is detected, of metastatic nature. The CT scan shows a right paramedian pelvic mass attributable to the uterus, hypodense, that at the PET scan shows intense cellular activity, with underactive area contained within, which is due to colliquation. The right ovary is highly increased in size, appears as hypodense, with fluid content and shows no pathological glucose metabolism at the PET

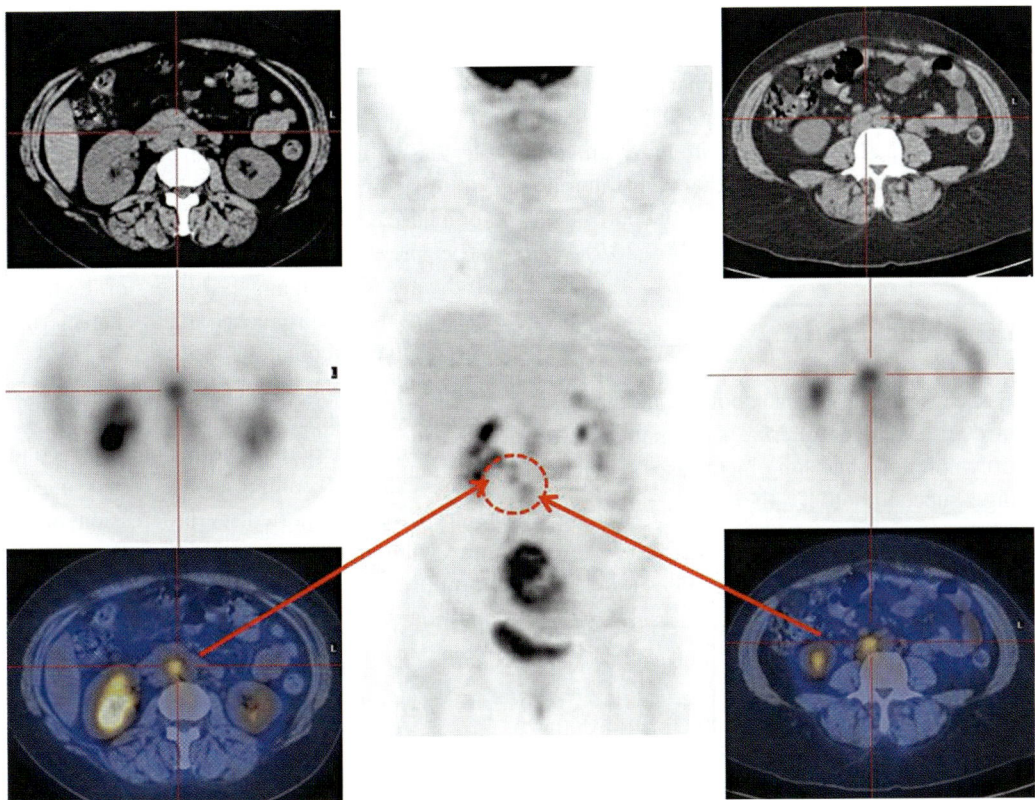

Fig. 26.2 CT-PET shows two lymph nodes increased in size, characterized by high metabolism of glucose, respectively, in the intercavo-aortic and iliac regions. This is associated with a moderate right hydronephrosis secondary to extrinsic nodal compression. Absence of obstruction in place

CT shows some subcentimetric pulmonary nodules bilaterally, the one characterized by higher metabolism is in the upper lobe of the right lung, adjacent to the fissure, SUV max 1.4. Non-pathological deposition of FDG in the image detected on CT in the right uterine appendages. Moderate right hydronephrosis is present, too (Fig. 26.1). See also Fig. 26.2.

26.4 Conclusions

The scan shows high metabolism at the PET scan due to a coarse uterine sarcomatous mass with lymph node and lung metastases, the latter being subcentimetric, therefore under the resolving limits of the technique.

26.5 Key Points

- The PET scan demonstrates and quantifies the high metabolism of the primary tumor and lymph node lesions, and this information is critical to assess the following response after chemotherapy.
- The limited glucose consumption of the lung lesions is to report at least in part to the resolutive limits of the PET. This needs to be emphasized in the report and its conclusions.
- The presence of multiple lung metastases indicates the high aggressiveness of the tumor and a poor prognosis that characterizes aggressive sarcomatous lesions.

The state of the urinary tract must always be evaluated in cancer patient; in particular, the presence of a moderate hydronephrosis secondary to extrinsic compression exerted on the ureter must be reported. A progression of the tumor volume, if not promptly treated, can cause an infiltration of the ureter and a secondary condition with obstructive renal parenchymal loss.

Cervical Cancer: Staging

27

27.1 Clinical History

Staging of cervical cancer with infiltration of the vagina and rectum in a 71-year-old woman.

- Abdomen MRI: gross lesion of the cervix that infiltrates the posterior wall of the vagina up to the lower third below, mesorectal fat on the rear, coming in close proximity to the anterior wall of the rectum. We appreciate some centimetric lymph nodes in the groin and surrounding tissues.

27.2 Diagnostic Question

Search for lesions with high glucose metabolism: Staging of cervical cancer.

27.3 Report

Mass characterized by abnormal glucose consumption at the cervix, SUV max 12. This mass is in contiguity with the anterior wall of the rectum (Fig. 27.1, *arrow*), infiltrates below the posterior wall of the vagina up to the inferior third and back, in the mesorectal fat.

There are not evident adenopathies characterized by pathological metabolism.

No areas of abnormal glucose consumption in the remaining parts of the body examined.

27.4 Conclusions

The PET scan shows a mass of the uterine cervix with infiltration of the surrounding tissues with high glucose metabolism (See Fig. 27.2).

27.5 Key Points

Knowledge of the precise distribution of the metabolic activity of the disease allows us to better understand what are the lines of progression of the tumor:

- locoregional infiltration of the rectum and the vagina is a key factor that influences the therapeutic approach. These data are useful in defining the possible surgical strategy and suggest a neoadjuvant chemotherapy;
- the quantization of the metabolic activity in the staging phase allows to evaluate the efficacy of neoadjuvant chemotherapy in subsequent PET scans;
- neoadjuvant chemotherapy may be useful to obtain a reduction in the mass and used to preserve sphincter function through a more conservative surgery;
- all of these options must be related to the overall clinical condition and age of the patient to avoid an unnecessary aggressive approach.

P. F. Rambaldi, *Whole-Body FDG PET Imaging in Oncology*,
DOI: 10.1007/978-88-470-5295-6_27, © Springer-Verlag Italia 2014

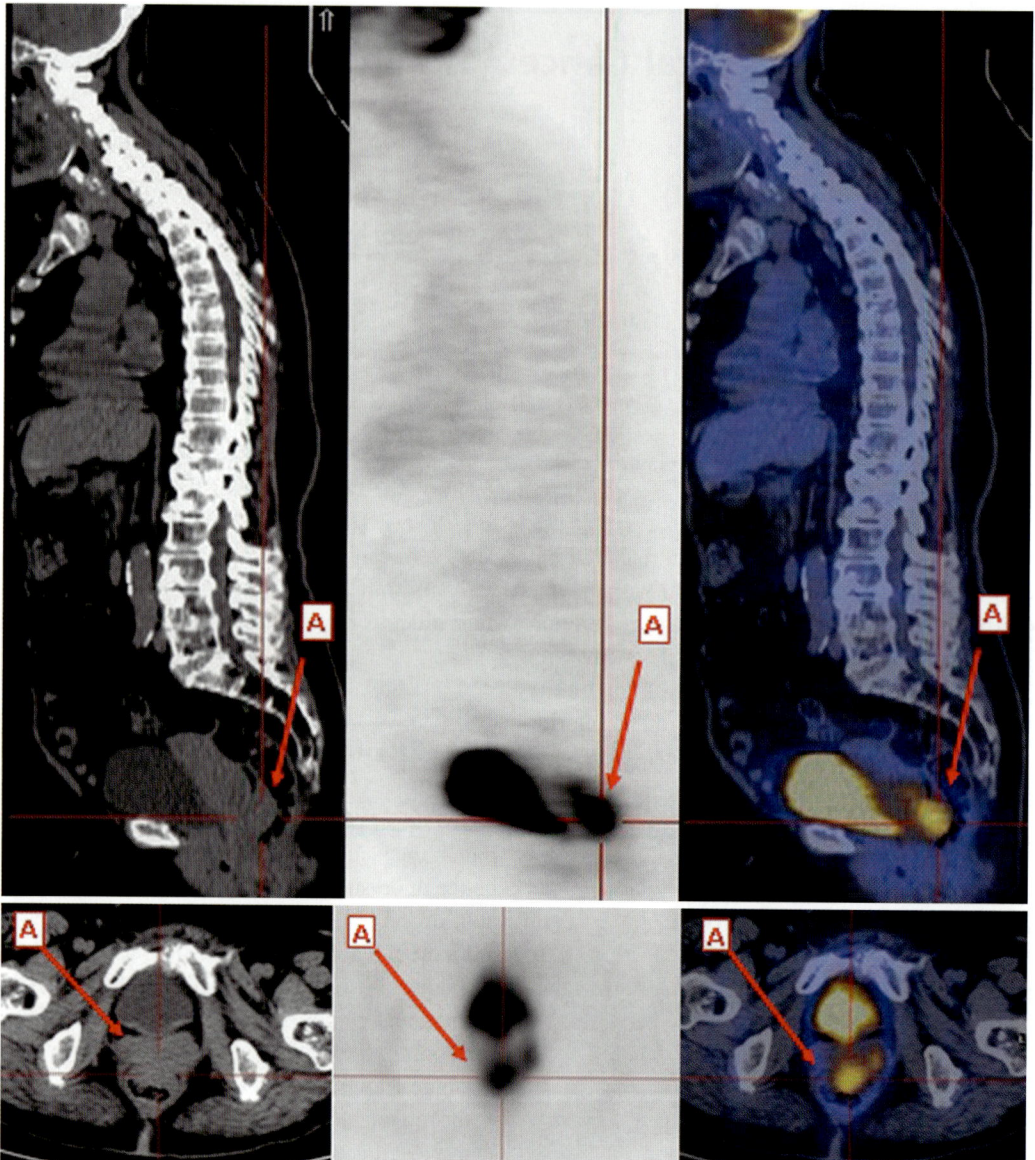

Fig. 27.1 Mass characterized by abnormal glucose consumption at the cervix, SUV max 12. This mass is in contiguity with the anterior wall of the rectum (*arrow*), infiltrates below the posterior wall of the vagina up to the inferior third and back, in the mesorectal fat

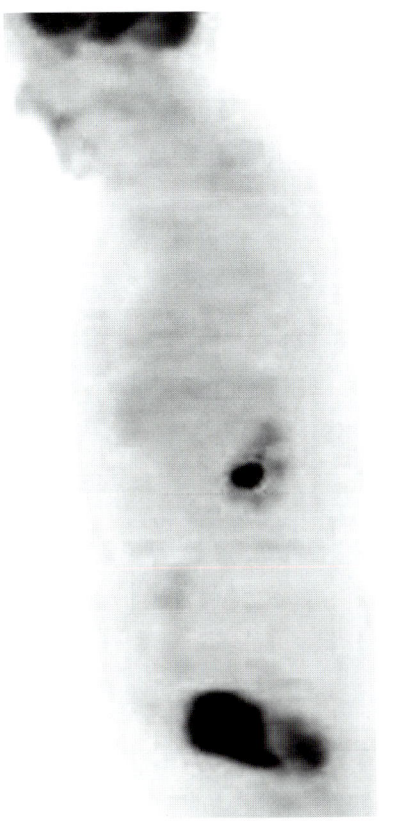

this finding is nonspecific when evaluated solely on the basis of volumetric criteria;

size "alone" is not an element of benignity/malignancy; therefore, whenever possible, the radiologist must provide a detailed description of the suspicious nodes found;

often traumatic, vascular, lymphatic, and inflammatory dystrophic leg or pelvis phenomena lead to an increase in volume and nonspecific reactive inguinal lymph nodes. Even when the inflammatory process stops, the involved lymph node does not resume its original volume for the presence of significant fibrosis or chronicity of the process;

inguinal lymph nodes measuring more than a centimeter are metastatic when at the CT; they appear as dysmorphic, hypodense, confluent, coalescing and are characterized only by modest impregnation after contrast; in such cases generally, the PET lesion documented high metabolism;

subcentimetric nodal metastasis can present a poor metabolism of FDG due to the resolving limits of the PET scan; only an increase in the volumetric and metabolic activity in the course of follow-up allows a correct diagnosis.

Fig. 27.2 The MIP image shows the intense glucose-consumption of the pelvic mass fingerprinting the posterior wall of the bladder

27.6 Reflections

In this woman, the RM describes the presence of pelvic subcentimetric lymph nodes:

Peritoneal Cancer Recurrence

28

28.1 Clinical History

Radical hysterectomy and bilateral salpingo-oophorectomy for peritoneal cancer in 43-year-old woman. Adjuvant chemotherapy was then performed.

After 12 months:
- total peritonectomy, cholecystectomy, the remaining epiploon was removed, colic double wedge resection, intraoperative chemo-hyperthermia with oxaliplatin. Removal of glissonian liver lesions. Bilateral pleural drainage. Adjuvant chemotherapy was then performed.

After 24 months:
- total body CT and abdominal ultrasound negative for focal lesions.
- CA 125 = 40 IU/ml (nv < 35).

After 30 months:
- total body CT and abdominal ultrasound negative for focal lesions.
- CA 125 = 120 IU/ml (nv < 35).

28.2 Diagnostic Question

Search for focal lesions with high glucose metabolism in woman with increase in the value of the CA 125, suspect for peritoneal recurrence of cancer.

28.3 Report

Presence of mass characterized by modest consumption of glucose in the small pelvis in correspondence of the bladder trigone in the left paramedian region, SUV max 2.8 (Fig. 28.1b, *arrow*). Serous metabolically active nodule at the left upper abdominal quadrant, coated on the medial surface of the spleen, hypodense at the CT scan, SUV max 2.6 (Fig. 28.1a, *arrow*).

Absence of pathological glucose consumption in the remaining parts of the body examined.

P. F. Rambaldi, *Whole-Body FDG PET Imaging in Oncology*,
DOI: 10.1007/978-88-470-5295-6_28, © Springer-Verlag Italia 2014

Fig. 28.1 The small
pelvis in correspondence of
the bladder trigone in the
left paramedian region
(See description in the text
(Report))

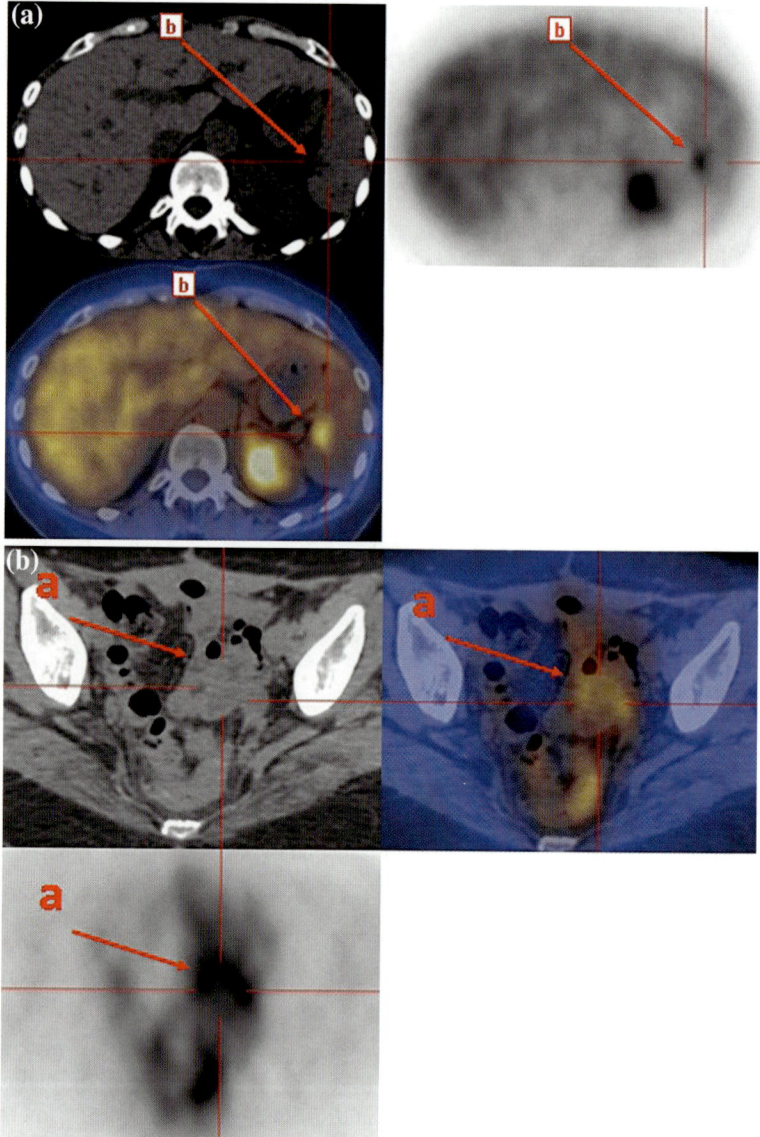

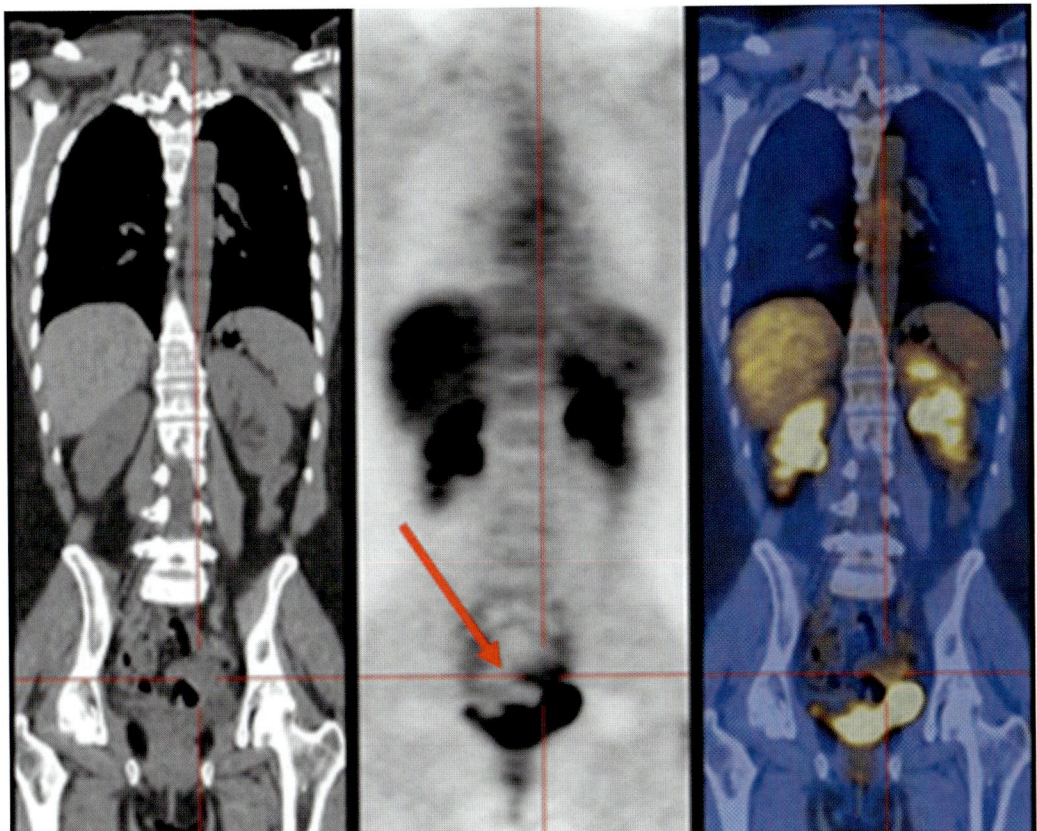

Fig. 28.2 At the bladder trigone in the left paramedian region, the CT-PET shows the presence of inhomogeneously hypodense, irregular tissue, with a limited deposition of glucose. This element is best seen in the coronal reconstructions

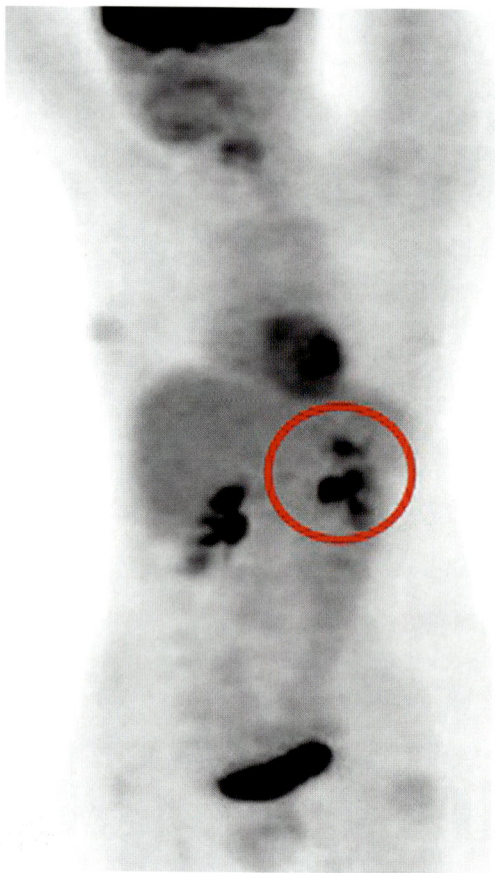

Fig. 28.3 MIP reconstruction of the serous splenic nodule is masked by the physiological stasis of the tracer at the level of higher goblets of the left kidney

28.4   Conclusions

The PET scan shows slight increase in glucose metabolism reported for peritoneal carcinomatosis due to pelvic lesion and the lesion on the splenic surface (See Figs. 28.2, 28.3).

28.5   Key Points

• A peritoneal recurrence can be characterized by restricted carbohydrate metabolism, so especially when the uptake is low, an accurate study of the CT images is due, particularly when in the ongoing follow-up, there is a clearly progressive increase in the values of CA 125 and suspicion of recurrence is high.

• In cases of doubt, MRI and/or a laparoscopic revision is suggested.

Vaginal Adenocarcinoma: Restaging After Chemoradiotherapy

29

29.1 Clinical History

73-year-old woman with locally advanced primitive adenocarcinoma of the vagina, with involvement of the vaginal fornix, treated with RT, brachyradiations and concomitant chemotherapy.

Follow-up three months after radiotherapy:

- Pelvis MRI: thickening of the vaginal walls, especially to the left where a nodular pelvic area with impregnation and inhomogeneity of the fat can be seen.
- PET-FDG: nuanced deposition of the tracer at the vaginal fornix in the left paramedian area.
- CT: fibrotic striae and scars in the lower lobe of the right lung. Uterus moderately bumpy and irregular. Thickening of the vaginal loggia, that is irregular.

Follow up twelve months after radiotherapy:

- PET-FDG: presence of disease with high carbohydrate metabolism at the vagina.
- pelvis MRI: volumetric increase of the uterine body and fundus with distension of the endometrial signal due to fluid; millimetric vegetations can be seen. Intense impregnation of the cervical region, the largest in the posterior- left paramedian where you can see irregular spiculature of the outer margin, which is very difficult to separate from the contiguous fat and the ipsilateral pararectal fascia. Fluid in the Douglas space.

Chemotherapy was then performed.

29.2 Question Diagnostic

Restaging of locally advanced vaginal cancer, which has already undergone chemotherapy, after one month from the end of the treatment: Determination of glucose metabolism.

29.3 Report

Abnormal glucose consumption of the vagina with cranial extension at the uterus, SUV max 11 (Fig. 29.1).

No areas of abnormal glucose consumption in the remaining parts of the body examined.

29.4 Conclusions

The PET scan shows cell activity of the pelvic mass compatible with the persistence of loco-regional disease after chemotherapy (Fig. 29.2)

P. F. Rambaldi, *Whole-Body FDG PET Imaging in Oncology*,
DOI: 10.1007/978-88-470-5295-6_29, © Springer-Verlag Italia 2014

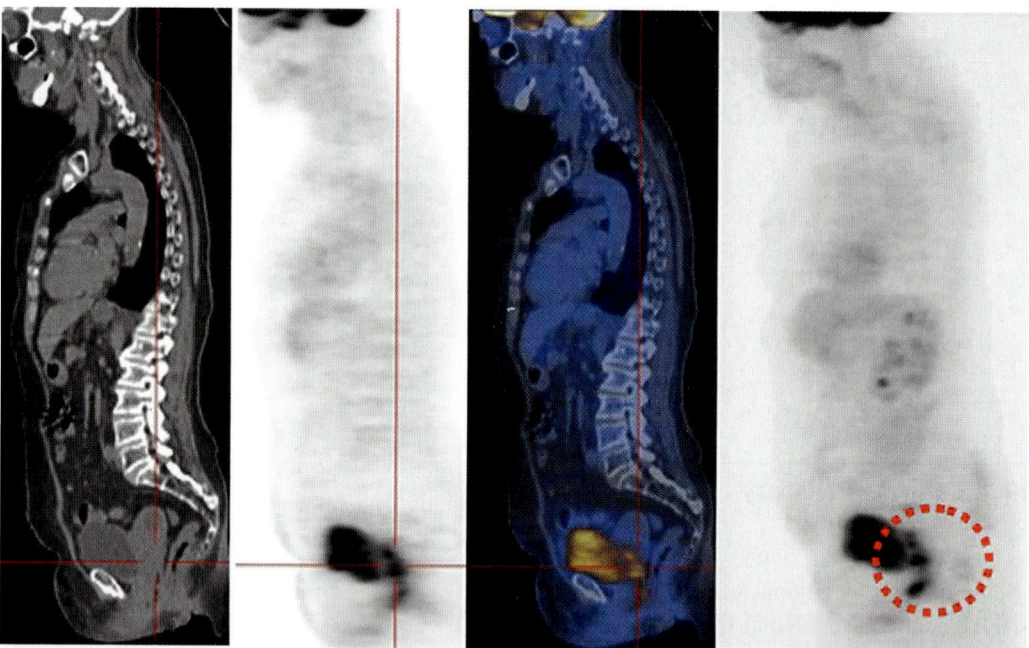

Fig. 29.1 Abnormal glucose consumption of the vagina with cranial extension at the uterus

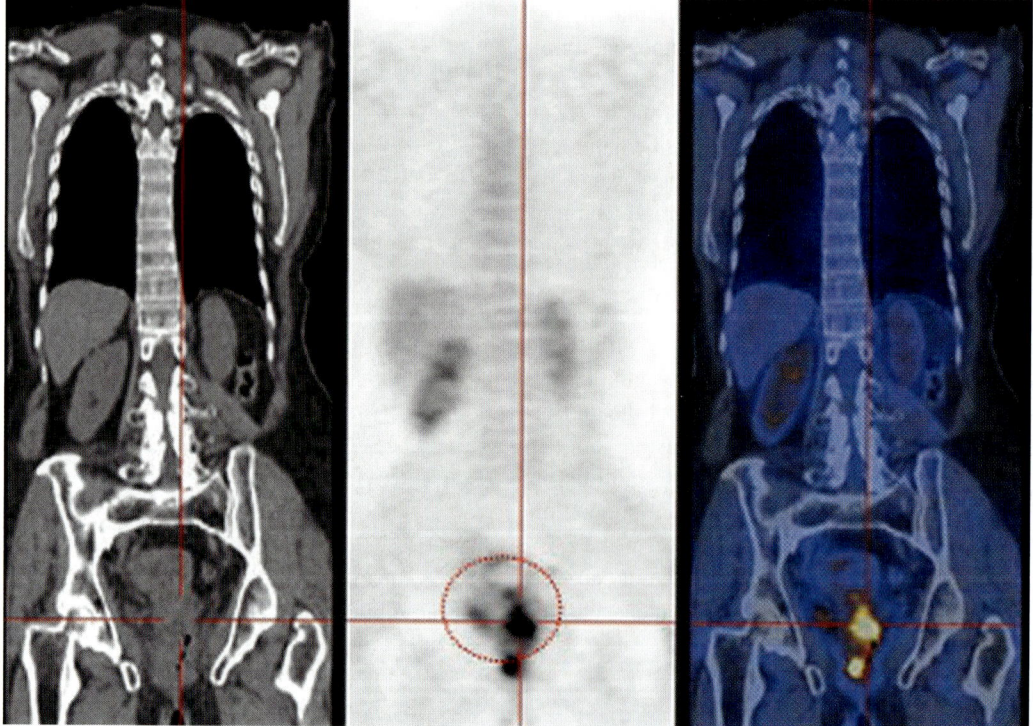

Fig. 29.2 The PET scan shows cell activity of the pelvic mass compatible with the persistence of locoregional disease after chemotherapy

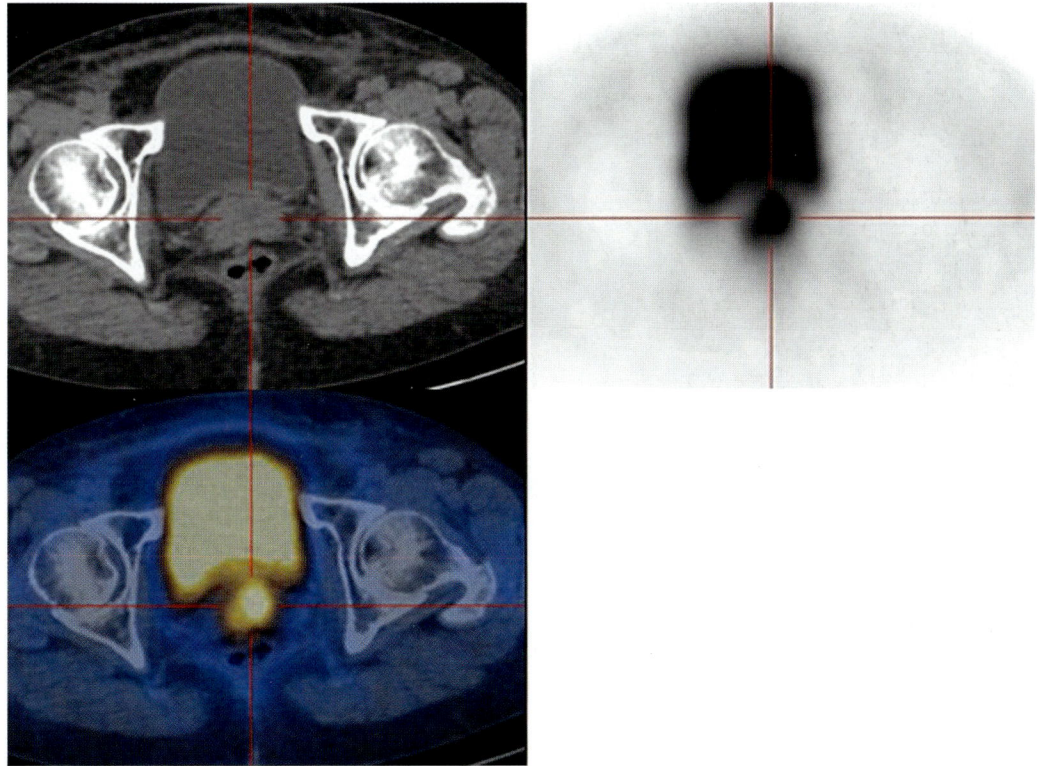

Fig. 29.3 CT-PET demonstrates volume increase of the body and fundus of the uterus that appears bumpy and irregular

The cervix is not separable from the vaginal loggia, that is thickened. The lesional metabolism is increased.

Mild bone marrow activation is due to post-chemotherapy rebound (See also Fig. 29.3).

29.5 Key Points

After chemoradiotherapy, PET is the best technique that allows us to obtain information on cell activity of the tumor, so it is critical:

- for accurate restaging,
- for subsequent treatment planning.
  - The absence of metastasis suggests a surgical approach.
  - The sagittal scans allow you to get an overview of the biological activity and the extent of locoregional disease.

Recurrence of Left Ovarian Adult-Type Granulosa Cell Tumor

30.1 Clinical History

Laparoscopic radical hysterectomy and bilateral salpingo-oophorectomy for left ovarian adult-type granulosa-cell tumor in a 59-year-old woman.

Follow-up after one year:
- Ultrasound: in the pelvic cavity an iso-hypo-echoic mass is detected, with bumpy margins, measuring 104 x 57 x 76 mm.
- CT: symmetric lung fields with centimetric nodule in the right upper lobe, lesion of possible repetitive nature. Voluminous solid irregular formations, largely necrotic and confluent within the peritoneum at the pelvic cavity (max = 15 x 10 cm), in the upper abdominal quadrants especially in the median and paramedian areas, left hypochondrium and the ipsilateral side (max = 10 x 6 cm). These lesions lead to widespread compressive effect on the gastrointestinal structures. After contrast injection, marked increase in density and large portions of necrotic contained within can be seen. The findings suggest extended peritoneal recurrence (diffuse carcinomatosis). Liver moderately increased in volume and irregular, with small hypodense formations in the right segments. Lumbar-aortic and celiac-mesenteric lymph nodes measuring 3 cms.

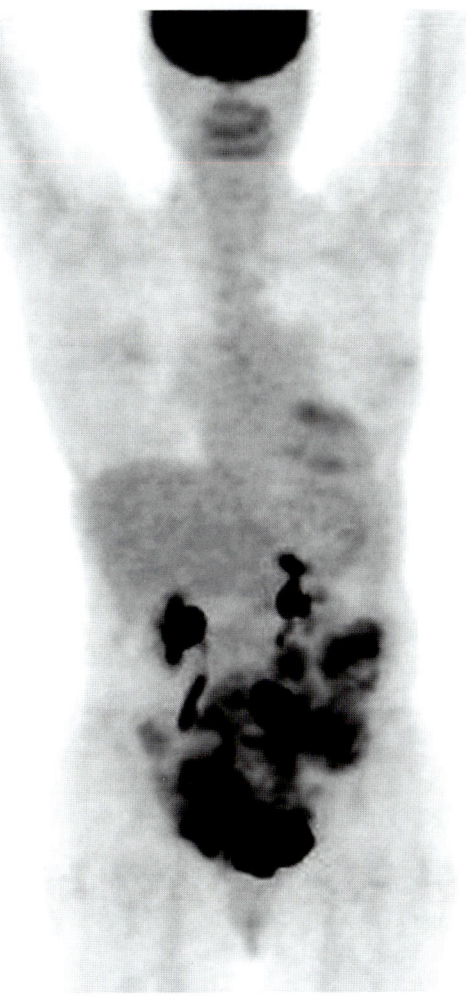

Fig. 30.1 The MIP image shows the extent of the disease in the pelvis and the intensity of the metabolic activity of the numerous metastatic masses. In this reconstruction, the pulmonary nodule is not seen because the limited metabolism of the lesion is masked by the physiological activity of the mammary glands

P. F. Rambaldi, *Whole-Body FDG PET Imaging in Oncology*, DOI: 10.1007/978-88-470-5295-6_30, © Springer-Verlag Italia 2014

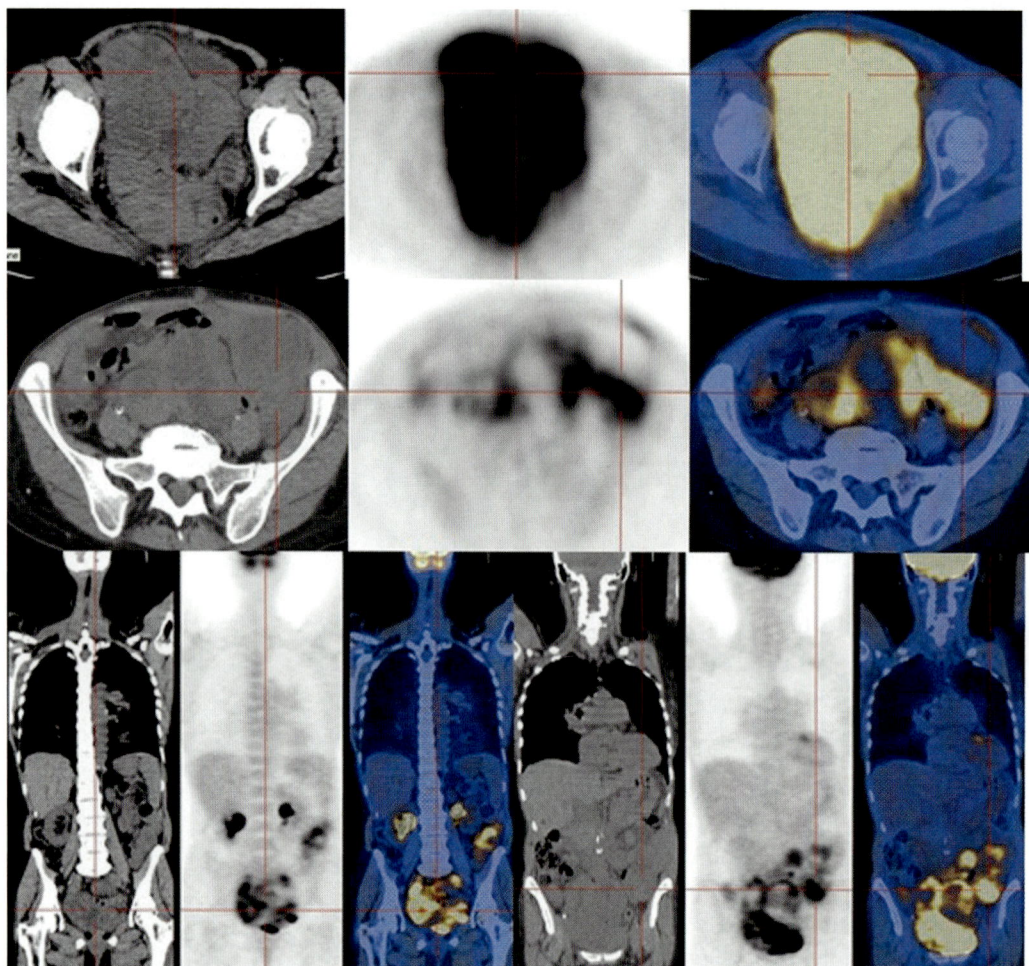

Fig. 30.2 CT shows the voluminous homogeneous, partly liquid and solid, widely confluent and necrotic masses occupying the pelvis. The coronal reconstruction shows the extension of the upper abdominal disease, especially to the left. The PET shows increased consumption of glucose with contextual areas with low metabolism contained within, due to the presence of liquid and or colliquative component

30.2   Diagnostic Question

Search for focal lesions with high glucose metabolism in patient with peritoneal carcinomatosis.

30.3   Report

Intense and irregular increase in the consumption of glucose in the pelvic area due to multiple, complex irregular masses already seen at CT, which also extend to the upper abdominal quadrants, especially to the left, SUV max 12.1.

The centimetric nodule seen at the upper lobe of the right lung reported by previous CT scan, shows limited consumption of glucose, SUV max 1.2.

The hepatic nodules detected by CT and reported in history have not pathological concentration of FDG. Modest bilateral hydroureteronephrosis du to extrinsic compression of the ureters in the middle and distal thirds.

30.4 Conclusions

The PET scan shows extensive peritoneal carcinomatosis with high carbohydrate consumption and a metastatic pulmonary nodule (See Figs. 30.1, 30.2).

30.5 Key points

- Cancers of the ovary in advanced stages determine peritoneal carcinomatosis;
- Often the lesion is chemosensitive, and therefore, before treatment, it is important to define the basal metabolic activity to be compared to that of PET which will be performed during the restaging;
- unlike the CA 125, PET-FDG has the advantage of identifying the locations, size, and extent of recurrence;
- CT does not define the metabolic activity of individual lesions, and it is not always able to differentiate normal anatomic alterations by outbreaks of postsurgical recurrence on PET scans that have high metabolism.

Pulmonary subcentimetric nodules that have a metabolism higher than that of normal parenchyma (SUV max > 0.8) are suspicious for metastatic disease.

Surgically Treated Endometrial Cancer: Bilateral Nodal Recurrence

31

31.1 Clinical History

Radical hysterectomy, bilateral salpingo-oophorectomy and systematic pelvic lymphadenectomy for endometrial cancer in 67-year-old woman.

Follow-up twelve months after:

- Elevation of the markers.
- CT: negative for focal lesions.
- MRI: colliquated lymph nodes in the bilateral iliac-obturatory stations, more evident on the left (max. 3 cm).

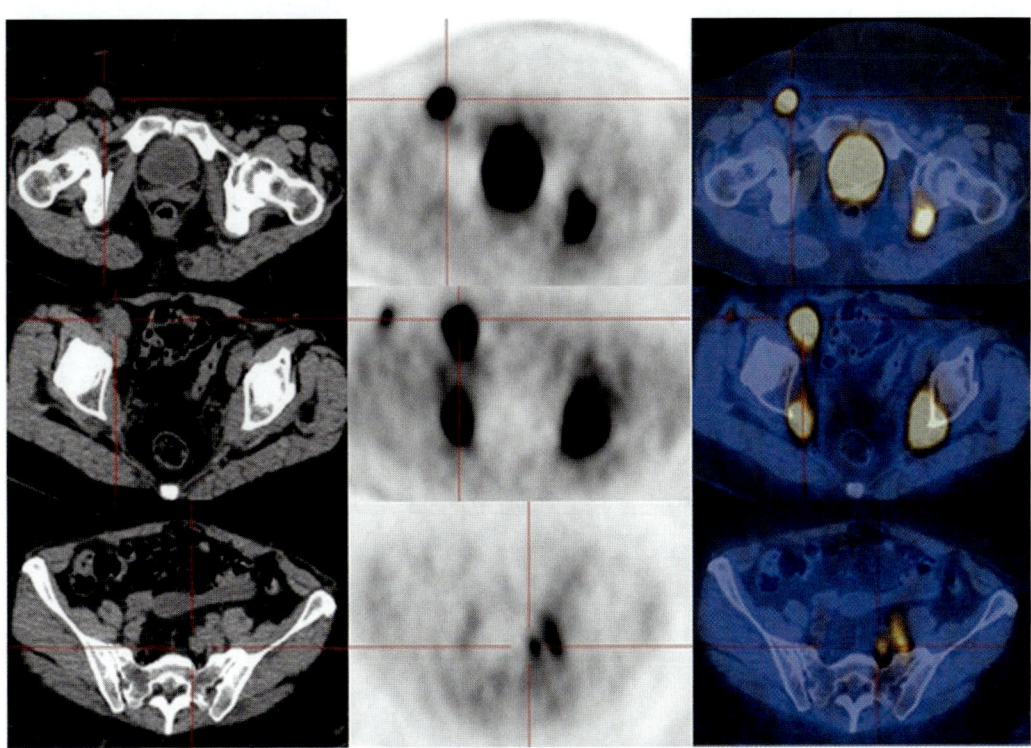

Fig. 31.1 Axial PET-CT images show some enlarged lymph nodes increased in size in the presacral left region

P. F. Rambaldi, *Whole-Body FDG PET Imaging in Oncology*,
DOI: 10.1007/978-88-470-5295-6_31, © Springer-Verlag Italia 2014

31.2   Diagnostic Question

Search for focal lesions with high glucose metabolism in woman with recurrent endometrial carcinoma: restaging.

31.3   Report

Abnormal glucose consumption of multiple lymph nodes in the intercavo-aortic, iliac and obturator bilaterally, left presacral, superficial and deep inguinal to the right, SUV max 14.

31.4   Conclusions

The PET scan shows altered glucose metabolism for extended recurrence of lymph node disease.

Axial PET-CT images show some enlarged lymph nodes increased in size in the presacral left region (Fig. 31.1). See also Figs. 31.2, 31.3.

31.5   Key Points

CT is good for the determination of the parameters T and N in advanced pelvic neoplasms,

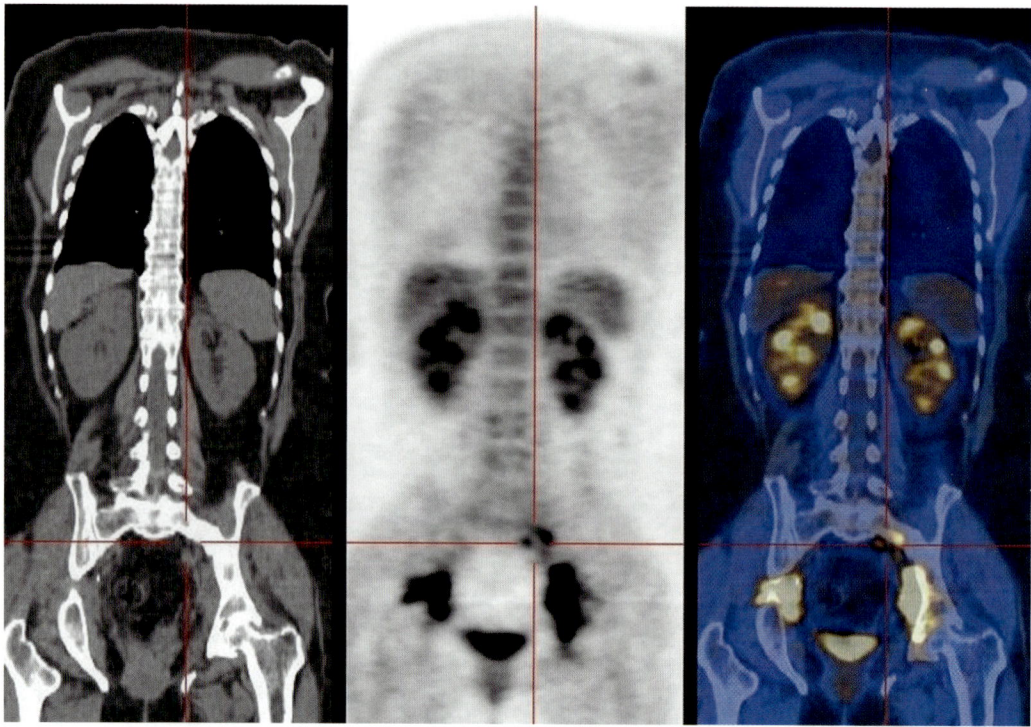

Fig. 31.2 The coronal reconstructions confirm the presence of adenopathy in the presacral and better demonstrate the involvement of the obturatory stations on both sides, also characterized by high metabolism (see also Fig. 31.3)

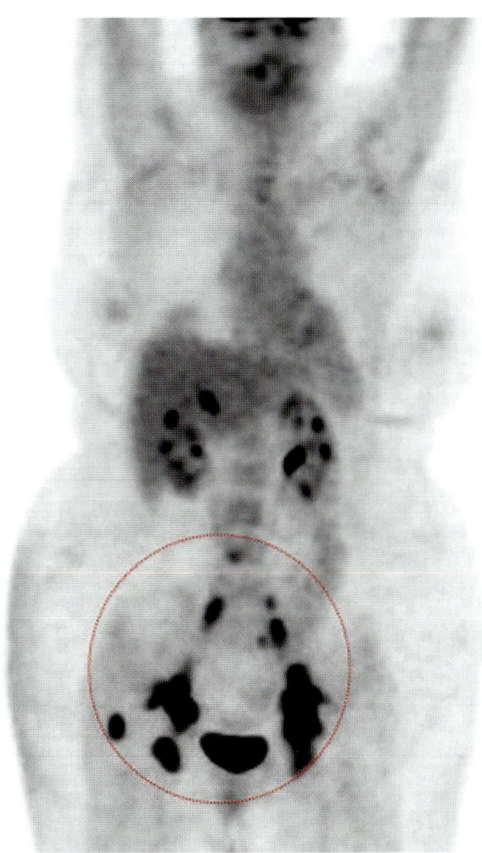

Fig. 31.3

providing important anatomical elements and volume of lymph nodes involved: inguinal, obturator, retroperitoneal, etc.

MRI, though, studies much better the extension of the primary tumor, and in particular, the relationship and the locoregional infiltration of the rectum, bladder and vagina.

PET is critically important:

- in radiological doubts;
- when the cancer markers are high, and the other techniques do not show recurrence of pathology;
- quantization of metabolic lesions before chemotherapy;
- in the definition of grading and prognosis.

Follow-up of Carcinoma of the Uterus: Left Lower Limb Lymphedema Due to Fibrous Scar

32

32.1 Clinical History

Radical hysterectomy, bilateral salpingo-oophorectomy and systematic pelvic lymphadenectomy for uterine cancer in 61 year old woman.

Previous bilateral saphenectomy.

Follow-up two years after: left lower limb lymphedema showed up.

- Bone scan: hyperaccumulation of the radio compound at the level of the lumbar spine (L1–L2), sacrum and coxofemoral joints.
- Pelvis MRI: widespread structural alteration of the bone elements of the pelvis, especially at the level of the sacral wings, the iliac wings, ischio-pubic branches, left acetabulum and trochanteric region of the femur and both ipsilateral femoral diaphysis.
- Pelvis CT: extensive areas of morpho-structural alteration with a 'map' appearance, which are characterized by alternating portions of osteolytic bone resorption with areas of thickening and sclerosis of the iliac wings bilaterally, the sacral wings, the ischio-pubic branches and the right ilio-pubic branch adjacent to the symphysis. In particular, at the right ilio-pubic branch, greater structural remodeling is observed with focal interruption of the cortical bone.

32.2 Diagnostic Question

Search for focal lesions with a high metabolism in woman with a history of cancer of the uterus in clinical remission and recent onset of left lower limb lymphedema.

32.3 Report

Moderate increase in the consumption of glucose in left coxofemoral articulation and pelvis, more evident to the ischio-pubic branches, symphysis in the right paramedian region and the left sacroiliac synchondrosis, SUV max 3.6.

Evidence of slight and widespread increase in the consumption of glucose to the soft tissues of the left thigh and ipsilateral gluteus due to lymphedema. Absence of significant areas of pathological metabolism in the remaining parts of the body examined. See Figs. 32.1, 32.2.

32.4 Conclusions

The PET scan does not show focal areas of pathological consumption of glucose in the body areas examined indicating a recurrence of disease.

P. F. Rambaldi, *Whole-Body FDG PET Imaging in Oncology*,
DOI: 10.1007/978-88-470-5295-6_32, © Springer-Verlag Italia 2014

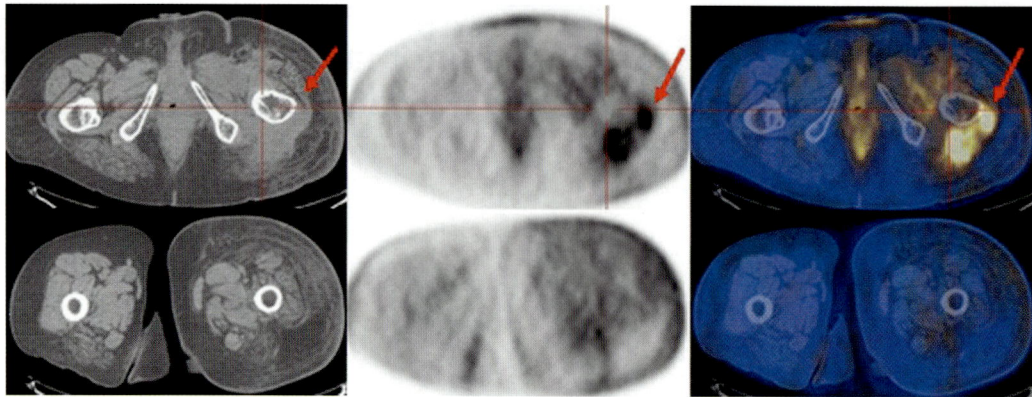

Fig. 32.1 The CT scan shows marked thickening of tissue in the left groin and ipsilateral thigh (*arrow*). There were no focal nodular changes. Absence of lymphadenopathy. At the PET scan, widespread increase of the deposition of glucose to the soft tissues of the lower left (*arrow*) by edema secondary to altered lymphatic drainage

Fig. 32.2 The MIP images evaluated with double window show nonspecific deposition glucose at the soft tissues of the left lower limb, by impaired lymphatic drainage. There are not clear focal lesions to relate to recovery of pathology in other parts of the body

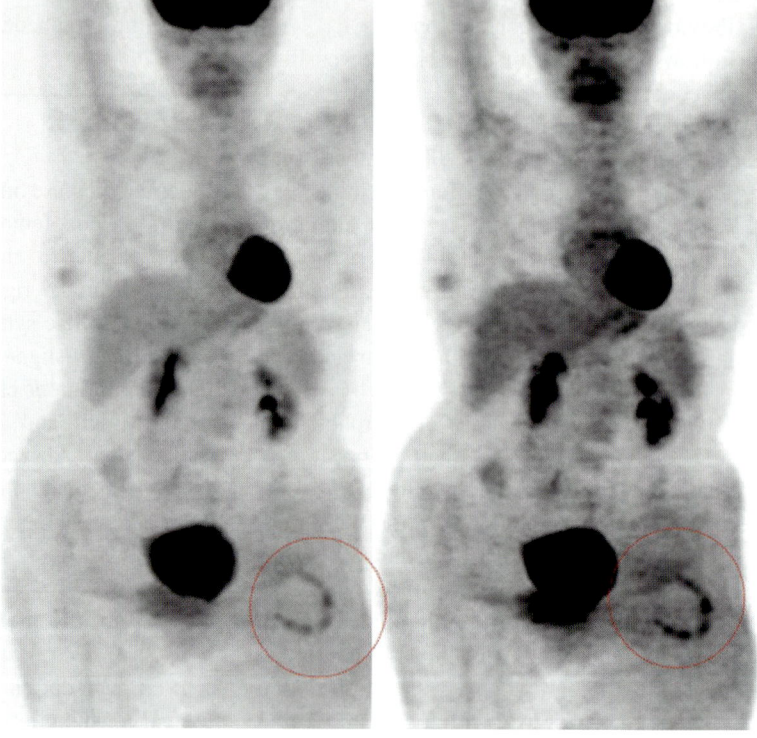

32.5   Key Points

- CT-PET has high sensitivity and specificity in defining etiology of patients with lymphedema.

- A negative CT-PET excludes a tumor recurrence and suggests a lymphedema by insufficient lymphatic drainage in primary or secondary lymphadenectomy. Sometimes, the cause is a vascular disease.

Squamous Cell Vulvar Surgically Treated Carcinoma: Nodal Recurrence of Disease

33

33.1 Clinical History

Radical vulvectomy and bilateral inguinal lymphadenectomy for moderately differentiated keratinizing type squamous cell carcinoma, pT2, pN1, PMX, in a 76-year-old woman. The patient underwent radiotherapy treatment but not adjuvant chemotherapy.

Follow-up after six months:

- Bone scan: negative for focal lesions.
- Ultrasound: presence of some dysmorphic hypoechoic lymph nodes in the groin bilaterally, with a maximum diameter of 14 mm to the right, 25 mm to the left.
- Cancer Markers: normal.

33.2 Diagnostic Question

Search for focal lesions with high glucose metabolism in patient with carcinoma of the vulva who underwent surgery and adjuvant radiotherapy.

33.3 Report

Multiple lymph nodes measuring more than a centimeter, characterized by intense carbohydrate consumption in the right iliac and inguinal-femoral regions on both sides, the most evident on the left, SUV max 12.

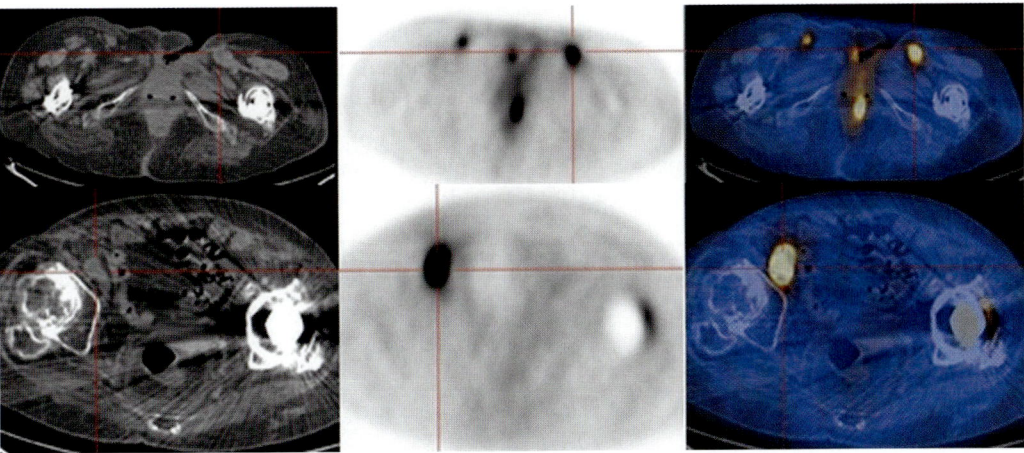

Fig. 33.1 PET-CT scan shows multiple, heterogeneously hypodense, enlarged lymph nodes with a high carbohydrate metabolism that can be seen also in the coronal reconstructions

P. F. Rambaldi, *Whole-Body FDG PET Imaging in Oncology*,
DOI: 10.1007/978-88-470-5295-6_33, © Springer-Verlag Italia 2014

Fig. 33.2 On CT-PET it is evident an alteration of the pubic bones at the symphysis bilaterally with cortical interruption. Not observed contextual newly formed tissue replacement. The increase in glucose metabolism does not suggest a neoplastic condition but is compatible with bone remodeling determined by a post-actinic fracture

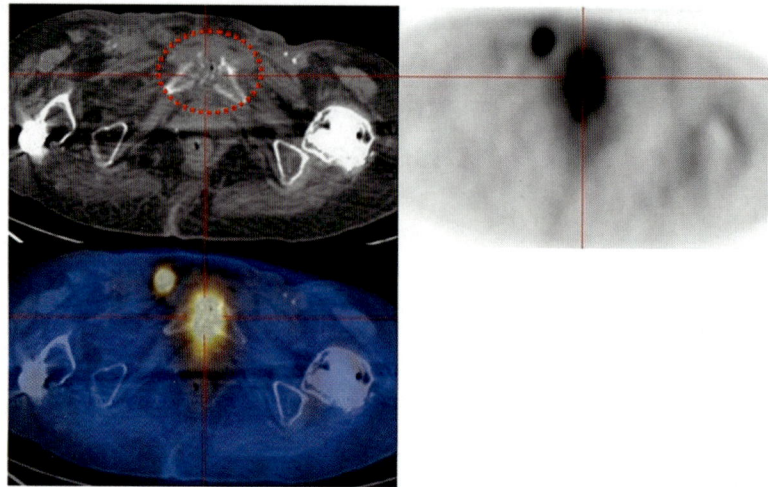

Increased metabolism of glucose, SUV max 5.6, at the pubic symphysis, that CT shows to be a clear morphostructural alteration. This element is correlated to osteoblastic reparative dystrophic remodeling.

Goiter with a nodule with high metabolism at the base of the left lobe, SUV max 13, to be compared with the hormonal profile and ultrasound.

33.4 Conclusions

The PET scan shows lymphadenopathy with high glucose metabolism supporting a diagnosis of recurrent disease.

In the right iliac and bilateral inguinal-femoral stations, PET-CT scan shows multiple, heterogeneously hypodense, enlarged lymph nodes with a high carbohydrate metabolism that can be seen also in the coronal reconstructions (Fig. 33.1). See also Figs. 33.2, 33.3, 33.4, 33.5.

33.5 Key Points

Carcinoma of the vulva frequently determines inguinal–femoral and pelvic lymph node metastases, mono—or bilaterally.

Locoregional bone and adjacent tissues infiltration is much rarer.

In this patient, the fracture of the pubic symphysis is a condition secondary to dystrophic post-actinic damage. This impression is also supported by the absence of newly formed tissue at this level.

The thyroid nodule with high glucose metabolism requires an endocrinologic evaluation:

- in patients with euthyroid activity or hypothyroidism with normal or high TSH, you should perform a FNAB;
- in hyperthyroid patients with inhibited TSH, a thyroid scan is suggested to define the self adenomatous component of the goiter.

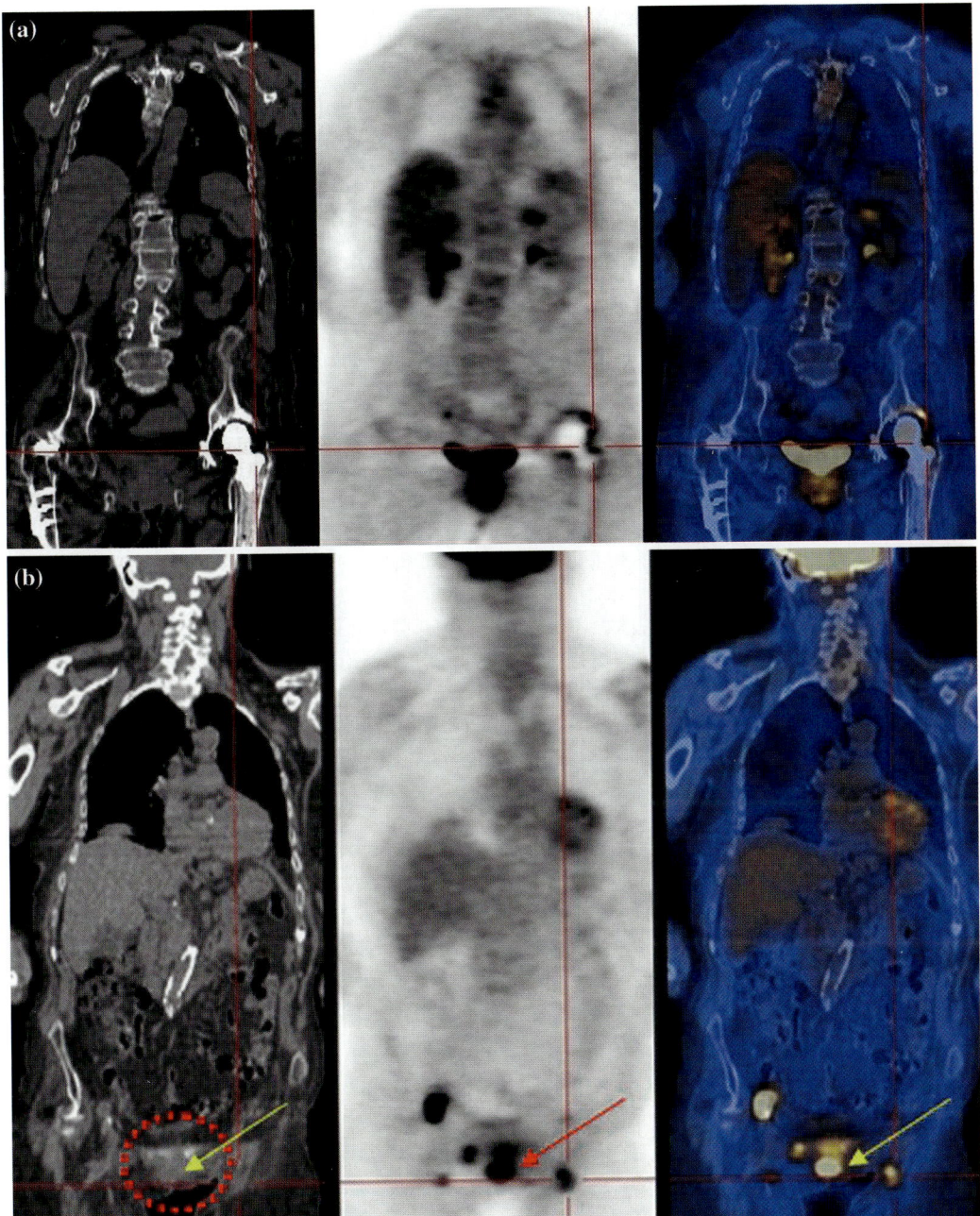

Fig. 33.3 The coronal CT reconstructions show typical artifacts caused by the presence of metallic prosthesis to the right femur and left hip. The low carbohydrate periprosthetic consumption is nonspecific and is not suggestive of infection

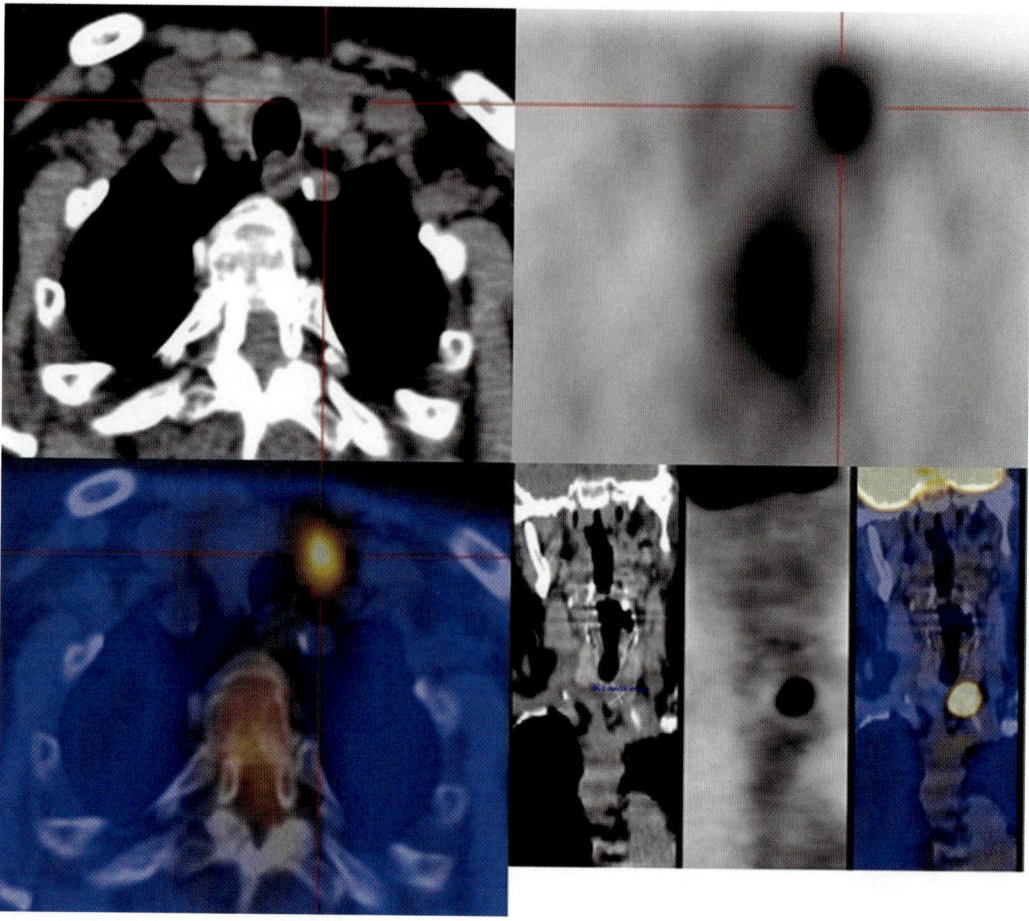

Fig. 33.4 CT-PET shows a hypodense nodule at the base of the left thyroid lobe consuming large amounts of glucose

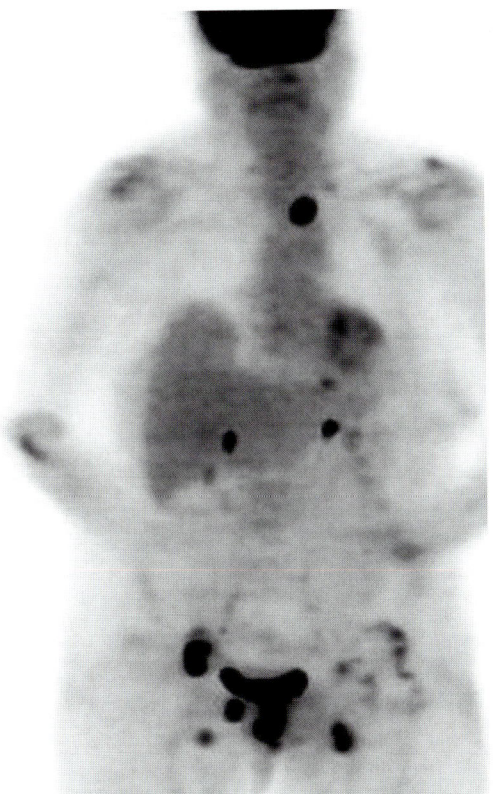

Fig. 33.5 CT-PET shows a hypodense nodule at the base of the left thyroid lobe consuming large amounts of glucose

Post-actinic Fracture of the Pubic Symphysis in Woman with a History of Cancer of the Uterus and Vulva

34

34.1 Clinical History

Radical hysterectomy, bilateral salpingo-oopho-rectomy and systematic pelvic lymphadenectomy for carcinoma of the uterus in a 70-year-old woman.

Eight years after, surgery is performed for vulvar carcinoma and underwent subsequent adjuvant radiotherapy.

Follow-up after one year:
- Pelvis CT: Irregular vulvo-perineal resection. Structural alteration of the pubic symphysis where inhomogeneous, solid tissue with a max. 4 cm diameter and calcified inclusions can be seen; modest diastasis of the ileo-pubic branches.
- The patient complains of persistent low back and pubic pain. Absence of pain in other skeletal sites.

34.2 Diagnostic Question

Patient with a history of cancer of the uterus and the vulva, showing structural lesion of the pubic bones: study of the lesional glucose metabolism.

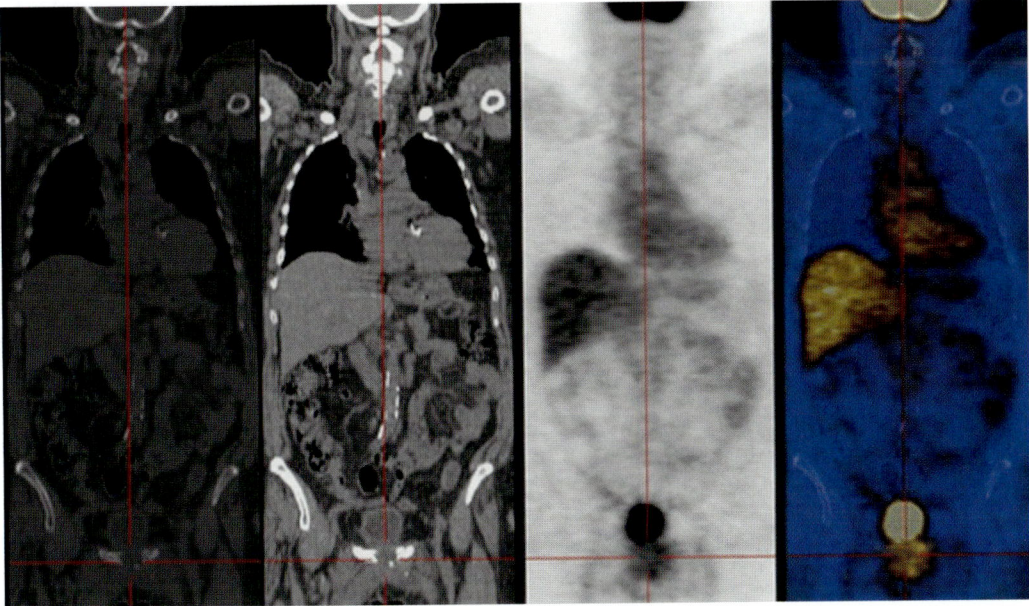

Fig. 34.1 Structural alteration of the pubic symphysis and surrounding soft tissue

P. F. Rambaldi, *Whole-Body FDG PET Imaging in Oncology*,
DOI: 10.1007/978-88-470-5295-6_34, © Springer-Verlag Italia 2014

Fig. 34.2 CT shows evidence of a morpho-structural bone alteration at the pubic symphysis, with obvious burst fracture and centrifugal extrusion of multiple fragments. Thickening of the bladder wall with altered compliance to draining, ''stress bladder'', is better evident in the coronal CT reconstruction. At the PET scan the modest increase in metabolism is caused by bone and soft tissue remodeling. In some cases the uptake of the soft tissues is determined by urinary contamination. See also Fig. 34.3

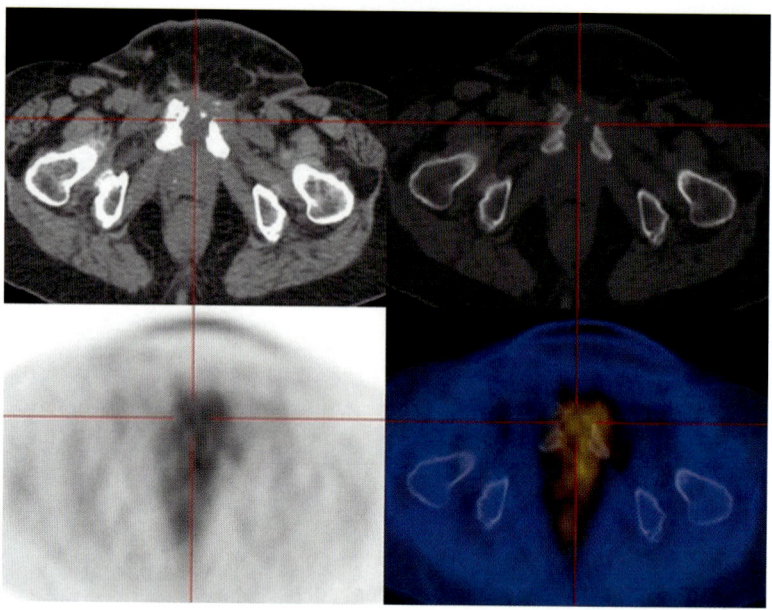

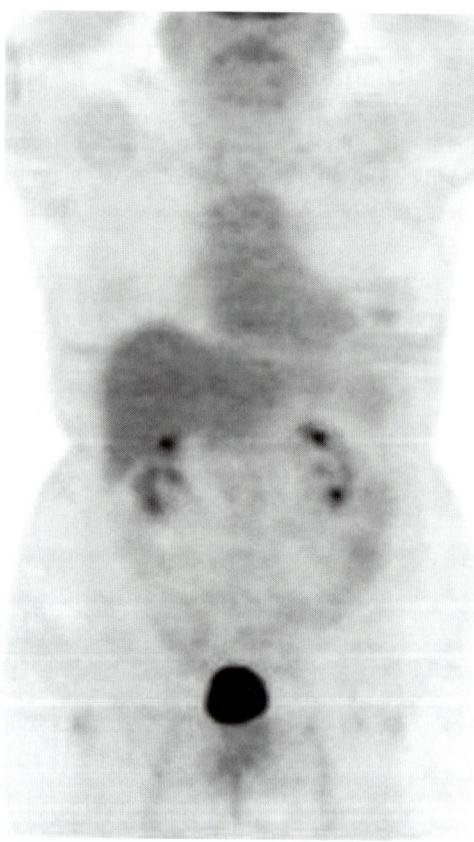

Fig. 34.3

34.3 Report

The PET scan shows no areas of abnormal glucose consumption in body areas examined.

The gross structural alteration of the pubic symphysis and surrounding soft tissue, described by CT reported back in medical history, is characterized by modest consumption of glucose due to a fracture and dystrophic- healing phenomena, SUV max 3.2 (Fig. 34.1).

34.4 Conclusions

The PET scan revealed no significant focal areas of pathological consumption of glucose in the body areas examined indicating a resumption of pathology, within biological and resolving limits (Fig. 34.2).

34.5 Key Points

- In this patient, the PET excludes recurrence of locoregional disease and the presence of distant metastases.

- Radiotherapy is responsible for the dystrophic bone alterations. The skeleton at this level is sensitive to fractures, also often determined by occult microtrauma.

- The glucose consumption measured by PET is due to osteoblastic cell reparative and reactive inflammation.

Part VI
Lymphomas and Thymomas

Non-Hodgkin Lymphoma: Diagnosis

35

35.1 Clinical History

43-year-old female with recurrent thrombophlebitis, presenting with chest pain and dyspnea. The patient is admitted into hospital on the clinical suspicion of pulmonary embolism.

CT: 16 mm solid nodule in the posterior segment of the superior lobe of left lung. The nodule shows irregular margins and is connected to the parietal pleura via thin branches; the lesion shows contrast enhancement. Multiple enlarged lymph nodes, largest width being 17 mm in the Barety lodge, in a pre-vascular, bilateral hilar, subcarinal and left peribronchial areas.

Comorbidities: thyroidectomy for nodular goiter.

35.2 Diagnostic Question

Search for focal lesions with high glucose metabolism in patients with pulmonary nodule and mediastinal adenopathy diagnosed during hospitalization for suspected pulmonary embolism secondary to thrombophlebitis.

35.3 Report

Adenopathy characterized by high deposition of FDG in the bilateral clavicular and mediastinal areas, with multiple nodal stations involved, the most evident in the Barety lodge, the

aortopulmonary window, pre and subcarinal, hilar areas of both sides and left peribronchial, SUV max 8.6.

The pulmonary nodule indicated by CT scan, reported in the clinical history to be in the posterior segment of the upper lobe of the left lung, shows modest increase in glucose metabolism, SUV max 3.

35.4 Conclusions

The PET scan shows extensive mediastinal lymph node commitment and involvement of nodal stations in the clavicular fossa bilaterally, suggestive of lymphomatous disease. Histological confirmation required. The left lung nodule has restricted consumption of glucose and therefore appears to be of inflammatory nature, even though malignancy cannot be thoroughly excluded. CT scans useful for screening (Figs. 35.1, 35.2, 35.3).

35.5 Key Points

In this young patient, there are some diagnostic hypotheses to be verified histologically:
- Lung cancer with nodal metastases
- Lymphoma with mediastinal and pulmonary involvement
- Double neoplasia (lymphoma and lung cancer)

P. F. Rambaldi, *Whole-Body FDG PET Imaging in Oncology*,
DOI: 10.1007/978-88-470-5295-6_35, © Springer-Verlag Italia 2014

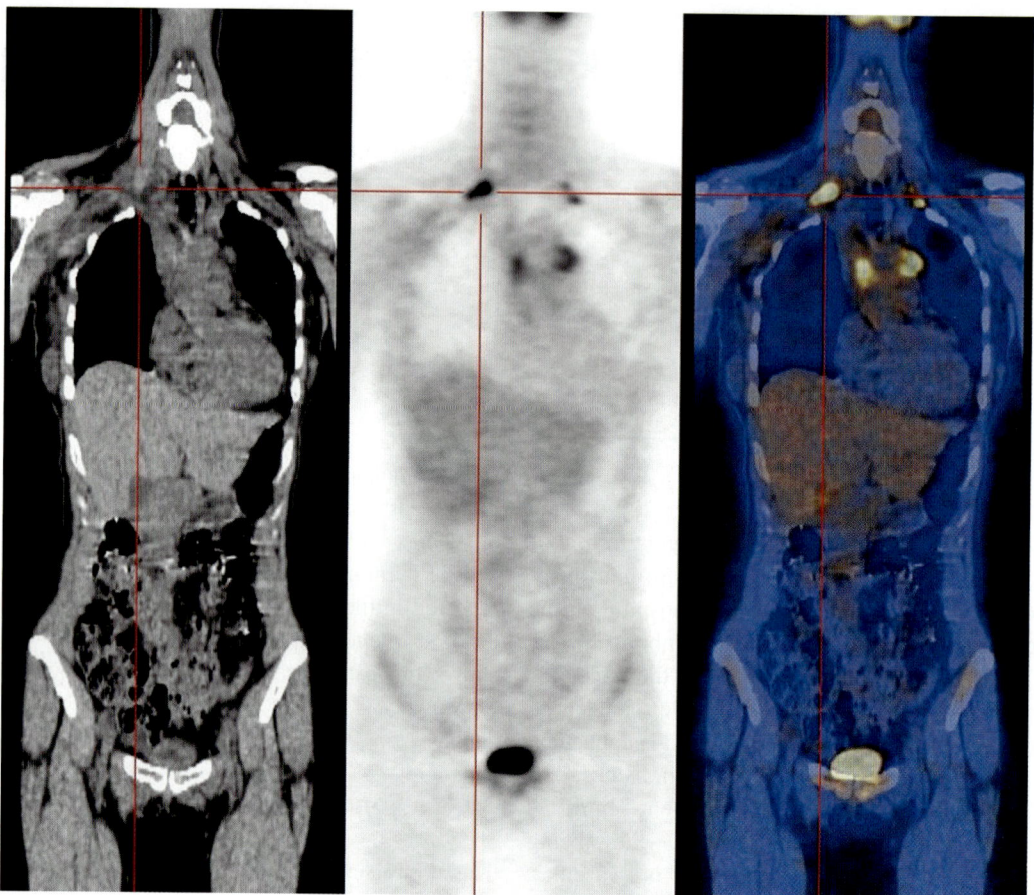

Fig. 35.1 MIP Image: mediastinal lymphadenopathy with elevated glucose metabolism

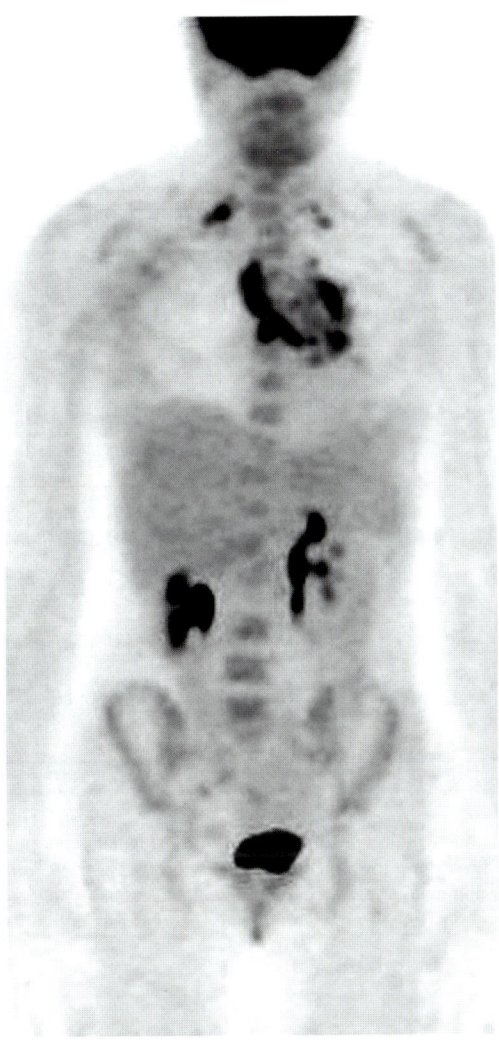

Fig. 35.2 MIP Image: mediastinal lymphadenopathy with elevated glucose metabolism

- Mediastinal lymphoma in a patient with secondary pulmonary remodeling due to recent embolism.

A careful analysis of the metabolic data shows that the left pulmonary nodule has a limited consumption of glucose; conversely lymph nodes have a more intense increase in FDG uptake. This element suggests the presence of a dual pathology: lymphoma was diagnosed occasionally after an episode of pulmonary embolism.

Definitive diagnosis after lymph node biopsy: non-Hodgkin lymphoma.

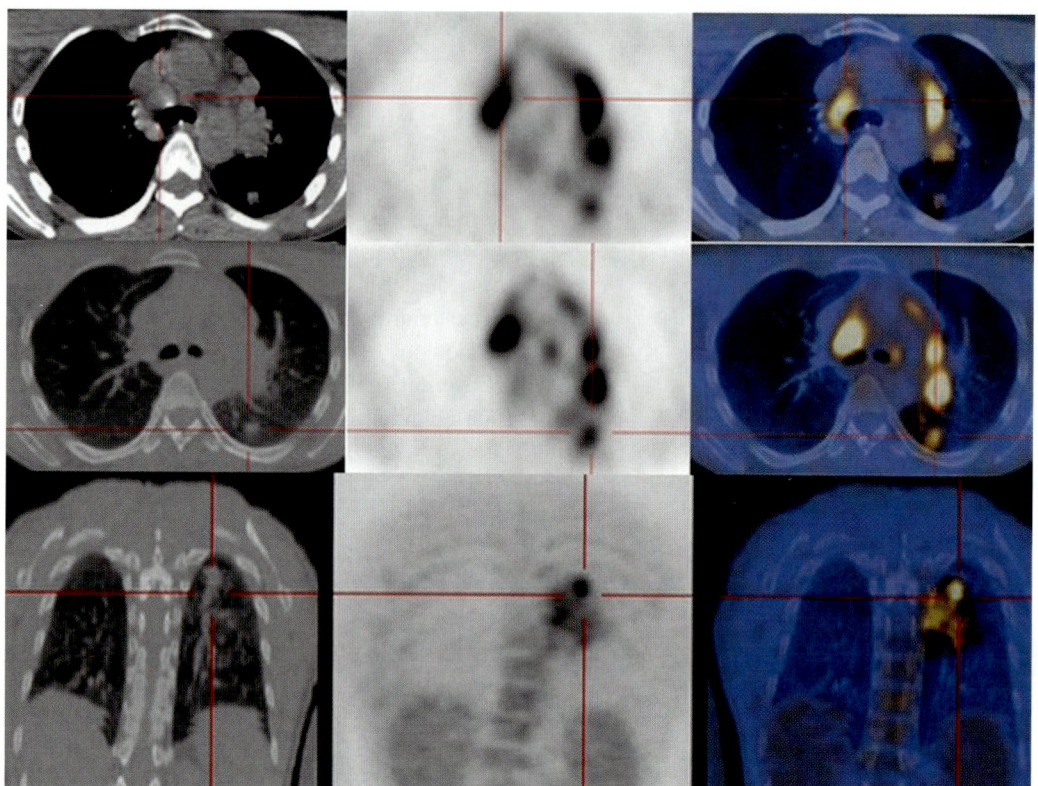

Fig. 35.3 PET-CT in the axial sections shows diffuse involvement of mediastinal lymph nodes, characterized by a high metabolism. At the posterior segment of the upper lobe of the left lung, the coronal reconstruction documents an ill-defined, inhomogeneous coarse parenchymal consolidation, with irregular margins, which has low metabolic activation resulting from inflammatory reactive rearrangement, probably due to embolism. A primary pulmonary neoplasm is unlikely

Follow-up of T-lymphoblastic Lymphoma During Chemotherapy, in Patient Who Underwent Radiotherapy and Talc Pleurodesis

36

36.1 Clinical History

36-year-old man with chest pain, fatigue and shortness of breath and a chest X-ray that detects a bulky mediastinal mass.

- Videothoracoscopy right: massive chest intensely vascularized mass compressing the mediastinal structures, infiltrating the parietal pleura and visceral fat, which has large friable knolls and bleeding easily. Partial parietal pleurectomy partial, talc plurodesis and biopsy of the tumor and the mediastinal pleura were practiced.
- Clinical and histologic diagnosis: Small cell undifferentiated carcinoma or very undifferentiated malignant neoplasm of the mediastinum, with pleuropulmonary massive spread and pleural effusion in a patient with mediastinal syndrome.

Mediastinal radiotherapy (ten sessions) is then performed, followed by chemotherapy (cisplatin and etoposide), that is suspended after the first cycle.

The review of the previously practiced histological biopsy of the mediastinal mass and of the parietal pleura allows definitive diagnosis of "T-lymphoblastic lymphoma", meaning it requires a re-evaluation diagnosis and treatment.

- BMB: bone marrow normocellular with good representation of hematopoietic precursors.
- FDG-PET performed 5 days before chemotherapy: negative for focal lesions with high metabolism, meaning good response to treatment.

Chemotherapy according to the hyper-CVAD scheme.

- CT: in the anterior superior prevascular mediastinum, a thickening of the adipose cellular tissue is found, measuring 47 × 24 mm, remnant and/or outcome of the disease, which does not show infiltrative aspects. Mediastinal lymph node stations are normal. The right lung is hypoexpanded compared with the contralateral; evidence of hyperdense plaques at the mediastinal pleura is found, likely following the previous partial pleurectomy and talc plurodesis. Sporadic and shaded microfoci of parenchymal thickening are present in the right lung, which are associated with scissural thickening and disventilatory phenomena in the lingular and postero-basal areas, probably of post-actinic nature. Submantellar nodule measuring 7 mm is found in the postero-basal segment of the left lower lobe.

P. F. Rambaldi, *Whole-Body FDG PET Imaging in Oncology*,
DOI: 10.1007/978-88-470-5295-6_36, © Springer-Verlag Italia 2014

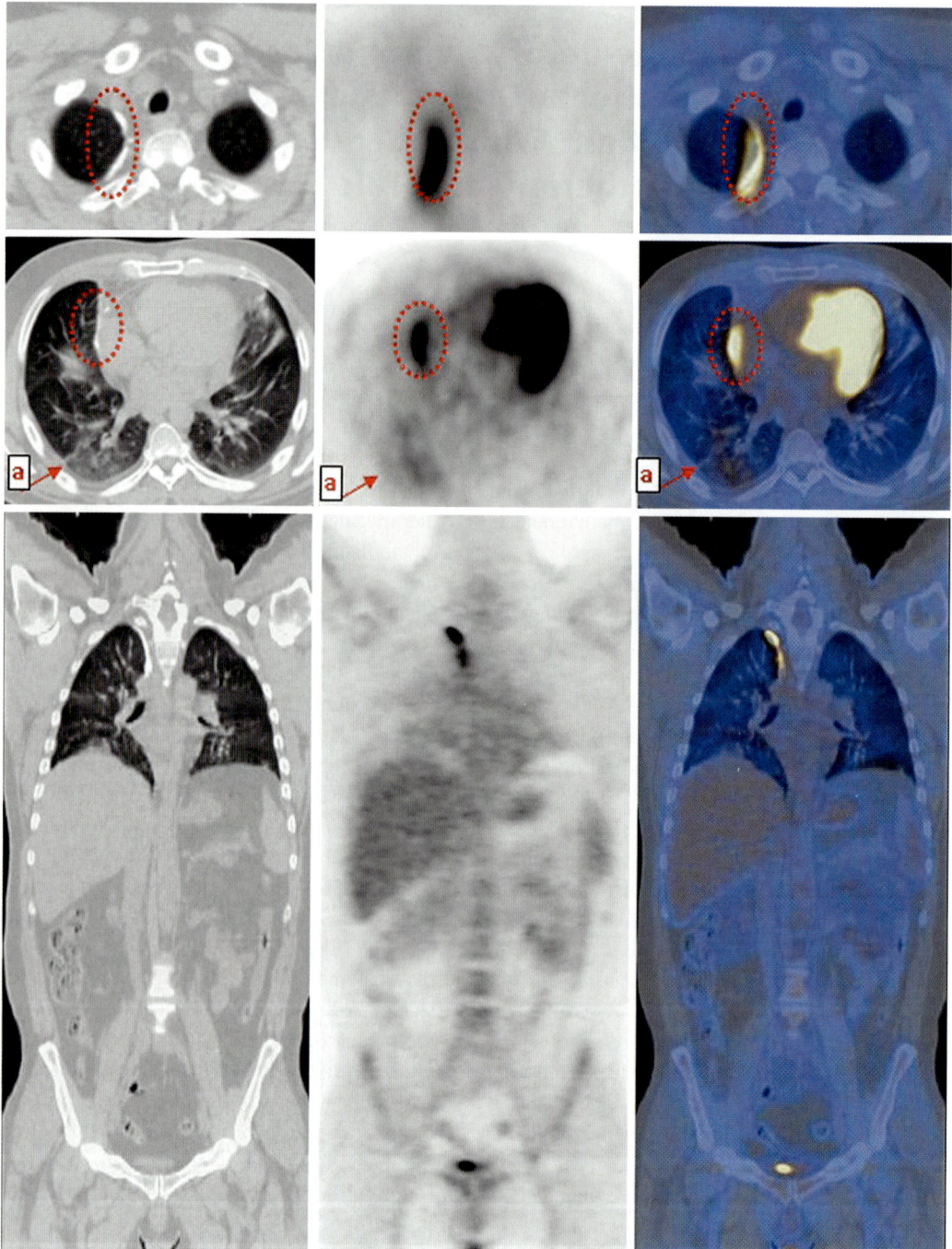

Fig. 36.1 On CT-PET, two hyperdense pleural plaques in the left upper lobe and in the cardio-phrenic ipsilateral area due to previous pleurectomy and talc pleurodesis are shown. The high metabolism is related to the granulomatous reaction. The parenchymal lung right lung nodule and the scissural thickening do not have pathological glucose consumption and are attributable to post-actinic disventilatory phenomena

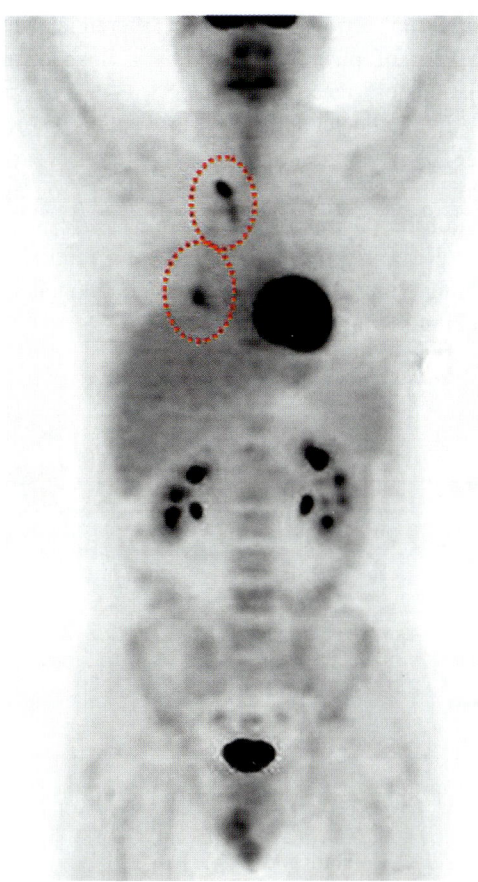

Fig. 36.2 MIP: pathological glucose consumption of the mediastinal pleura, in the superior lobe and in the cardiophrenic area, due to granulomatous reaction. No other focal areas of pathological metabolism were found

36.2   Diagnostic Question

Evaluation of therapeutic response in a patient with T-lymphoblastic lymphoma receiving chemotherapy: search for lesions with high glucose metabolism.

36.3   Report

Intense glucose consumption in some hyperdense plaques at the mediastinal pleura in correspondence of the upper lobe and in the cardiophrenic area, SUV max 6.2. These formations are visible on the images acquired with mitigation technique and they appear unchanged compared to the CT reported in history.

No pathological glucose consumption observed at the parenchymal nodule in the anterior superior prevascular mediastinum, which was described by the same CT. The images show some attenuation areas of parenchymal thickening bilaterally that have no pathological metabolism and were thus was related to fibrotic post—actinic disventilatory phenomena. Absence of pathological glucose deposition in the remaining parts of the body examined.

Fig. 36.3 The CT-PET shows a thickening tissue in the right anterior mediastinum that does not infiltrate the surrounding tissues and presents no pathological glucose consumption as a response to the treatment. Adenopathies with an altered metabolism are not found

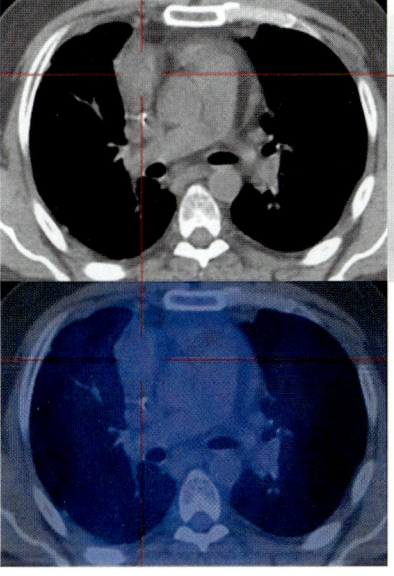

36.4   Conclusions

The PET scan shows no focal lesions characterized by high consumption of FDG, meaning there was a good response to radio-chemotherapy. The presence of granulomatous pleural reaction with high metabolic activity was determined by the talc pleurodesis. See Figs. 36.1, 36.2, 36.3.

36.5   Key Points

The talc pleurodesis determines a granulomatous inflammatory reaction that in the active phases is characterized by high metabolism of glucose.

It is not always possible to differentiate the recovery of pleural diseases by a nonspecific inflammatory reaction.

After radiochemotherapy, this patient shows a good metabolic response of pulmonary and mediastinal lesions, so it is unlikely a progression of the pleural lesions alone.

We can say that the disease is in remission although there is a coexisting granulomatous reaction secondary to talc pleurodesis.

NHL: Evaluation of the Response to Chemotherapy

37.1 Clinical History

70-year-old man with mediastinal large B-cell NHL, diagnosed after excision of a voluminous anterior mediastinal swelling, is in remission after chemotherapy.

Follow-up after one year.

- PET-FDG: pathological glucose consumption in the upper mediastinum due to right paratracheal lymphadenopathy, which extends in the retrocaval area, compatible with recurrence of pathology, SUV max 9.
- Chest and abdomen CT: conglomerate lymphadenopathy measuring 3 cm in the right paratracheal area that extends caudally to the lodge of Barety. Smaller swollen lymph-nodes are adjacent to the aortic arch (17 mm) and on the right side of the seam front (20 mm) (Fig. 37.1a).

Chemotherapy is thus performed.

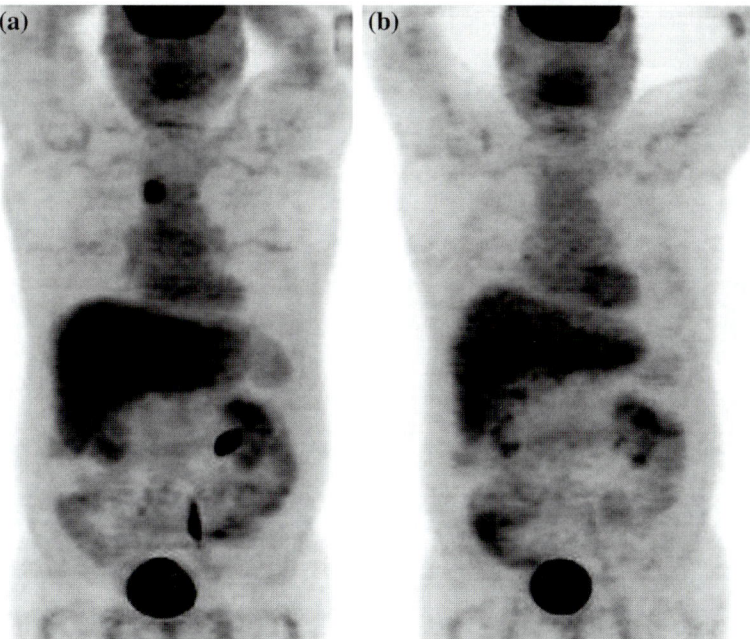

Fig. 37.1 a. Smaller swollen lymph-nodes are adjacent to the aortic arch. **b**. No focal lesions

P. F. Rambaldi, *Whole-Body FDG PET Imaging in Oncology*,
DOI: 10.1007/978-88-470-5295-6_37, © Springer-Verlag Italia 2014

37.2 Diagnostic Question

Search of focal lesions with high metabolism of glucose in a patient with NHL after chemotherapy.

37.3 Report

The PET scan shows no focal lesions characterized by pathological consumption of glucose in the body segments examined (Fig. 37.1b).

37.4 Conclusions

The PET scan today shows no pathological glucose consumption at the adenopathy reported by the previous scan, demonstrating the response to the treatment performed. See Figs. 37.2, 37.3.

37.5 Key Points

- The CT-PET may be performed in the course of chemotherapy to allow the evaluation of the extent of the response to treatment and/or persistence of pathology.
- The complete remission is documented only when the PET examination performed four - weeks after chemotherapy is negative.
- The complete remission is documented only when the PET scan performed three months after radiotherapy or radioimmunotherapy is negative.
- In lymphomas, strict supervision of clinical and instrumental data is always advisable, especially when there is a mismatch between morphologic and metabolic findings.
- The careful collection of the clinical history allows us to understand how frequent is the

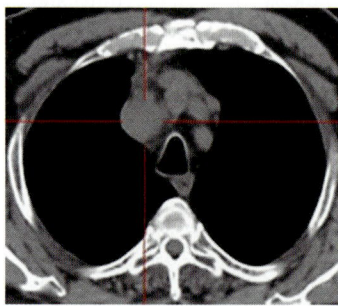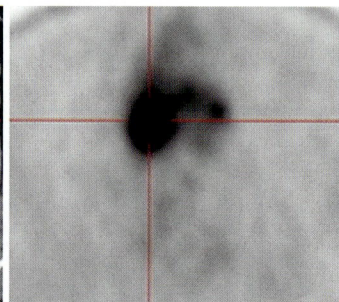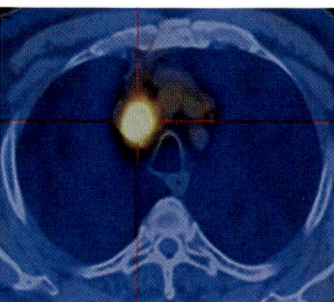

Fig. 37.2 CT-PET scan performed before chemotherapy shows the presence of dishomogeneous, solid tissue, that looks like an adenopathy in the right paratracheal area extending caudally down to the lodge of Barety and in the retrocaval area. The glucose consumption of the lesion is high

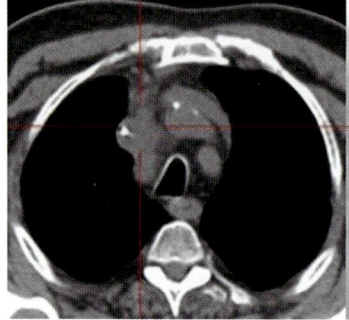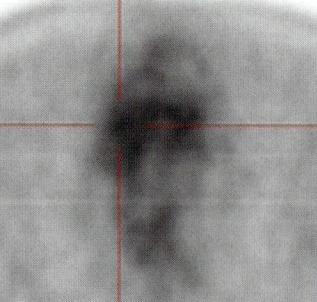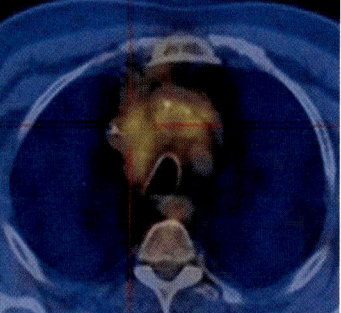

Fig. 37.3 Follow up after chemotherapy: CT scan shows some adenopathies measuring less than 1 cm in the anterior mediastinum, in the lodge of Barety and prevascular area, that do not have pathological metabolism of glucose, as shown in the PET scan

finding of a mismatch between the morphologic image and the metabolic one.

- A PET-FDG that does not show pathological carbohydrate consumption, in effect indicates metabolic activity in relation to:

specific pathophysiological conditions,

interfering therapies (chemotherapy, radiation therapy, and other drugs),

absence of disease.

Mediastinal Mass: Thymic Carcinoma   38

38.1 Clinical History

44-year-old man with increasing dyspnea:
- Chest X-ray: enlargement of the anterior superior mediastinum to the right.
- CT: gross swelling of solid nature resembling an adenopathy that develops occupying the anterosuperior mediastinum asymmetrically and extending to the lodge of Barety. No lymph-nodes along the jugular chain on both sides and in the abdominopelvic region are found to be enlarged.

38.2 Diagnostic Question

Search for focal lesions with high glucose metabolism in patients with mediastinal mass of nature yet to be defined.

38.3 Report

Abnormal glucose consumption in the right anterior superior mediastinal mass previously reported in history, SUV max 15 (Fig. 38.1).

Presence of a metabolically inactive pulmonary nodule measuring less than a centimeter, in middle lobe of the right lung.

No areas of abnormal glucose consumption in the remaining parts of the body examined.

38.4 Conclusions

The PET scan shows mediastinal disease with a high carbohydrate metabolism, suspicious for cancer of the thymus, to be confirmed histologically.

Diagnosis is then confirmed histologically. See Fig. 38.2.

38.5 Key points

- The differential diagnosis of solitary mediastinal masses includes many diseases, and a young man in the presence of high glucose metabolism mass suggests lymphoma or thymoma. The probability of a lung cancer or other neoplastic conditions is lower.
- In the suspected clinical diagnosis of lymphoma, FNAB is not recommended (or contraindicated) because the result is often indeterminate and therefore does not allow a full diagnosis.
- Samples obtained through wide excision biopsies allow a rigorous assessment of cytology and immunohistochemistry of the tumor, both necessary to have an accurate diagnosis and prognosis.

The FDG-PET is crucial in defining the grading of thymomas; extensive metabolism correlates with more aggressive forms and a worse prognosis.

P. F. Rambaldi, *Whole-Body FDG PET Imaging in Oncology*,
DOI: 10.1007/978-88-470-5295-6_38, © Springer-Verlag Italia 2014

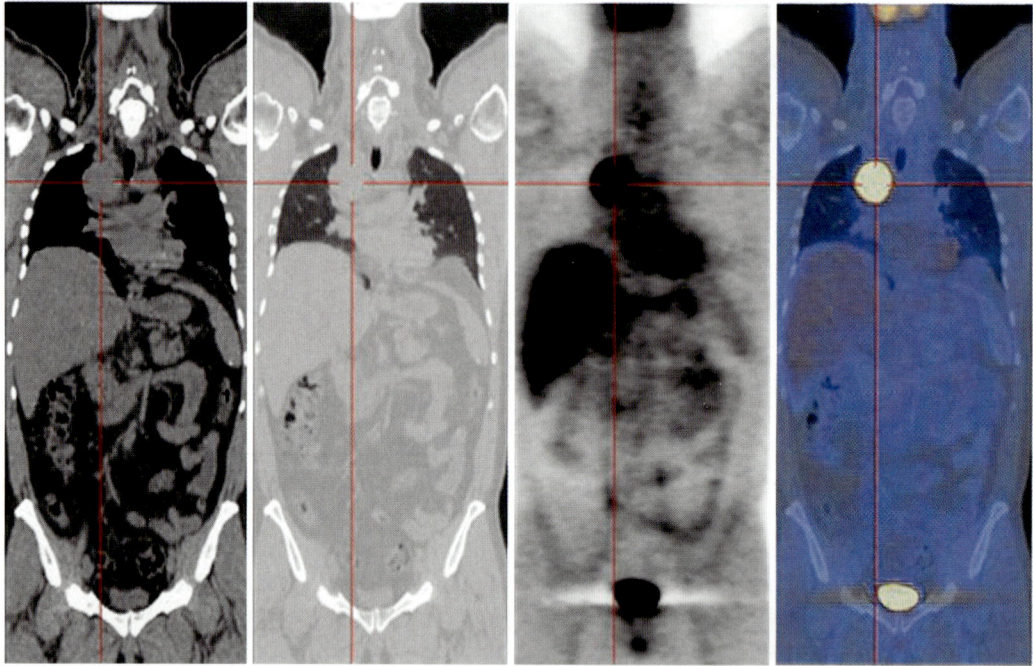

Fig. 38.1 The PET scan shows mediastinal disease with a high carbohydrate metabolism, suspicious for cancer of the thymus

Fig. 38.2 The PET-CT scan shows a solid mass in the lodge of Barety. This mass is rounded and characterized by homogeneous density, regular margins and high glucose metabolism

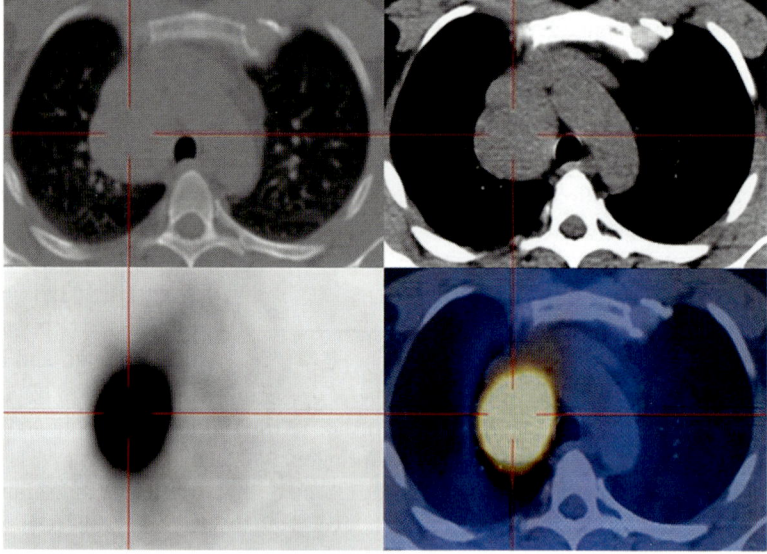

- Some authors have demonstrated that FDG uptake is significantly higher in invasive thymomas than in encapsulated;
- It seems that the level of carbohydrate consumption, SUV max, is lower in the less aggressive histological types (type A, AB, and B1) and significantly higher in the thymic carcinomas (type C).

Hodgkin's Lymphoma: Response to Chemotherapy

39

39.1 Clinical History

19-year-old woman with mediastinal large cell B lymphoma, histologically diagnosed. The patient underwent two cycles of chemotherapy.

- CT neck, chest, abdomen, pelvis (baseline study): bulky solid mass, inhomogeneous, which occupies the thymic lodge, extending to the right in the middle mediastinum with a maximum diameter of 15 cm. The mass surrounds the adjacent vascular structures, including anonymous veins, the superior vena cava, the ascending aorta, the aortic arch and but not the pericardium wall.
- PET-CT (baseline study): bulky mediastinal mass characterized by high consumption of glucose (SUVmax 13).

39.2 Diagnostic Question

Search for focal lesions with high glucose metabolism in patients with mediastinal LH during chemotherapy, II cycle (interim PET).

39.3 Report

The mediastinal lymphoma described by CT scan and reported in history shows limited consumption of glucose, SUVmax 1.7.

Absence of pathological metabolism in the remaining body segments examined.

39.4 Conclusions

The PET scan shows significant response to treatment in progress (Fig. 39.1). See also Figs. 39.2, 39.3.

39.5 Key Points

The early assessment of response by CT-PET after the second cycle of chemotherapy (interim PET) is difficult when there are no pictures of a baseline examination as in this case. Progression of disease is unlikely when the activity is low in the lesion.

- A thymic reactive hyperplasia in the active phase, due to post-chemotherapy rebound, can be excluded because it is generally characterized by high metabolism and has an 'inverted V' morphology.
- The SUVmax is not always realizable as it does not always provide a precise estimate of the actual carbohydrate lesional consumption, and in relation to the high incidence of technical artifacts, it is preferable to trust more in a qualitative assessment of the images.
- Generally, lymphomas have high consumption of FDG, so when the interim PET documents an SUVmax of 1.7 at the dominant lesion, which is an activity lower than that of the liver, the response to treatment in progress may be considered good.

P. F. Rambaldi, *Whole-Body FDG PET Imaging in Oncology*,
DOI: 10.1007/978-88-470-5295-6_39, © Springer-Verlag Italia 2014

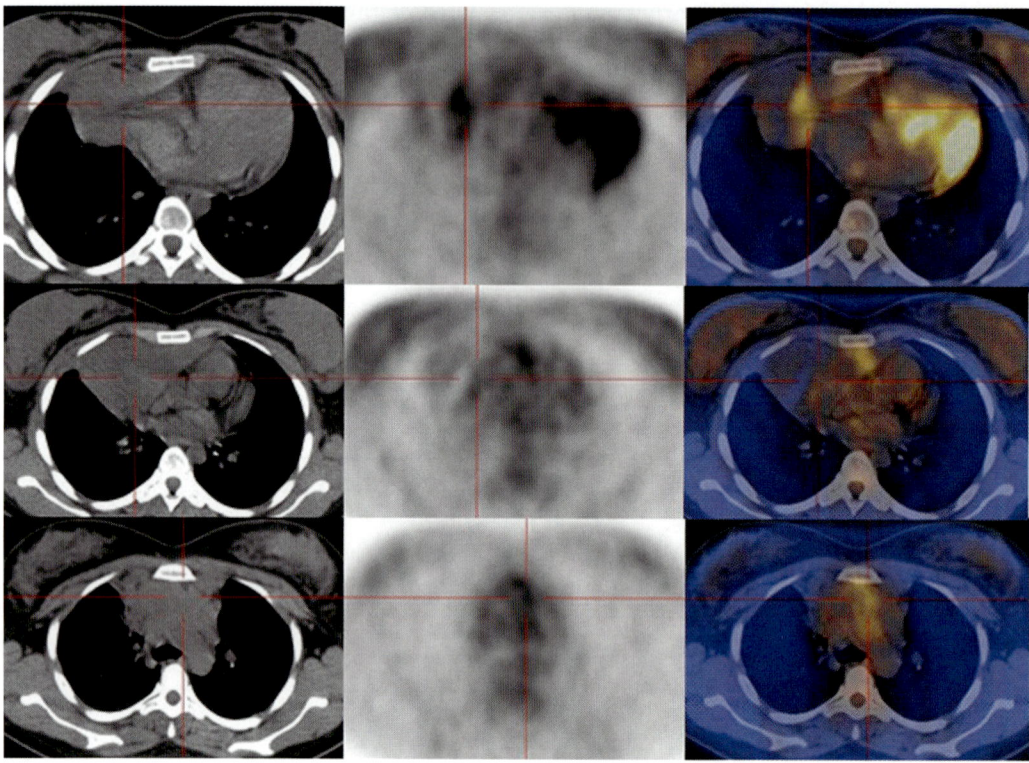

Fig. 39.1 CT-PET: gross solid, inhomogeneous mass occupying the right anterior and medium mediastinum, with limited glucose metabolism

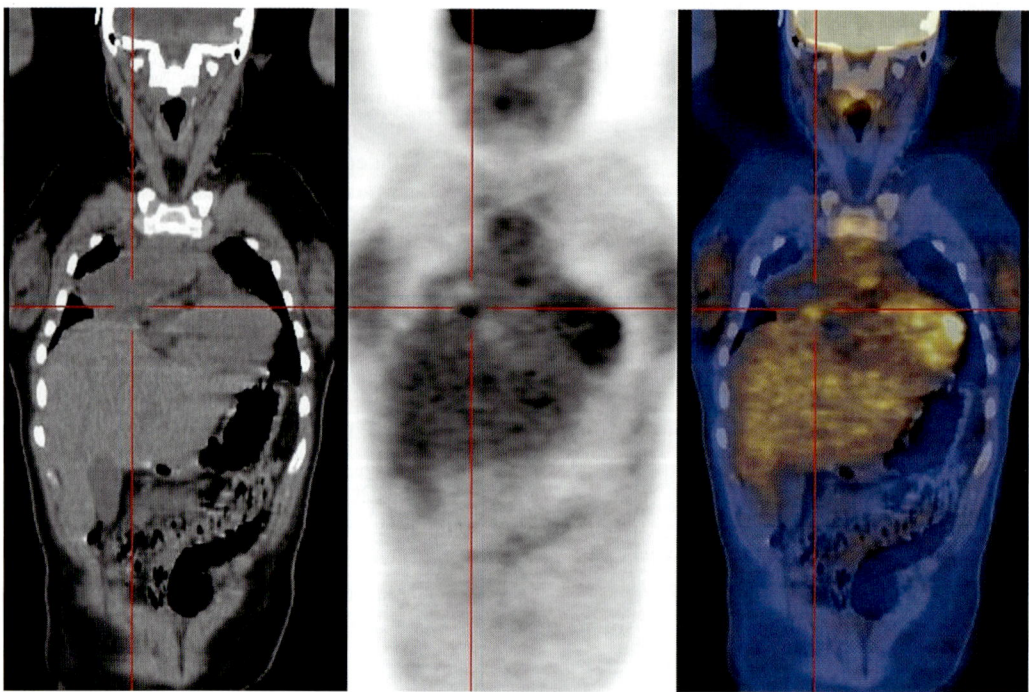

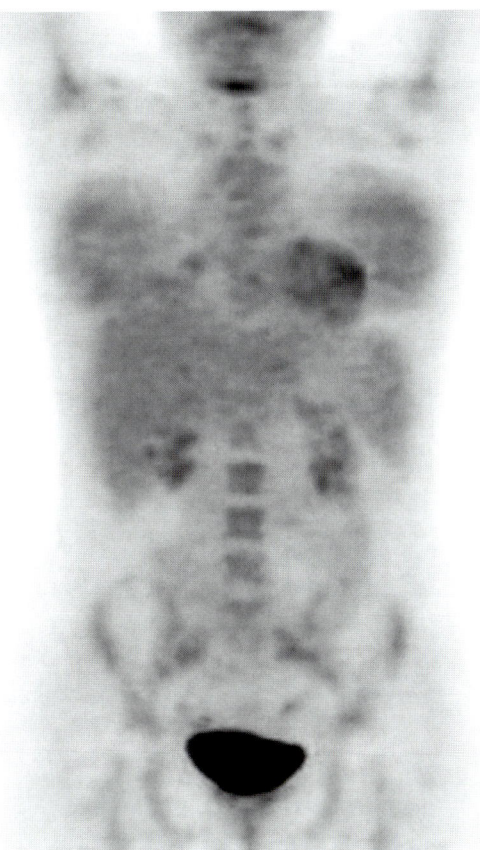

Fig. 39.3

• After chemotherapy, the concentration of FDG is a function:
  – of the vitality of tumor cells,
  – the remnant cellular pool associated with neoplasia,
  – involutive and/or necrotic-colliquative phenomena that characterize the volumetric reduction in the lymphomatous mass in case of a good response to treatment.

Before reaching a final conclusion, it is essential to assess a comprehensive study of the images that takes into account:
– CT attenuation;
– the morphology of the accumulation;
– inhomogeneities and focal metabolic activity;
– the average tumor/liver uptake comparison considered the reference point below which the interim PET is documenting a good response to chemotherapy, a low probability of persistence of disease and a good prognosis.

◀ **Fig. 39.2** The coronal CT-PET image shows the solid mediastinal mass, with limited carbohydrate deposition (Fig. 39.2). In the MIP reconstruction focal lesions with a high uptake of glucose are not shown, in particular the mediastinal mass presents metabolic activity comparable to that of the liver (Fig. 39.3). Also observed widespread fixation of glucose in the bone marrow due to post-chemotherapy rebound. Clear increase in the metabolism of the mammary glands, typical of young women

Granulomatosis

40

40.1 Clinical History

41-year-old foundry worker, performs Chest CT after presenting with dyspnea.

- Chest CT: micronodules in the centrilobular and sub-pleural areas, especially in the upper and middle lung regions bilaterally, with mild dilatation of a subsegmentary distal lobar upper branch. Peribronchial cuffing at the hilar and perihilar areas on both sides. Minimal thickening of the pleural layers that look 'wrinkled', particularly the visceral pleura, due to traction. Hilar-mediastinal lymph-nodes are found.

40.2 Diagnostic Question

Patient with mediastinal lymphadenopathy to be defined: characterization of the glucose metabolism of the lesion.

40.3 Report

Multiple nodules measuring more than a centimeter and of adenopathic nature, characterized by modest consumption of glucose, the most evident are found at the paratracheal, subcarinal and aortopulmonary window, in the lodge of Barety, prevascular and parahilar bilateral regions, SUV max 3.3.

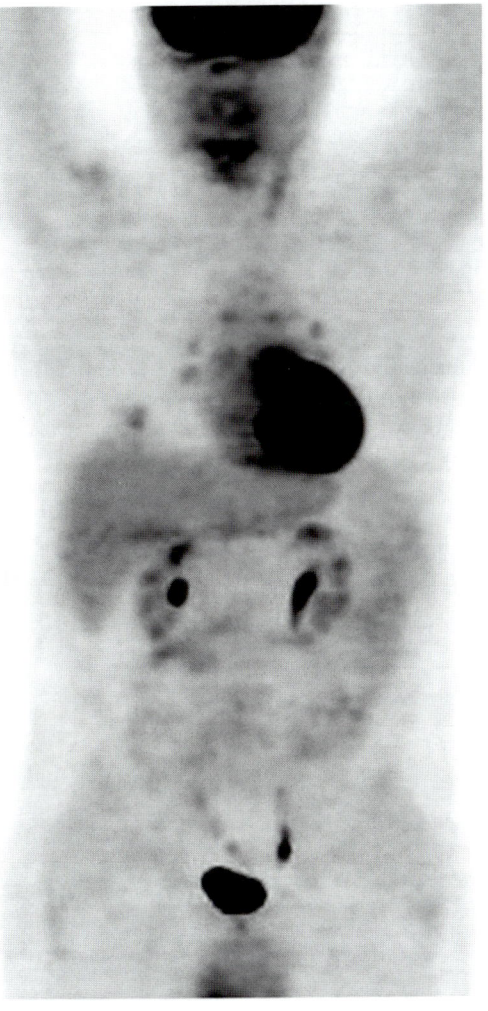

Fig. 40.1 No areas of abnormal metabolism

P. F. Rambaldi, *Whole-Body FDG PET Imaging in Oncology*,
DOI: 10.1007/978-88-470-5295-6_40, © Springer-Verlag Italia 2014

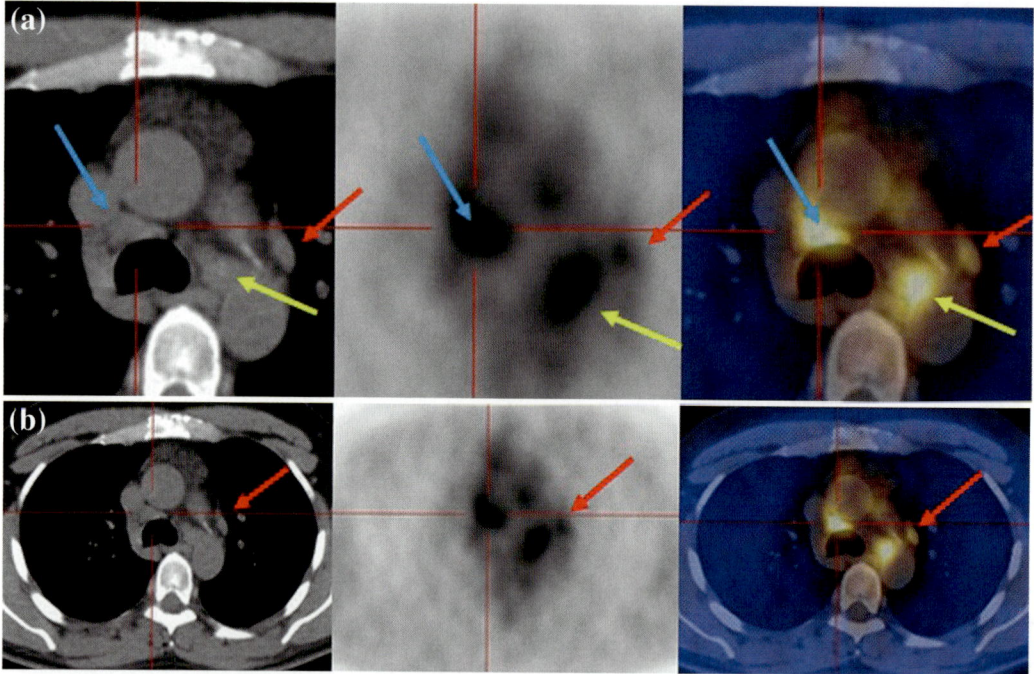

Fig. 40.2 The CT shows some mediastinal lymph node size of increased dimension in the pre-tracheal (a, blue arrows), the aorto-pulmonary window (**a**, *yellow arrows*) and in the prevascular area (**a**, **b**, *red arrows*)

Increased deposition glucose is found in the anterior costal arch of the 5th rib, due to skeletal alteration caused by post-traumatic fracture, SUV max 3.7.

No areas of abnormal metabolism in the remaining parts of the body examined (Fig. 40.1).

Fig. 40.3 Modest increase in glucose metabolism

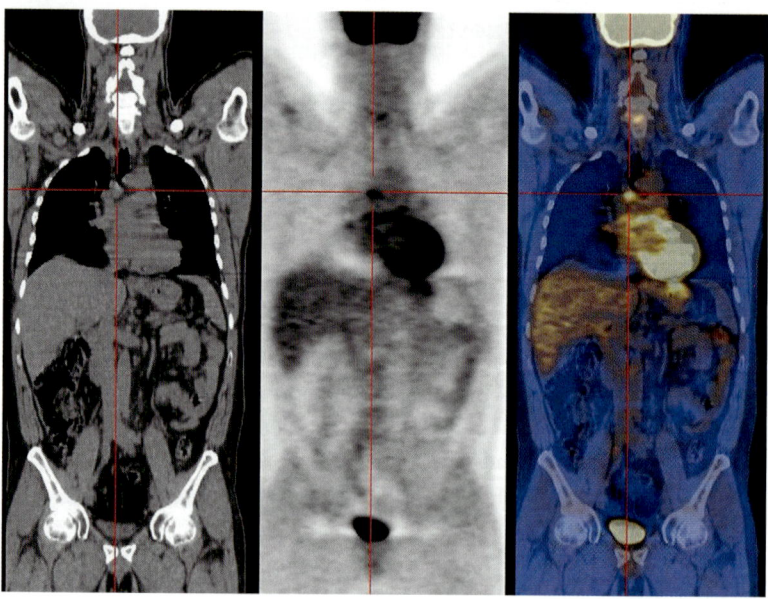

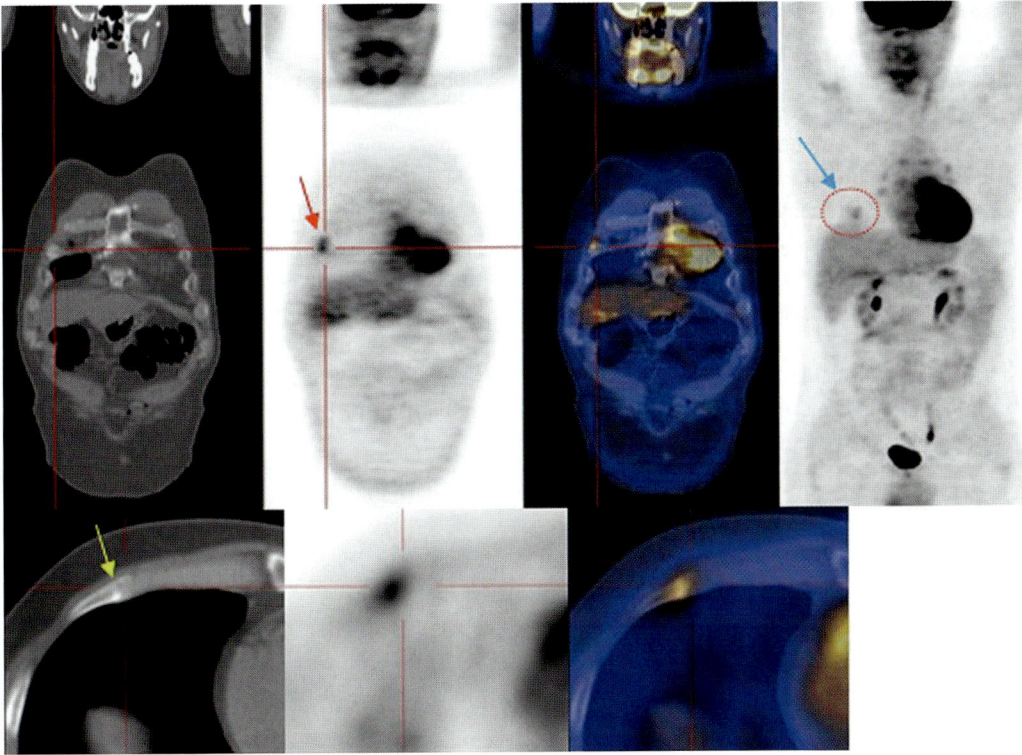

Fig. 40.4 The CT-PET demonstrates increased glucose consumption at the anterior right costal arch of the fifth rib (*blue arrow*) at the level of which is not observed newly formed tissue (*yellow arrow*). The absence of osteolytic images suggests the lesion to be post-traumatic

40.4   Conclusions

The scan shows mediastinal lymphadenopathy, probably of granulomatous nature.

Histological exam is necessary to define the treatment program and completely exclude a neoplastic condition.

Mediastinoscopy was then performed and allowed the removal of two lymph nodes, on which a nonspecific granulomatous process was demonstrated.

The CT shows some mediastinal lymph node size of increased dimension (Fig. 40.2), in the pre-tracheal (Fig. 40.2a, *blue arrows*), the aortopulmonary window (Fig. 40.2a, *yellow arrows*) and in the prevascular area (Fig. 40.2a, b, *red arrows*). See also Figs. 40.3, 40.4.

40.5   Key Points

The presence of widespread involvement of mediastinal stations opens up a large and difficult differential diagnosis.

- Some evidence suggests the occupational disease:
  - the patient worked in a foundry;
  - the finding reported in CT and clinical history was of centrilobular and subpleural micronodules, in particular of the upper and

middle lung regions, typical of benign pathologies;

– the symptom of wheezing reported by the patient is not pathognomonic of a neoplastic disease, but can also be determined by a benign condition that involves diffusely pulmonary parenchyma;

– lymph node involvement detected by CT-PET does not justify the patient's dyspnea and is probably due to other pathological conditions;

– CT-PET lymph nodes are small and have only a modest increased glucose consumption, and this element suggests a disease characterized by limited aggression (see MIP image).

The conclusions of our report are important as follows:

– It can suggest a benign disease,

– recommends a biopsy because it is the only way to allow definitive diagnosis.

– The tissue sample to be taken must be quantitatively and qualitatively aimed at a specific cyto-histological typing, so mediastinoscopy or another invasive procedure is indicated.

– A tissue sample is frequently insufficient and it is often of indeterminate diagnosis.

Microscopically and Macroscopically Capsulated Stage IA Thymoma

41.1   Clinical History

42-year-old woman with a history of papillary thyroid carcinoma in situ measuring 2 mm, occasionally diagnosed after thyroidectomy performed for nodular goiter, pT1, pneumothorax, PMX - Stage I/UICC 2002. Radical treatment completed with I-131.

Follow-up after two years.

- Test with recombinant TSH: normal.
- CT: hypodense solid tissue in the anterosuperior left mediastinum measuring 8 × 5 cms specifically in the prevascular area, showing slight enhancement after contrast, looking like a swollen lymph node conglomerate. Liver of normal size, irregular density, showing at the sixth segment a 7 cm hypodense lesion, that shows peripheral enhancement in the early phase and centripetal progression in the late, after contrast injection. This finding, unchanged from the examination of three years ago, is compatible with an angioma. Spleen within the limits of size, dishomogeneous in density, shows multiple hypodense nodular areas (max = 4 cm), without enhancement after contrast, unchanged from previous scans and defined as cysts.

Bronchoaspirate of the mediastinal mass: cells of chronic inflammatory type, negative for atypical cells.

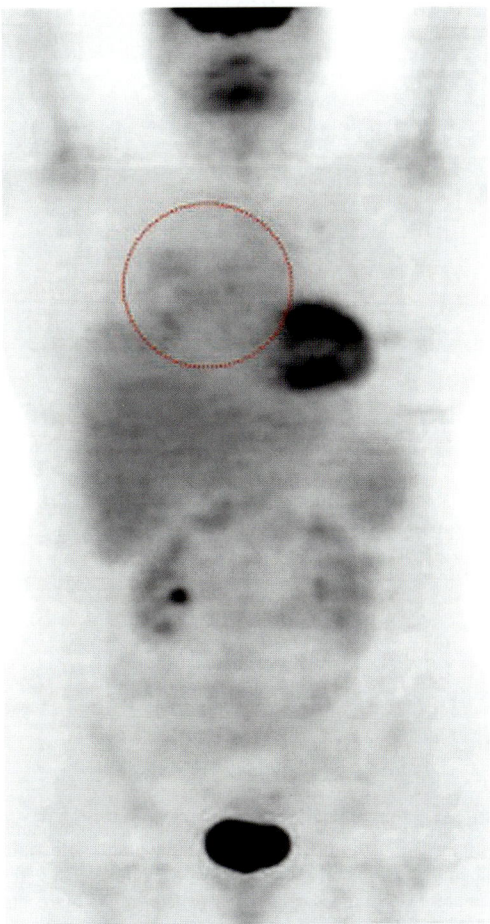

Fig. 41.1 MIP reconstruction: there are no focal lesions with a high glucose uptake, in particular the mediastinal mass shows metabolic activity comparable to that of the liver

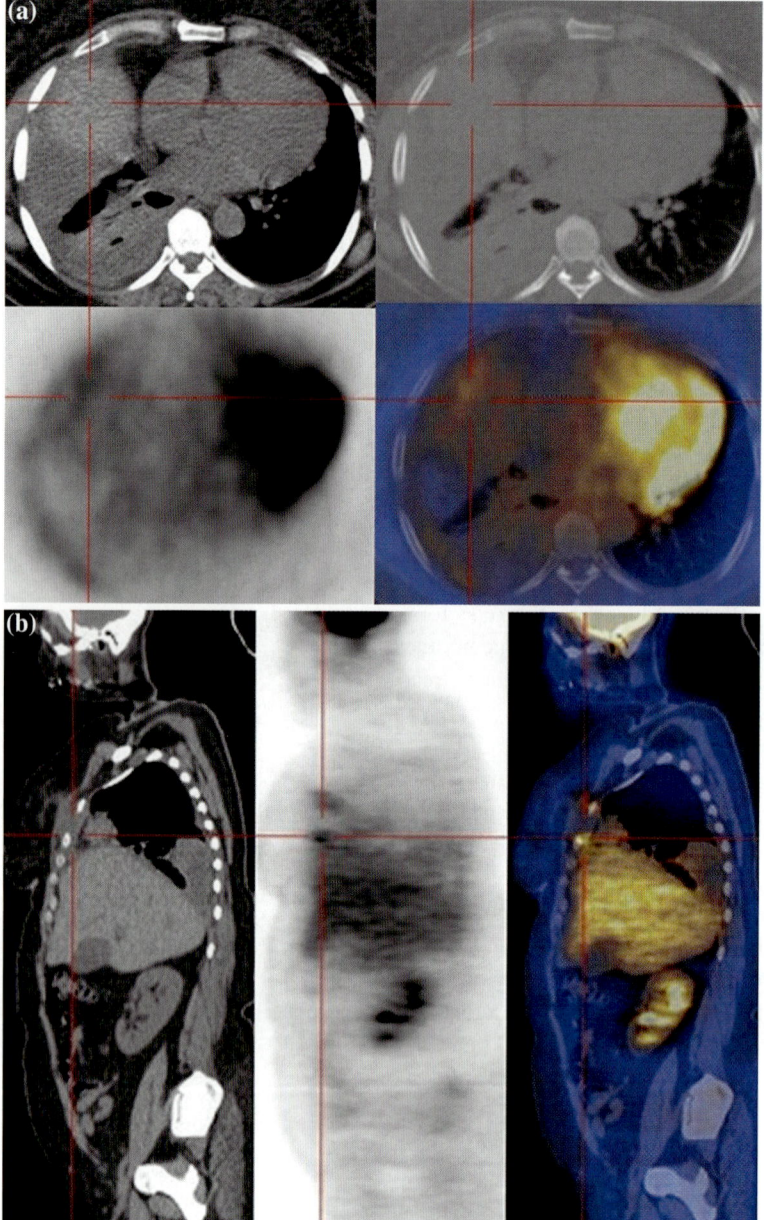

Fig. 41.2 The PET-CT scan shows opacification of the pulmonary medium and basal fields average with right pleural effusion, characterized by irregular density for the presence of areas of atelectasis determined by recent FNAB, with reduced expansion of the right hemithorax and hemidiaphragm lifted upwards (**a**). The recent fine-needle aspiration path is best evident in the sagittal reconstruction of the CT-PET, documenting the increased density of the soft tissues of the anterior wall of the ipsilateral hemithorax (**b**). The lesion carbohydrate consumption is low, comparable to that of the mediastinal background

- Bronchial washings: cytologic exam shows a serum-proteinaceous fluid mixed with a few inflammatory elements.

- FNAB: nondiagnostic cytology, featuring only blood.

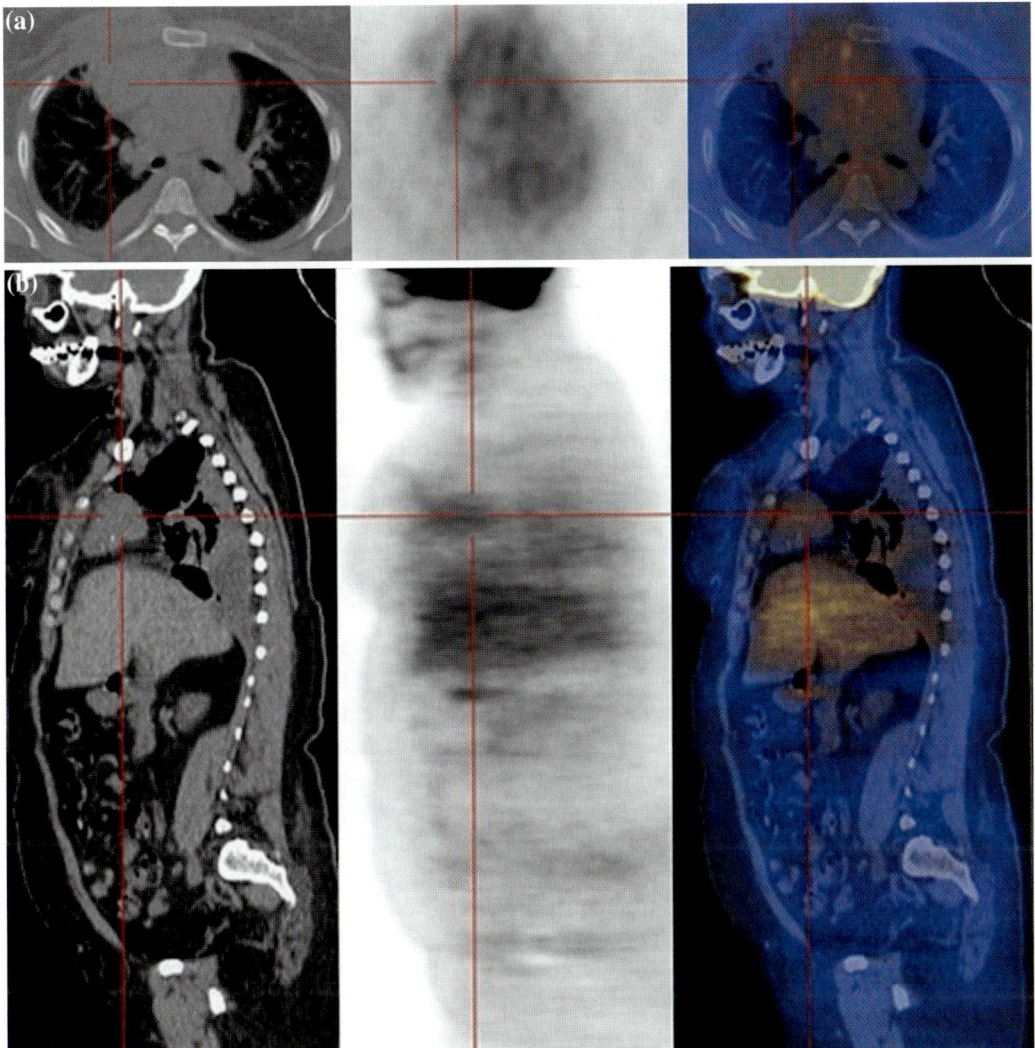

Fig. 41.3 In correspondence of the anterior and prevascular mediastinum, CT-PET shows a solid homogeneous, multilobed mass, characterized by limited carbohydrate consumption (**a**). In the sagittal scan this mass is well dissociated from the vascular structures and the sternum (**b**)

- CT: opacification of the lung medium and basal fields, with mixed densities due to the presence of areas of atelectasis and an anterior mediastinal retrosternal mass, characterized by altered density.

41.2 Diagnostic Question

Search for focal lesions with high glucose metabolism in patient with mediastinal mass to be defined.

41.3 Report

The gross mass shown at the anterior superior left paramedian mediastinum, demonstrates restricted carbohydrate consumption, SUVmax 1.6. No areas of abnormal metabolism in the remaining parts of the body examined.

41.4 Conclusions

The mediastinal mass shows limited carbohydrate metabolism as a thymoma of low malignant potential; histological confirmation has to be performed.

Subsequently the mass was excised and a definitive diagnosis of thymoma microscopically and macroscopically capsulated, stage IA was made. See Figs. 41.1, 41.2, 41.3.

41.5 Key Points

CT-PET allows a metabolic characterization that shows low glucose consumption, and limited cell vitality and aggressiveness.

- The gross mediastinal mass:

  - It is not of thyroid nature, because the thyroid test with recombinant TSH is normal;
  - It is asymmetric, so it has not the morphological characteristics of thymic hyperplasia.
- When bronchoscopy is negative, the FNAB is indeterminate and imaging does not show elements of aggressiveness of the tumor, and the oncologist should suggest a mediastinoscopy or surgical removal because:
  - you need a definitive diagnosis,
  - a decompression of the mediastinum is needed,
  - the patient is young.

Tumors of the thymus account for the 0.2–1.5 % of all cancers, so they are rare with an incidence of approximately 0.15 cases per 100,000 people. They are the most common tumors of the mediastinum, accounting for 20 % of tumors in this district and 50 % of those located at the anterior mediastinum. Over 90 % of tumors of the thymus are located in the anterior mediastinum, and the others are located in the neck or in other compartments of the mediastinum.

Ocular Lymphoma

42

42.1 Clinical History

51-year-old woman with an endorbitary right retrobulbar lesion compatible with NHL, undergoing staging.

42.2 Question Diagnostic

Search for lesions with a high carbohydrate metabolism and staging.

Fig. 42.1 In the MIP reconstruction, the endorbitary formation is masked by physiological brain glucose consumption. Focal lesions in other parts of the body are not detected

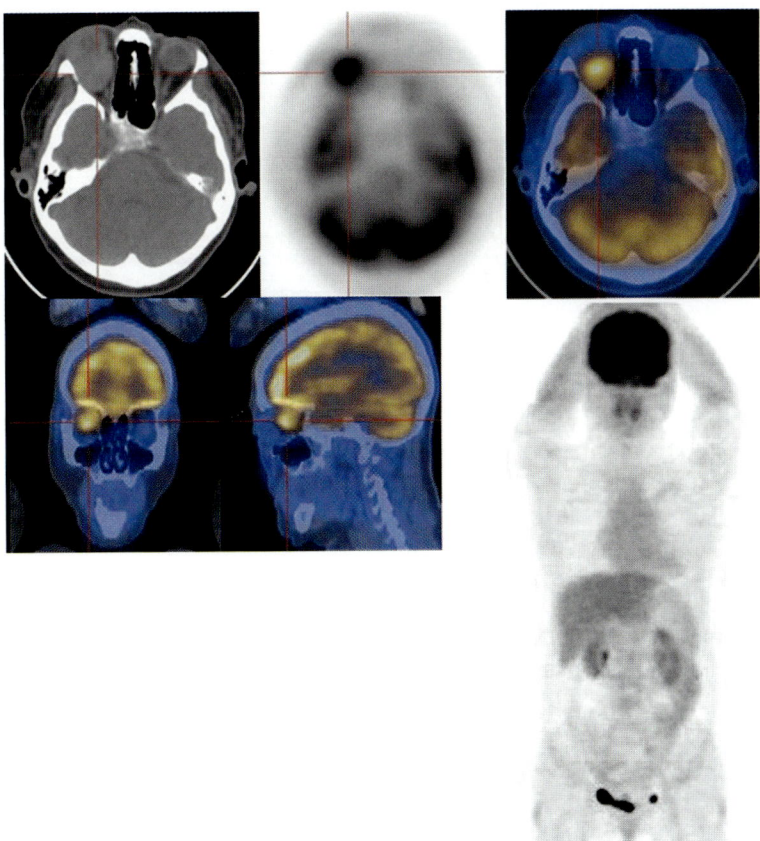

P. F. Rambaldi, *Whole-Body FDG PET Imaging in Oncology*,
DOI: 10.1007/978-88-470-5295-6_42, © Springer-Verlag Italia 2014

42.3   Report

The PET scan shows modest increase in glucose consumption at the endorbitary right retrobulbar mass seen at CT, SUVmax 6.6. No significant areas of pathological metabolism in the remaining body segments examined.

42.4   Conclusions

The scan today shows high metabolic activity in the lymphomatous right retrobulbar lesion (Figs. 42.1).

42.5   Key Points

- Always suspect a neoplastic condition in patients with unilateral ophthalmopathy of recent onset.
- CT-PET metabolism defines the district and excludes focal lesions of other organs and systems.

DIC of the Left Breast with Liver Metastases: Metabolic Response to Chemotherapy

43

43.1 Clinical History

45-year-old woman with DIC of the left breast who underwent neoadjuvant chemotherapy.

- Ultrasound: Liver size increased with inhomogeneous echotexture due to the presence of at least two hypoechoic nodules, with regular margins, located in segment II and VI, measuring 17 and 15 mm respectively, to be evaluated with contrast-enhanced CT.
- CT: presence of expansive solid mass in the inner quadrants of the left breast. Multiple hypodense hepatic nodules, with blurred margins and irregular contrastographic impregnation, resembling metastases.
  Control after neoadjuvant chemotherapy.
- CT: significant regression of multiple liver foci scattered in most segments, their current size varying from a few millimeters to 2 cms, characterized by necrotic center, irregular margins and modest marginal post-contrast-enhancement.

Left quadrantectomy left and adjuvant chemotherapy are then performed.

43.2 Diagnostic Question

Search for focal lesions with high glucose metabolism in woman who underwent left quadrantectomy for breast DIC with liver metastases: restaging.

43.3 Report

Slight focal concentration of FDG in the left breast and ipsilateral axillary area, SUV-max = 2.2, this element is to be referred to post-surgical scar remodeling. No areas of abnormal metabolism in the remaining parts of the body examined. See Fig. 43.1.

P. F. Rambaldi, *Whole-Body FDG PET Imaging in Oncology*,
DOI: 10.1007/978-88-470-5295-6_43, © Springer-Verlag Italia 2014

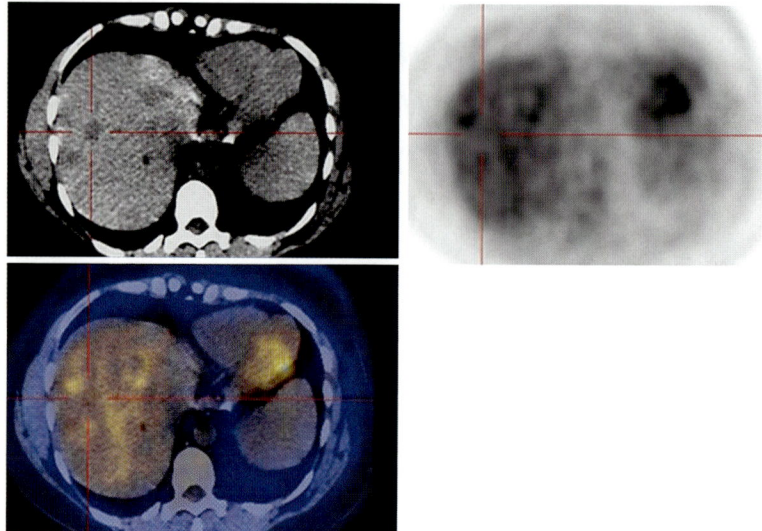

Fig. 43.1 Multiple hypodense hepatic nodules reported show no significant increase in the consumption of glucose

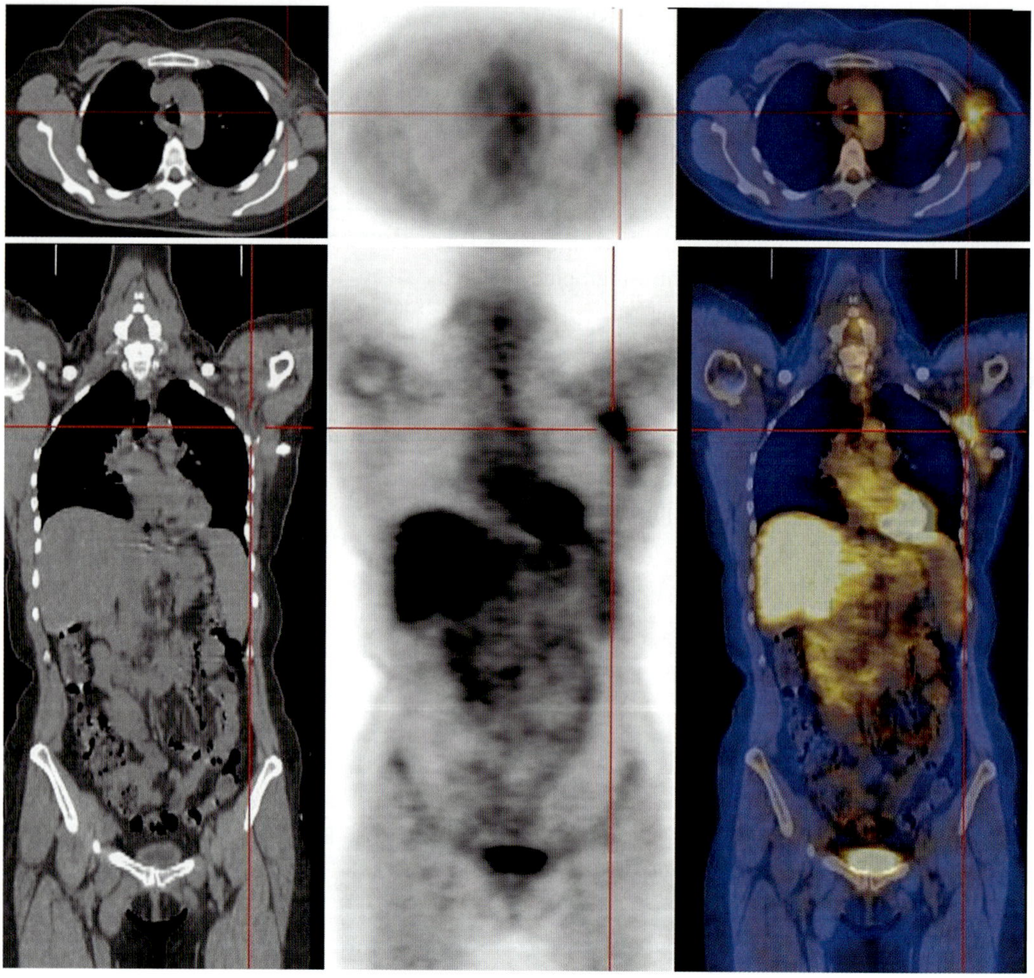

Fig. 43.2 CT-PET: in left armpit there are no mass lesions even if there is small portion of irregular solid tissue that has little carbohydrate metabolism. This element is to be referred to post-surgery scar remodeling. The absence of focal nodular lesions on CT confirms this hypothesis

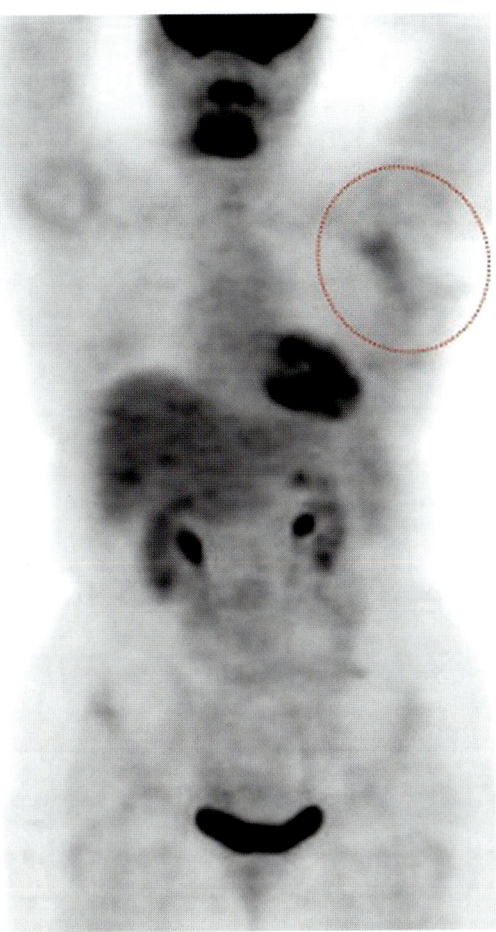

Fig. 43.3 The MIP image does not show nodular high glucose consumption typical of neoplastic lesions: the test is negative for recurrent disease with high metabolism

43.4 Conclusions

The PET scan shows positive metabolic response to chemotherapy of hepatic lesions, documented by previous CT scans and reported in history.

A close follow-up with CT-PET or contrast-enhanced CT is advisable at 3 months. See Fig. 43.2.

43.5 Key Points

The reporting of a PET in restaging after chemotherapy is complex, especially when there is no baseline examination for comparison. See Fig. 43.3.

Districts that have a vague and ill-defined concentration of FDG are related to unspecified conditions such as post-surgery remodeling, as in this case.

These elements suggest a systemic response to chemotherapy and hormonal treatment of maintenance.

You must remember that the PET

- has LOW accuracy in the study of focal breast lesions measuring less than a centimeter, due to resolution limits and respiratory motion artifacts.
- has LOW accuracy in the definition of liver metastases measuring less than a centimeter, due to the background metabolic activity of the liver and motion artifacts (respiratory excursion of the diaphragm),
- not all histological types of breast cancer uptake FDG (e.g., lobular neoplasia, papillary and mucinous carcinomas).

44.1 Clinical History

53-year-old woman who underwent left quadrantectomy with axillary drainage for DIC. Adjuvant chemo-radiotherapy was then performed.

The follow-up at 3 years and 6 months demonstrated a liver metastasis, that is subsequently is chemo-treated and then thermoablated.

The follow-up at 4 years and 6 months showed a left lung metastasis that was radio-treated afterwards.

The follow-up at 5 years and 6 months showed another liver metastasis, which was then thermoablated.

The patient undergoes evaluation after six years.

- CT: pulmonary nodule of the anterior segment of the left lower lobe measuring 13 × 17 mm. Lower mediastinal lymphadenopathy at the right cardiophrenic angle, measuring 20 × 15 mm. Hypodense liver mass in the third segment, measuring 50 × 46 mm. Hypodense paracholecystic nodule in the fifth segment measuring 29 × 23 mm, resulting from necrosis (due to previous ablation). Three millimetric hypodense nodules in the right lobe of the liver, of the microcystic type. 8 mm focal lesion in liver segments VII and VIII. Lymphadenopathy of the lesser omentum, hepatic hilum, cefalopancreatic and left paraortic regions.

44.2 Question Diagnostic

Restaging for treatment planning in patient with metastatic breast cancer: search for focal lesions

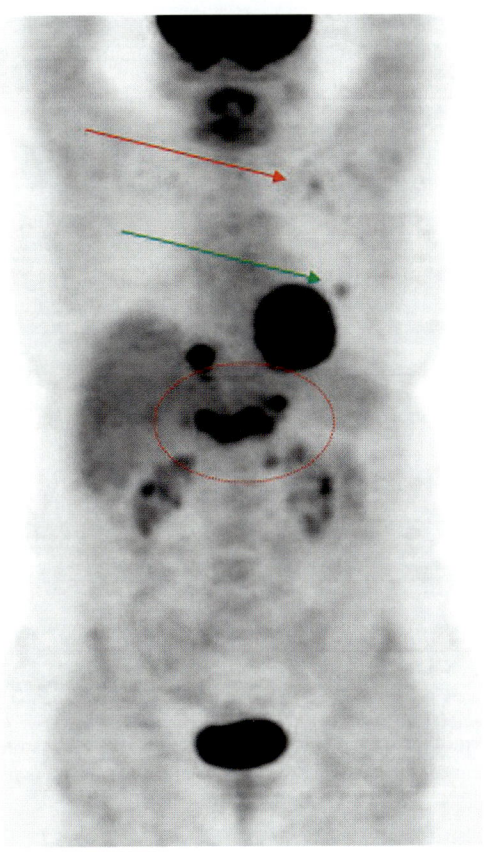

Fig. 44.1 Left subclavear adenopathy measuring less than a centimeter

P. F. Rambaldi, *Whole-Body FDG PET Imaging in Oncology*,
DOI: 10.1007/978-88-470-5295-6_44, © Springer-Verlag Italia 2014

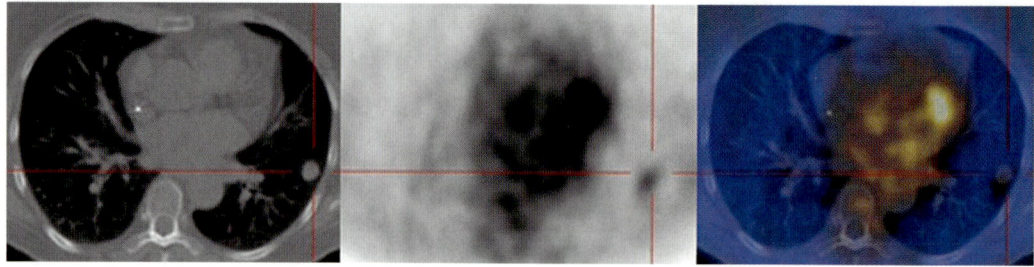

Fig. 44.2 CT scan shows, in the anterior segment of the lower lobe of the left lung, a metastatic mantle nodule, which had been previously radio treated (Fig. 44.2). The PET scan showed restricted carbohydrate consumption due to late post-actinic remodeling

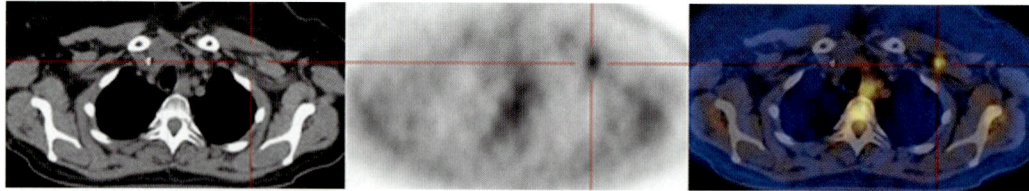

Fig. 44.3 CT-PET detects a small left subclavian lymph node, characterized by pathological glucose consumption (Fig. 44.3)

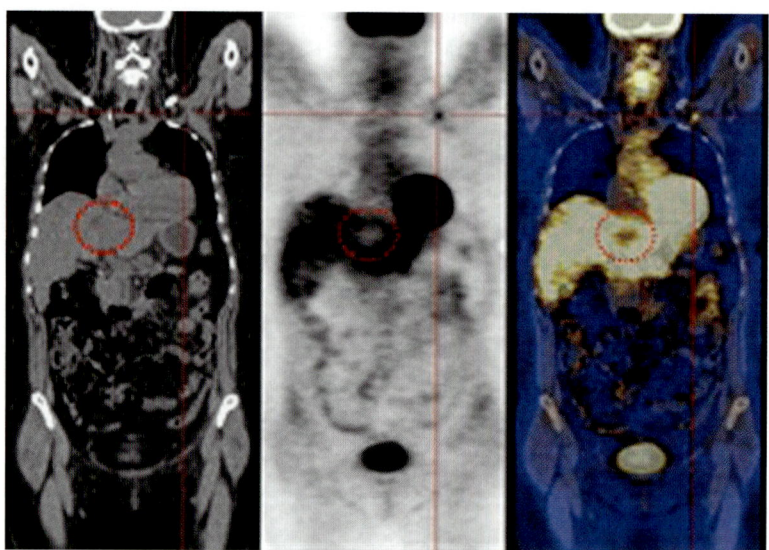

Fig. 44.4 In the coronal scans, the coronal reconstructions of the clavicular lymph node, there is a hypodense lesion in liver segment III, previously termoablated, which is seen as cold at the PET scan

with a high metabolism of glucose. Current therapy: "arimidex".

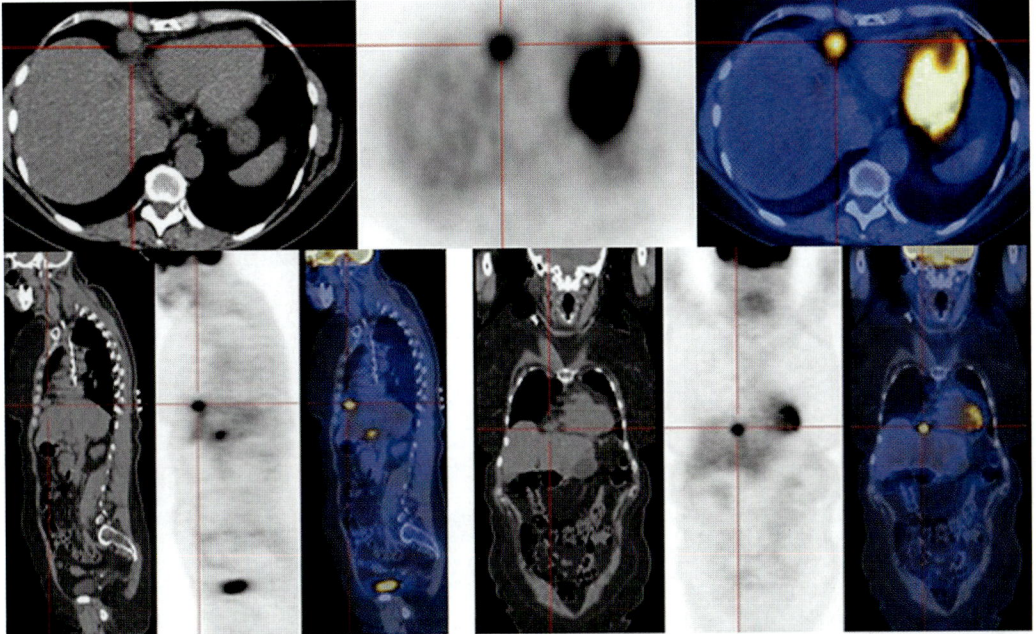

Fig. 44.5 Cold at the PET scan

44.3 Report

Lymphadenopathy with increased metabolic activity in the front right front cardio-phrenic angle and in the inter-hepato-diaphragmatic area, SUVmax 7.

Left subclavear adenopathy measuring less than a centimeter, SUVmax 2 (Fig. 44.1, *red arrow*).

In the left para-aortic and celiac-mesenteric areas and hepatic hilum, there are numerous confluent enlarged lymph nodes, characterized by high glucose metabolism, SUVmax 8.5.

The pulmonary nodule shown in the anterior segment of the left lower lobe and previously radio-treated, shows limited consumption of glucose due to actinic damage, SUVmax 1.8 (Fig. 44.1, *green arrow*).

Mild metabolic alteration to the thoracic spine (D6 and D10) due to benign disease, SUVmax 2.2.

44.4 Conclusions

The PET scan shows progression of disease due to extended lymph node involvement.

There were no focal lesions of the liver and lung with high metabolism. See Figs. 44.2, 44.3, 44.4, 44.5, 44.6.

44.5 Key Points

In metastatic breast cancer, the involvement of organ systems may have different development paths and times are not always predictable. Each diagnostic test must meticulously describe the different biological behavior of the disease in different districts.

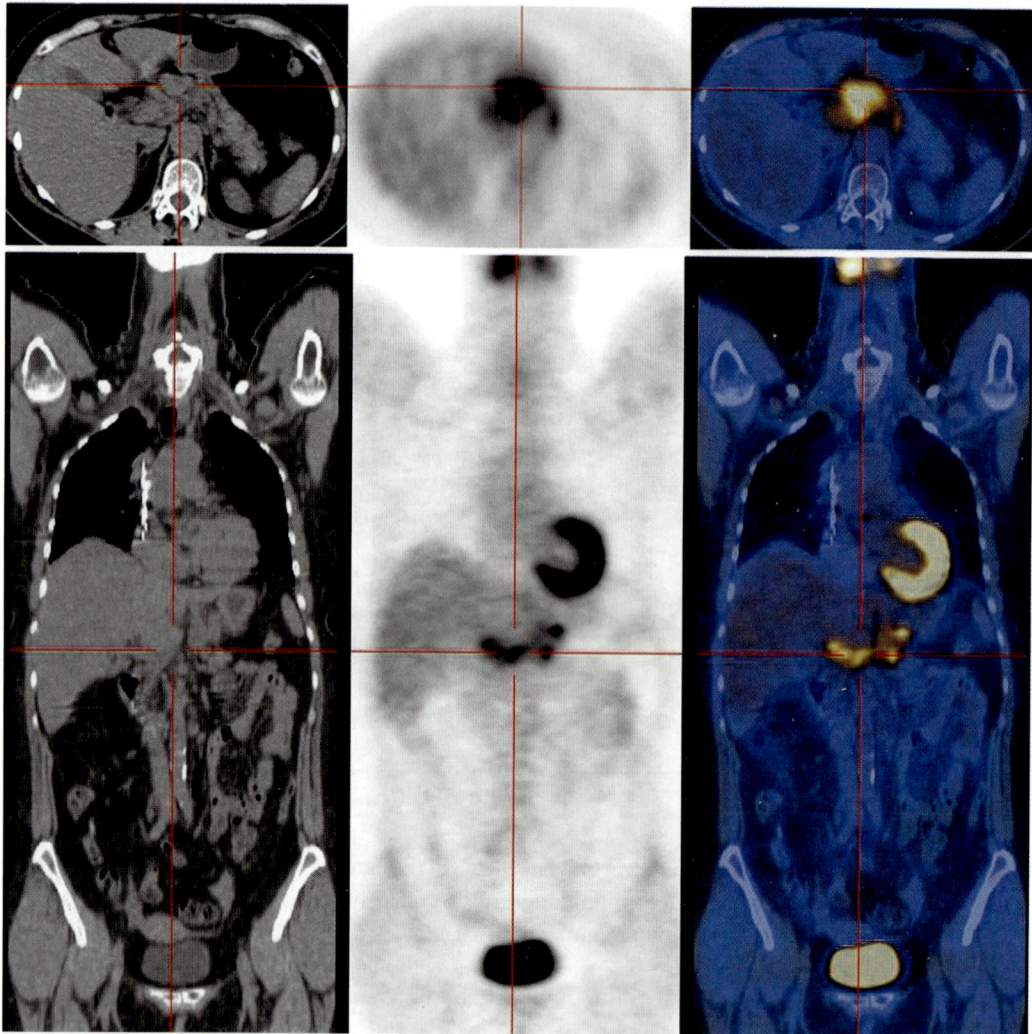

Fig. 44.6 CT-PET shows multiple fused lymph-nodes, the most evident at the lesser omentum, hepatic hilum and in the peripancreatic area

In patients with systemic disease, PET-FDG allows the clinician to understand what are the ways of progression of the disease, so we can say that in this woman,

- liver lesions are quiescent (remission);
- pulmonary nodule is off (remission);
- there is extensive lymphadenopathy (progression):
- not detected impaired bones and brain.

Note: The sensitivity of PET in the definition of subcentimetric pulmonary and liver nodules can be affected by resolution and biological limits or technical artifacts.

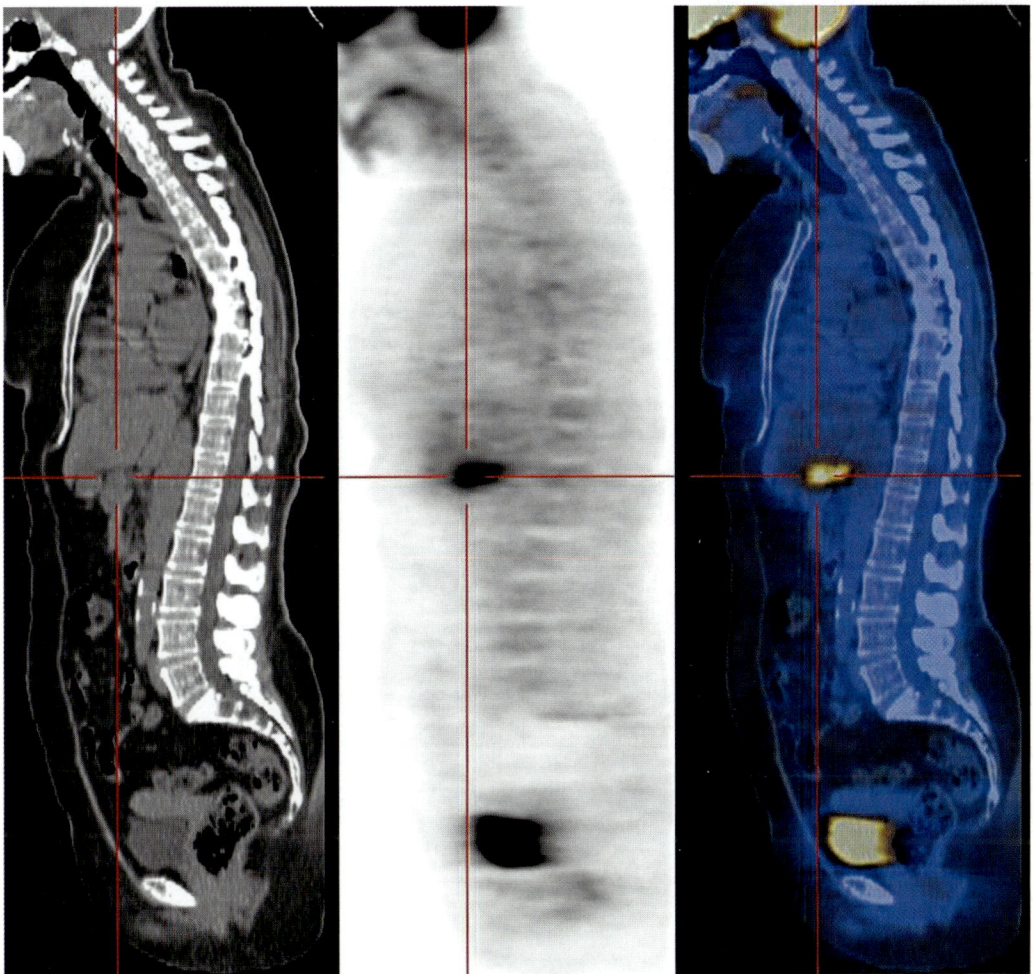

Fig. 44.6 (continued)

Infiltrating Ductal Carcinoma with Solitary Liver Metastasis

45

45.1 Clinical History

48-year-old woman, underwent left quadrantectomy and removal of two sentinel lymph nodes for infiltrating ductal carcinoma.

- After one month undergoes axillary lymphadenectomy for positive sentinel lymph node (G3, pT2, pN2, PM0).
- Radiotherapy is then performed.
  Follow-up two years after.
- Markers: CEA = 25.30 ng/ml (NV < 5).
- Total body CT: liver of normal dimensions, steatotic, with hypodense mass measuring 4 cm in the seventh segment that shows no post- contrastographic impregnation and coulb be identified with a secondary injury.
- Ultrasound: Subglissoniana, hypoechoic hepatic mass measuring 66 × 38 mm in segment VII; size is increased, compared to the previous scans, probably due to a focal lesion.

45.2 Diagnostic Question

Patient with a history of breast DIC shows liver lesion of uncertain nature: definition of the metabolism of glucose (diagnosis and restaging).

45.3 Report

The seventh segment of the liver characterized by a mass with high consumption of glucose,

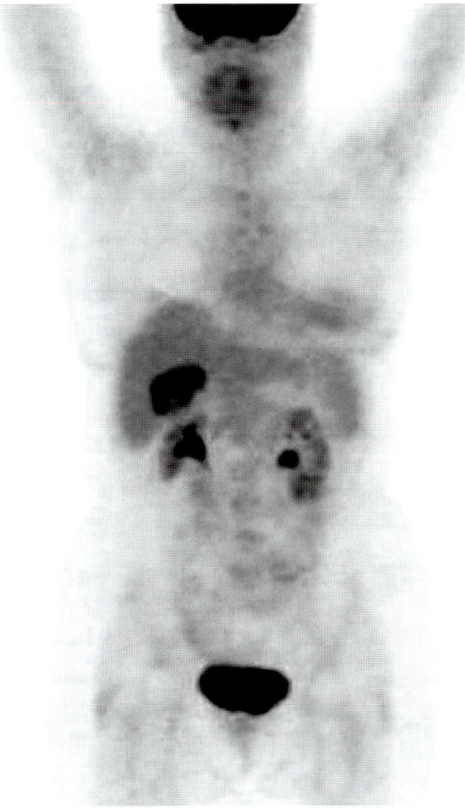

Fig. 45.1 Mass with a high glucose metabolism and underactive area on the inside, due to colliquation. SUV max 7.8

SUV max 7.8, with underactive area due to contextual colliquation. Absence of pathological metabolism in the remaining parts of the body examined (Fig. 45.1).

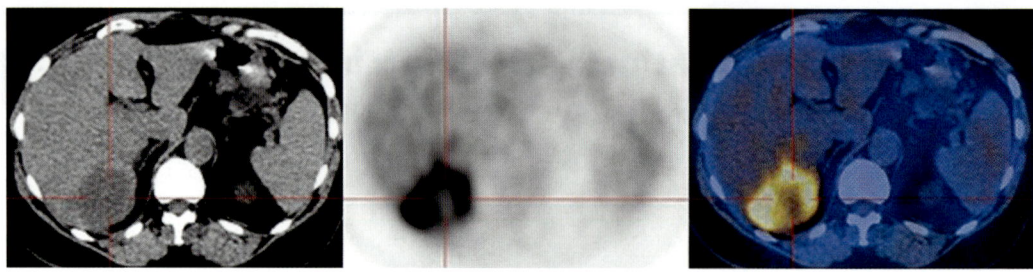

Fig. 45.2 Liver mass with high carbohydrate metabolism, probably caused by a recurrence of disease

45.4   Conclusions

The PET scan shows a liver mass with high carbohydrate metabolism, probably caused by a recurrence of disease. Histological confirmation is useful (Fig. 45.2).

- If the liver lesion shows intense metabolic activity, it suggests a recurrence of pathology.
- It is advisable to have a histological confirmation to exclude a primary liver tumor.
- The absence of metastatic lesions in other parts of the body suggests a possible surgical option.

45.5   Key Points

- The presence of axillary lymph node metastases in staging is a negative prognostic index.

46.1 Clinical History

53-year-old woman with breast cancer and a left axillary adenopathy and a bone lesion at the level of the left iliac wing.

- PET-FDG: hyperaccumulation of the tracer at the level of the left breast (SUVmax 6.4), in the ipsilateral axillary region (SUVmax 3.9) and at the left iliac bone (SUVmax 7.0).

  Neoadjuvant chemotherapy is then performed.

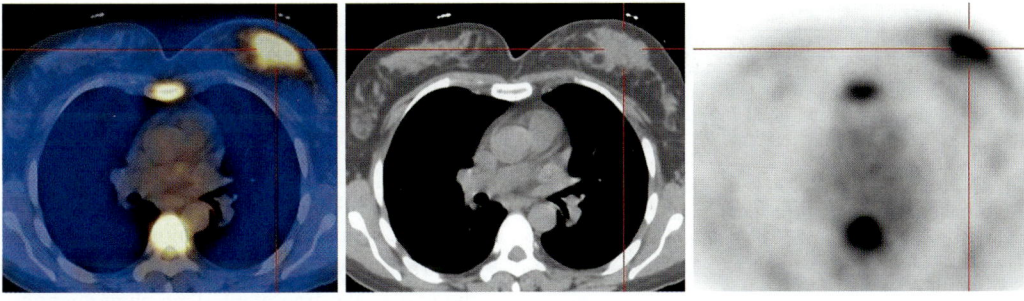

Fig. 46.1 PET-CT (Fig. 46.1): in the upper quadrants of the left breast a rough solid, irregular lesion, with modest increases in glucose metabolism is detected. Intense consumption of FDG at the level of a backbone metamer and the sternum due to post-chemotherapy rebound is also found.

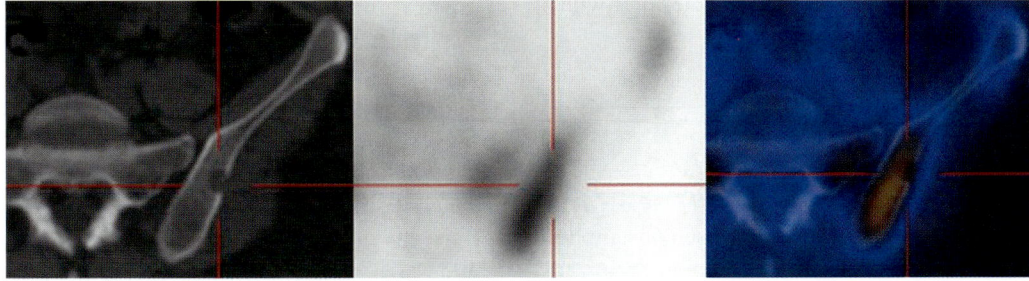

Fig. 46.2 CT-PET (Fig. 46.2): the left iliac bone presents a lytic roundish area with interruption of the cortical profile; this element is suggestive of a metastatic lesion although focal carbohydrate consumption is not shown. The dissociation between metabolism and morphology of the lytic lesion is determined by the response to neoadjuvant chemotherapy. This element is confirmed by the fusion image

P. F. Rambaldi, *Whole-Body FDG PET Imaging in Oncology*,
DOI: 10.1007/978-88-470-5295-6_46, © Springer-Verlag Italia 2014

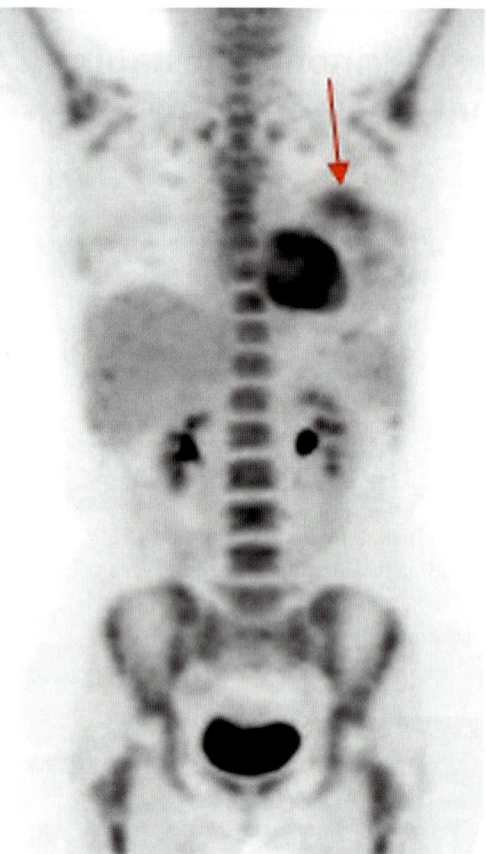

Fig. 46.3 The MIP image shows: widespread activation of bone marrow due to post-chemotherapy rebound; left mammary mass characterized by modest consumption of glucose (*arrow*)

46.2   Diagnostic Question

Restaging after neoadjuvant chemotherapy for breast cancer: search for focal lesions with a high metabolism of glucose.

46.3   Report

The clinically appreciable left breast lump shows modest increase in glucose consumption, SUVmax 3.8.

The recurrent lesions reported in history, evident on CT attenuation at the left axilla and ipsilateral iliac wing, showed no pathological metabolism.

No areas of abnormal FDG consumption in the remaining parts of the body examined. Widespread post-chemotherapy increase in metabolic activation at the bone marrow.

46.4   Conclusions

The PET scan shows persistence of disease in the nodule at the left breast.

Non-pathological glucose metabolism of other injuries reported in previous PET, due to positive response to chemotherapy. See Figs. 46.1, 46.2, 46.3.

46.5   Key Points

- The PET scan shows the good metabolic response of the lesions at the left axilla and ipsilateral iliac bone, even if the primary tumor has moderate persistence of residual biological activity.
- The apparent activation is secondary to bone marrow rebound post-chemotherapy activation that may persist for several months after the end of the treatment. This phenomenon is due to the high consumption of carbohydrate of the activated immunocompetent and hematopoietic cells residing in the bone.
- When there is marked activation of bone marrow, it is more difficult to assess the metabolic status of secondary bone lesions demonstrated by previous tests.
- The absence of focal accumulation of glucose suggests the positive metabolic response of the metastatic lesion characterized by osteolysis, which is still morphologically evident on CT.
- From the radiological point of view (CT), the lithic area repair, when possible, is a slower

event and requires apposition of new bone matrix, which in the late stages leads to crowding morphostructural thickening.

- In this case, bone scan will not help, because it demonstrates the persistence of focal consumption of phosphonates secondary to the repairing of osteolytic metastases.
- Never alert the clinician when you look at PET-FDG and see a widespread activation of the bone: this finding should not be supplemented by further unnecessary diagnostic procedures. The patient will go through the follow-up according to the protocol defined by the oncologist.
- These tips are to be integrated with clinical and laboratory data because, if necessary, we have to be always ready to re-evaluate the case (Fig. 46.3).

Staging of Breast Cancer with Axillary Lymphadenopathy

47

47.1 Clinical History

65-year-old woman with right breast cancer, measuring 5 cm in diameter, and axillary adenopathy and suspect commitment of the internal mammary nodal chain.

- Mammography integration with ultrasound: massive lesion in the supero-external quadrant of the right breast (5 cm), with irregular edges and consequent stromal reaction, cutaneous and subcutaneous edema. Presence of diffuse microcalcifications: finding relates to breast cancer. Some suspect lymph nodes can be found at the axilla (max width 5 cm) and at the level of the internal mammary chain.

47.2 Diagnostic Question

Staging of breast cancer: research for focal lesions with a high glucose metabolism.

47.3 Report

The PET scan shows a right breast mass characterized by abnormal glucose consumption, SUVmax 8, with nodal axillary involvement at all levels, SUVmax 9.

No abnormal metabolism in the lymph nodes of the internal mammary chain.

No pathological consumption in the L2 vertebra; CT shows that the structural alteration is of benign type (Fig. 47.1).

No areas of abnormal FDG deposition in other parts of the body examined.

47.4 Conclusions

The PET scan shows a right breast cancer with massive involvement of the axillary lymph nodes with a high carbohydrate deposition.

The MIP image shows a right breast focal lesion and two coarse ipsilateral lymph node packages with a high metabolism of glucose (Fig. 47.2).

The PET-CT scan shows an expansive mass in the right breast. The ipsilateral axilla is occupied by conglomerate lymph nodes. The glucose consumption of all these lesions is high (Fig. 47.3).

47.5 Key Points

The PET-FDG is not a routine examination in the staging of breast cancer.

P. F. Rambaldi, *Whole-Body FDG PET Imaging in Oncology*, DOI: 10.1007/978-88-470-5295-6_47, © Springer-Verlag Italia 2014

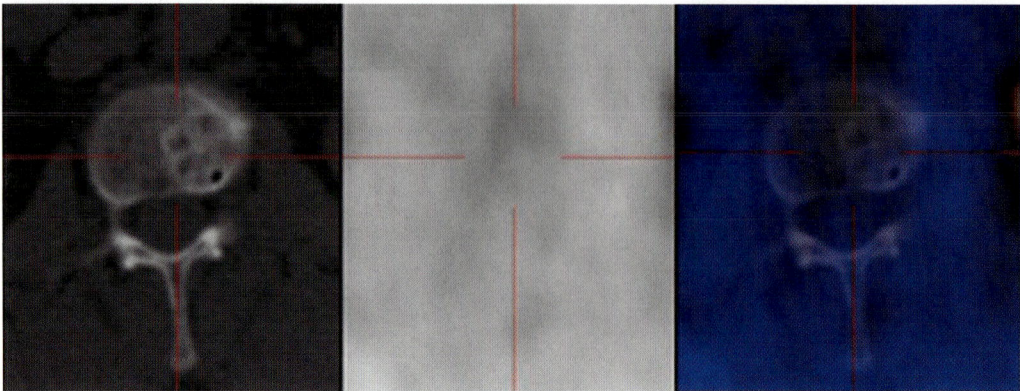

Fig. 47.1 CT shows that the structural alteration is of benign type

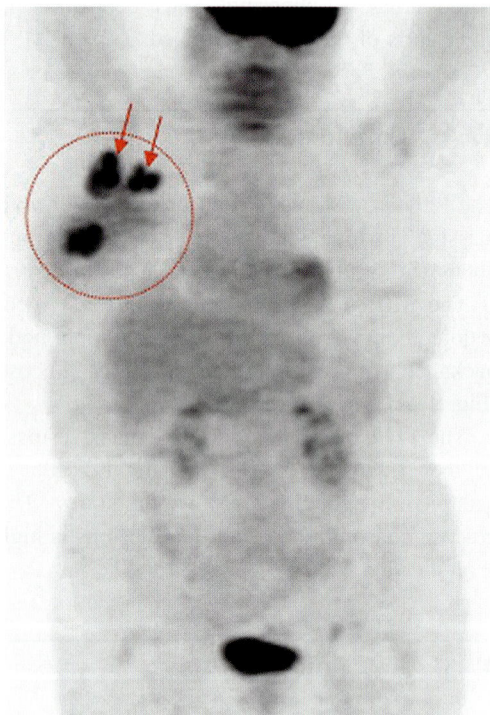

- In the presence of large primitive breast lesions associated with extended lymph node involvement, the metabolic data complement the morphological ones.
- When programming a neoadjuvant chemo-therapy, a baseline FDG-PET study is essential to properly assess the subsequent metabolic response to the treatment.
- The scan is useful to rule out the commitment of the internal mammary chain and the presence of distant metastases.

Fig. 47.2 MIP image shows a *right* breast focal lesion and two coarse ipsilateral lymph node packages

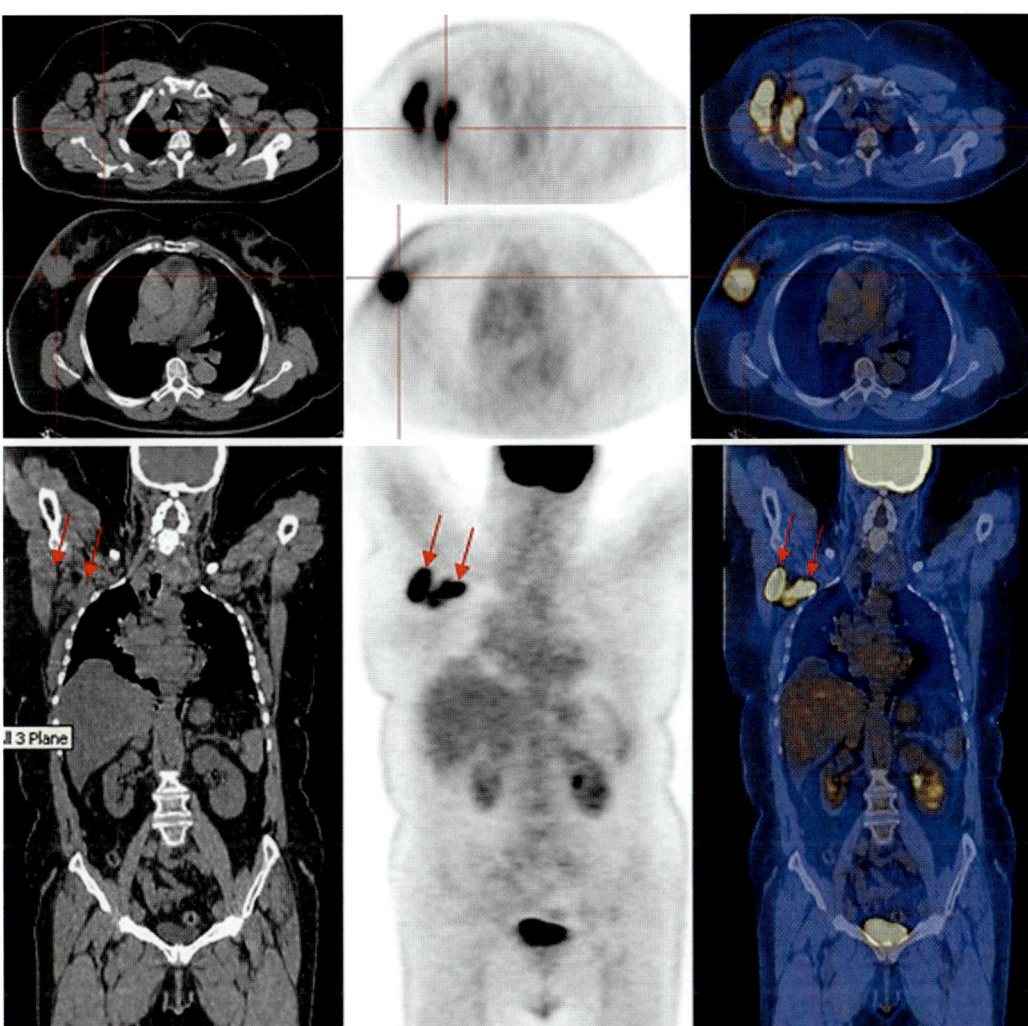

Fig. 47.3 **a** PET-CT scan shows an expansive mass in the *right* breast, **b** the ipsilateral axilla is occupied by conglomerate lymph nodes. The glucose consumption of all these lesions is high

Man with Breast Cancer Follow-Up After Surgery: Scar Glucose Uptake

48

48.1 Clinical History

Right radical mastectomy and axillary dissection for ICD in a 60-year-old man. Adjuvant chemotherapy was then performed.

Follow-up after one year.

- Bone scan: negative for focal lesions.
- FDG-PET: negative for focal lesions.
- CT: negative for focal lesions. Right mammary resection with tissutal thickening due to scarring. Presence of a hemangioma in the right hemisoma of L2.

Follow-up after a year and six months.

- FDG-PET: modest increase in glucose consumption at the right anterior chest surgical scar, SUV max = 1.9, to be clinically investigated and studied.
- Tumor markers: normal.

48.2 Diagnostic Question

Follow-up of breast cancer: search for focal lesions with a high metabolism of glucose.

48.3 Report

The PET scan shows no areas of abnormal glucose consumption in the body areas examined.

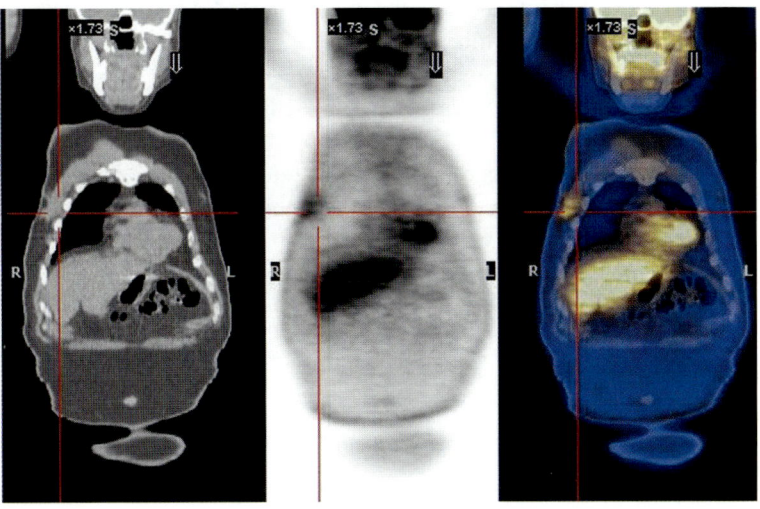

Fig. 48.1 Modest increase in metabolism at the surgical scar on the right chest, SUV max 1.6

P. F. Rambaldi, *Whole-Body FDG PET Imaging in Oncology*,
DOI: 10.1007/978-88-470-5295-6_48, © Springer-Verlag Italia 2014

Modest increase in metabolism at the surgical scar on the right chest, SUV max 1.6 (Fig. 48.1, 48.2).

48.4   Conclusions

The PET scan revealed no significant focal areas characterized by pathological consumption of glucose in the body areas examined relating to recurrence of disease, within the resolving limits. Mild metabolic remodeling at the right chest scar correlates to dystrophic scarring phenomena.

48.5   Key Points

- The scars are characterized by inflammatory, hypertrophic, and/or hyperplastic reactive phenomena; thus, expressing a nonfocal, diffuse, nonspecific, and limited in size glucose consumption that does not exceed that of the liver in the background.
- Rarely, there is a granulomatous reaction or an infection at the scar, events that lead to increased metabolic activation.
- A locoregional recurrence of disease has intense deposition of FDG, with metabolic activity that exceeds that of the mediastinum and the liver; it is infiltrative, focal, and its consistency is hard-wood to the touch and tends to increase over time.
- In cases of doubt, ultrasound-guided FNAB is indicated, a minimally invasive and low-cost procedure.
- A negative PET suggests a clinical and instrumental follow up in time, with a simple ultrasound of the lesion.

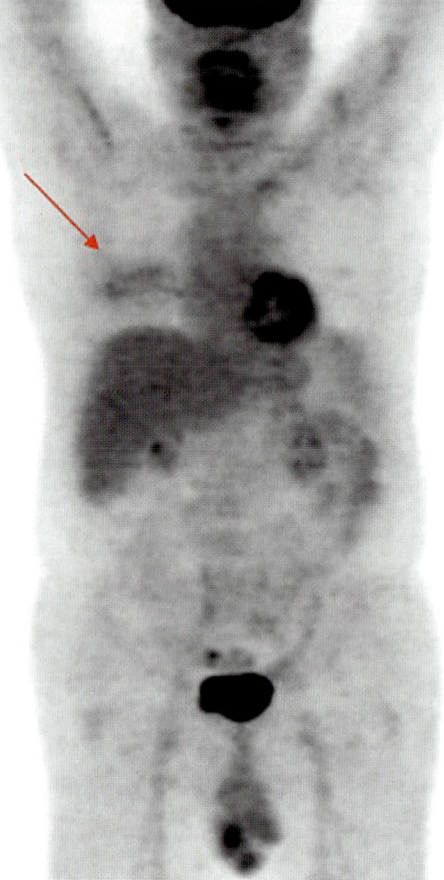

Fig. 48.2 Modest increase in metabolism at the surgical scar on the right chest, SUV max 1.6

- PET-CT is not suitable in the follow-up of these patients unless there is a real suspicion of disease progression in other districts.
- Tumor markers are nonspecific. Only their increase over time suggests the presence of locoregional recurrence or distant metastasis (Fig. 48.3).

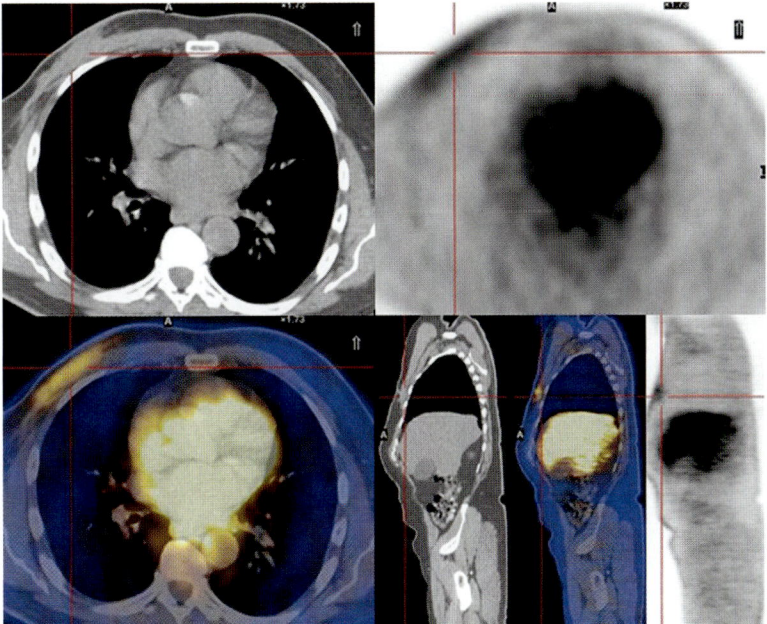

Fig. 48.3 In correspondence of the right anterior chest wall, the CT-PET demonstrates the presence of inhomogeneous tissue, extending from the surgical scar to the subcutaneous layer and the underlying muscle wall, from which it does not appear dissociable. The lesional consumption of glucose is low

Breast Cancer: Post-Surgical Brachial Plexopathy

49

49.1 Clinical History

59-year-old woman who underwent left mastectomy and right quadrantectomy, preceded by neoadjuvant chemotherapy for bilateral DIC.

Restaging after surgery:
- CT: inhomogeneous parenchymal density of the liver due to the presence of some lumps in the V, VII and VIII segments, faintly hypodense at the basal scan, with ring marginal enhancement after contrast, evocative of focal lesions.

Reassessment after adjuvant chemoradiotherapy.
- Total body CT: negative for focal lesions.
- Bone scan: negative for focal lesions.
- Ultrasound: Hepatic steatosis, with some nodules in the right lobe, the first measuring 24 mm hypoechoic with a hyperechoic central area within the fifth segment and at least two other strongly hypoechoic, respectively, measuring 13 and 9 mm and located at the VI–VII segments.

After surgery left brachial plexopathy appeared to worsen.

49.2 Diagnostic Question

Restaging after chemotherapy in woman with bilateral breast cancer, liver chemotreated metastases and recent left plexopathy, of nature

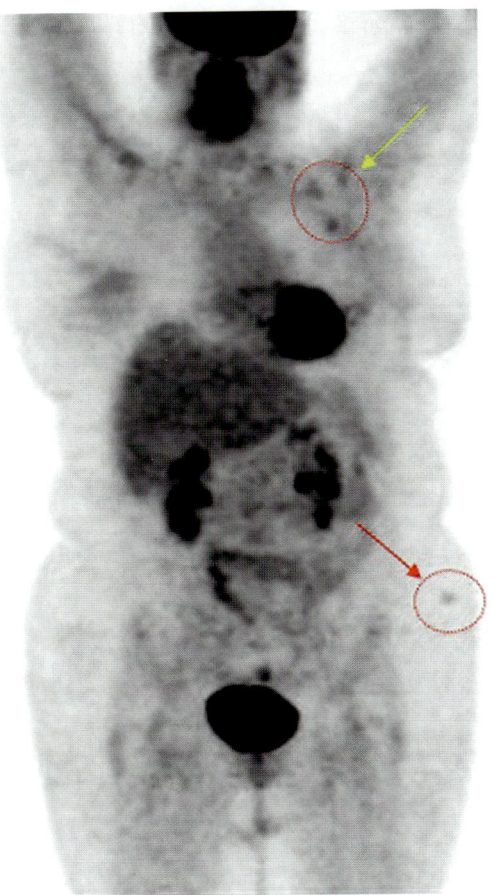

Fig. 49.1 MIP image: slight increase in the concentration of FDG in the left axilla with small nodes characterized by limited metabolism, therefore deemed as reactive (*yellow arrow*). The liver shows physiological glucose consumption and presents no metastatic disease. Slight focal nodular uptake in the left buttock due to a granuloma (*red arrow*)

P. F. Rambaldi, *Whole-Body FDG PET Imaging in Oncology*,
DOI: 10.1007/978-88-470-5295-6_49, © Springer-Verlag Italia 2014

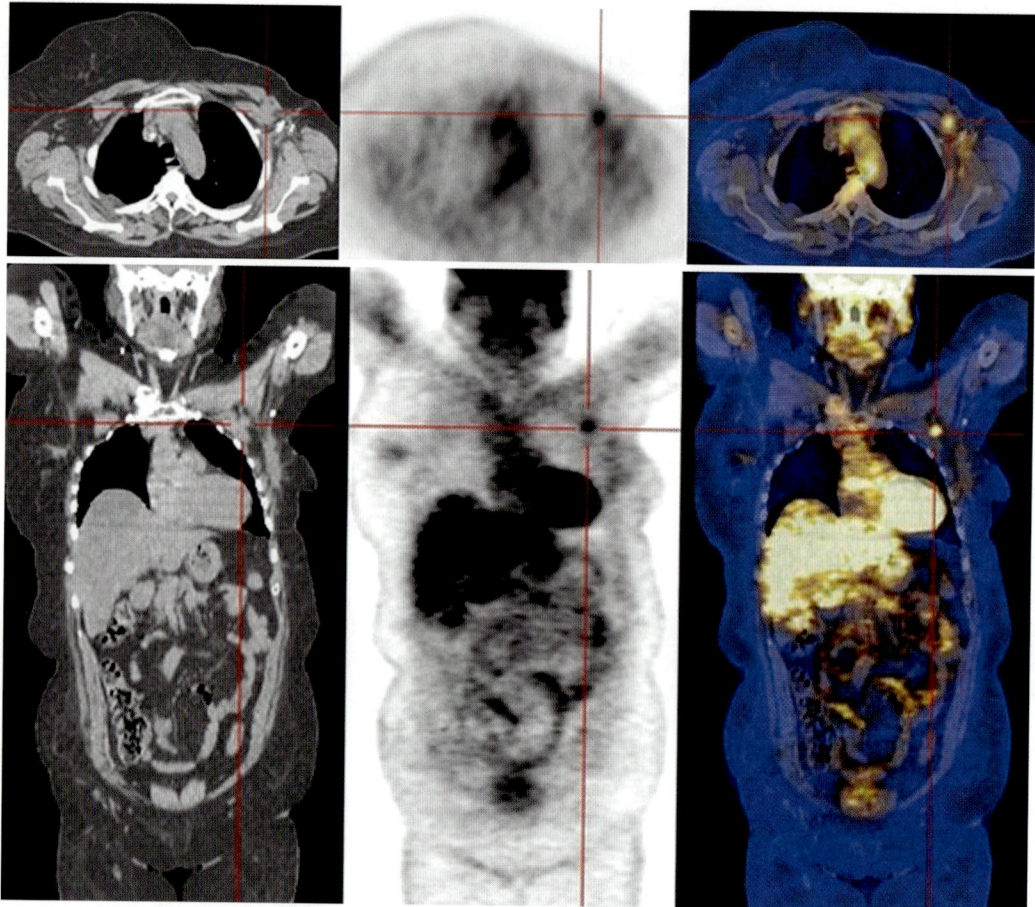

Fig. 49.2 The CT scan shows the previous left mastectomy with axillary dissection. Adjacent to the metal clips thickening of the pectoral muscle is evident and an axillary centimetric lymph node that shows a slight increase of glucose metabolism at the PET scan

yet to be determined: search for focal lesions with a high metabolism of glucose.

metabolism due to good response to the treatment performed.

49.3 Report

Small lymph nodes characterized by modest increase in glucose consumption in the left axill to post-surgical reactive remodeling, SUV max = 2.7. Absence of liver lesions with a high

49.4 Conclusions

The PET scan does not show focal areas of pathological consumption of glucose in the body areas examined to indicate a recurrence of disease within the resolving limits.

No evidence of pathological metabolism of the liver lesions that could be seen at CT as reported in history, due to good response to chemotherapy. See Figs. 49.1, 49.2.

49.5 Key Points

PET has high accuracy in defining the etiology of a brachial plexopathy that may also occur late in relation to an axillary dissection. This pathological condition may be secondary to insufficient lymphatic drainage or replacement of metastatic axillary lymph nodes.

- Only the massive neoplastic infiltration of the axilla determines a secondary plexopathy.
- The presence of some non-coalescing centimetric lymph nodes, characterized by limited glucose consumption suggests an inflammatory condition. Metastatic disease is unlikely.
- The axillary lymphadenectomy results in a fibrotic condition and insufficient subclinical lymphatic drainage. On this anatomic substrate, a post-surgical concomitant nonspecific inflammatory condition can cause a plexopathy. The axial and coronal reconstructions demonstrate the presence of some lymph nodes with limited metabolism with reactive characteristics that confirm this condition (a).

Follow-Up of Papillary Breast Cancer: Solitary Sacroiliac Benign Lesion

50

50.1 Clinical History

68-year-old woman who underwent left quadrantectomy for papillary carcinoma. Pathological stage: pT1c, pN0, PM0. Underwent radiotherapy.
  Follow-up after two years.

- Chest CT: absence of focal lesions.
- Bone scan: intense accumulation at the level of the right iliac bone crest and sacroiliac joint.
- Cancer markers: normal.
- Ultrasound of the abdomen: negative for focal lesions.
- Pelvis CT: structural remodeling of the right iliac bone and of the sacro-iliac joint, with presence of areas of osteosclerosis mixed with some hypodense areolas.

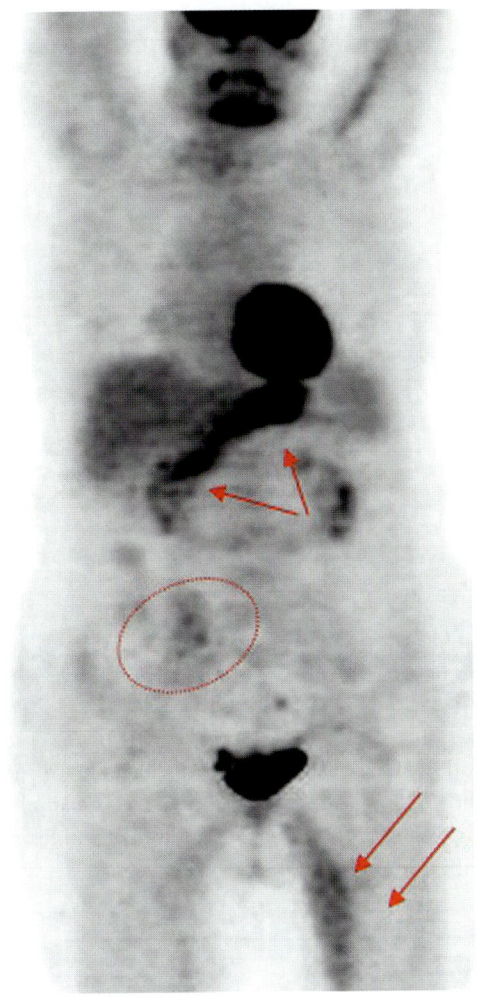

Fig. 50.2 MIP image: absence of focal lesions; metabolic activation of the adductors of the left thigh due to nonspecific post-traumatic inflammation, as reported by the patient. Presence of diffuse gastric paraphysiological uptake

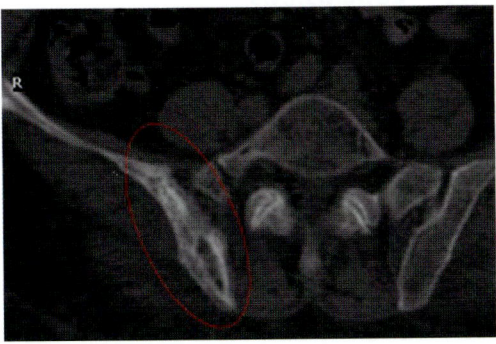

Fig. 50.1 PET scan shows a solitary lesion of the hipbone with limited carbohydrate metabolism

P. F. Rambaldi, *Whole-Body FDG PET Imaging in Oncology*,
DOI: 10.1007/978-88-470-5295-6_50, © Springer-Verlag Italia 2014

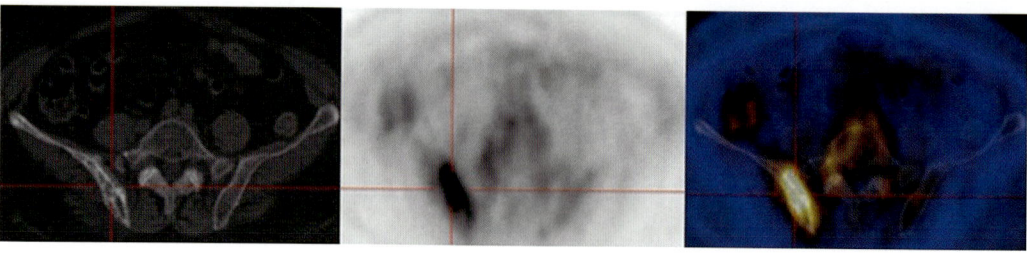

Fig. 50.3 The PET-CT image shows *right* iliac bone structural rearrangement with phenomena of osteosclerosis associated with images of trabecular bone resorption of dystrophic nature (Figs. 50.3, 50.4). No interruption of the cortex. Only a modest increase in glucose metabolism of the lesion can be seen

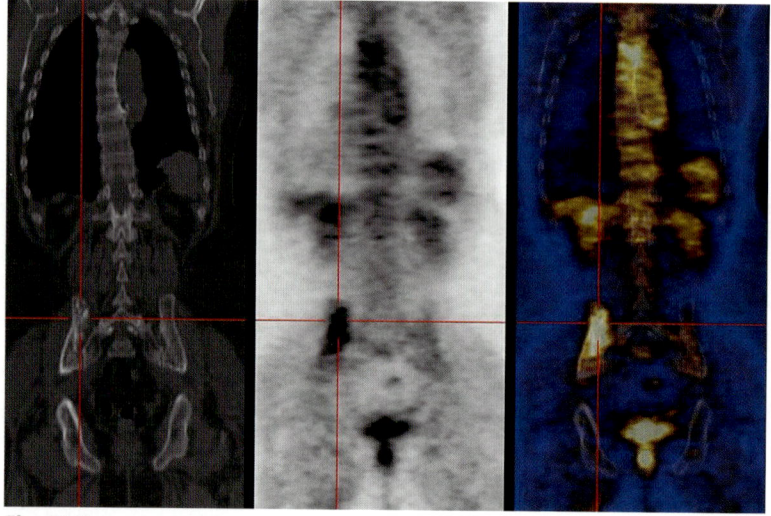

Fig. 50.4

50.2   Diagnostic Question

Follow-up of papillary breast cancer with morphostructural alteration of the pelvis, suspicious for recurrence of disease: search for focal lesions with a high metabolism of glucose.

50.3   Report

Slight increase in glucose consumption in the right hemipelvis, more evident at the hip bone, SUV max 2.2. No areas of abnormal metabolism in the remaining parts of the body examined.

50.4   Conclusions

The PET scan shows a solitary lesion of the hip bone with limited carbohydrate metabolism, painless when compressed, suggesting a benign disease (Fig. 50.1).

It suggests follow-up in time to exclude a focal lesion with low carbohydrate consumption. See also Figs. 50.2, 50.3, 50.4.

50.5 Key Points

- In a follow-up of cancer patients, it is not uncommon to identify solitary bone lesions of dubious nature. Not always the extended use of different imaging techniques allows a certain etiological diagnosis.
- In patients with breast cancer, solitary bone lesions are a difficult problem to solve, sometimes even the biopsy will not settle the question.
- When the techniques of diagnostic imaging are indeterminate and the lesion is clinically silent and is not at risk of pathologic fracture, instrumental control is recommended over time.
- Some authors have shown that the follow-up of solitary dubious bone lesions allows to document the progression of pathology, then the malignancy in 50 % of cases. The remaining 50 % of the lesions is stable in time, therefore, and is to be referred to benign conditions, in these situations, the patient continues the oncologic follow-up of the underlying disease as indicated by the guidelines.

In the analysis of this case, it must be considered that the patient had papillary carcinoma pT1c, pN0, and PM0, so a much lower chance of developing bone metastases.

In the critical evaluation of dubious images, the stage of the primary tumor of this woman is a discriminating factor and it is fundamental to suggest a less aggressive diagnostic and therapeutic attitude that leaves no room for follow-up over time.

Breast Cancer Follow-Up: Nodal and Skeletal Progression of Disease

51

51.1 Clinical History

45-year-old woman who underwent left quadrantectomy and ipsilateral axillary lymph node dissection for DIC—pT2, pN2, M0. Adjuvant radio-chemotherapy performed.

Follow-up two years after:

- PET-FDG: numerous areas of pathological accumulation of the marker in the skeleton, that is diffusely involved (clavicles, thoracic and lumbar spine, pelvis, femur). Pathological uptake of a retroclavear left lymph node.
- Total body CT: negative for focal lesions.
- MRI of the thoracic and lumbar-sacral spine: numerous dorsal and lumbosacral vertebrae (D1, D6, D10, D12, L1, L2, L3, S1) show an alteration of the bone marrow signal, patchy and irregular, probably metastatic in origin.
- Ophthalmology report: the clinical and instrumental examination showed the presence of 4 small lesions at the right iris, hypopigmented, localized in the upper sectors and involving in part the irido-corneal angle. The cytologic pattern is compatible with intraocular metastasis of known breast cancer.

Follow-up three years after:

- Cancer markers: CEA = 27.50 ng/ml (nv < 5), TPA = 100 IU/l (nv < 75).
- Bone scan: presence of scattered bone lesions.
- PET-FDG: multiple areas of abnormal increased consumption of glucose (SUV max 8.9) that spread to the skeleton and appear mainly as thickening. Modest increase in the consumption of glucose in the left clavicular fossa due to lymphadenopathy, SUV max 4.1.

51.2 Diagnostic Question

Patient with operated breast cancer and bone dissemination: evaluation of the metabolic progression of disease.

51.3 Report

Multiple secondary areas of pathological increase in the consumption of glucose that spread to the skeleton and appear mainly as thickening, SUV max 9.6.

Presence of two lymph nodes characterized by modest increase in deposition of FDG respectively in the left clavicular fossa and in the dorsal—retroscapolar area, SUV max 3.2.

There were no lung, hepatic and ocular lesions with high metabolism, within the resolving and biological limits of the technique.

51.4 Conclusions

The PET scan shows progression of disease for the presence of scattered bone lesions and two lymph nodes with high carbohydrate deposition (See Figs. 51.1, 51.2, 51.3).

P. F. Rambaldi, *Whole-Body FDG PET Imaging in Oncology*,
DOI: 10.1007/978-88-470-5295-6_51, © Springer-Verlag Italia 2014

51.5 Key Points

- In patients with breast cancer, metastatic bone disease sometimes shows a slow progression, especially when the tumor is hormone-dependent.

- In the presence of bone secondary dissemination, CT identifies thickening lesions, but it cannot tell apart the metabolically active one from the others and vice versa; the PET scan instead allows characterization of cell activity.
- Osteosclerotic lesions have a limited risk of pathologic fracture.

Fig. 51.1 CT scan shows multiple bone thickening lesions. The PET characterizes the lesions with a high metabolism of glucose. This information must be critically assessed

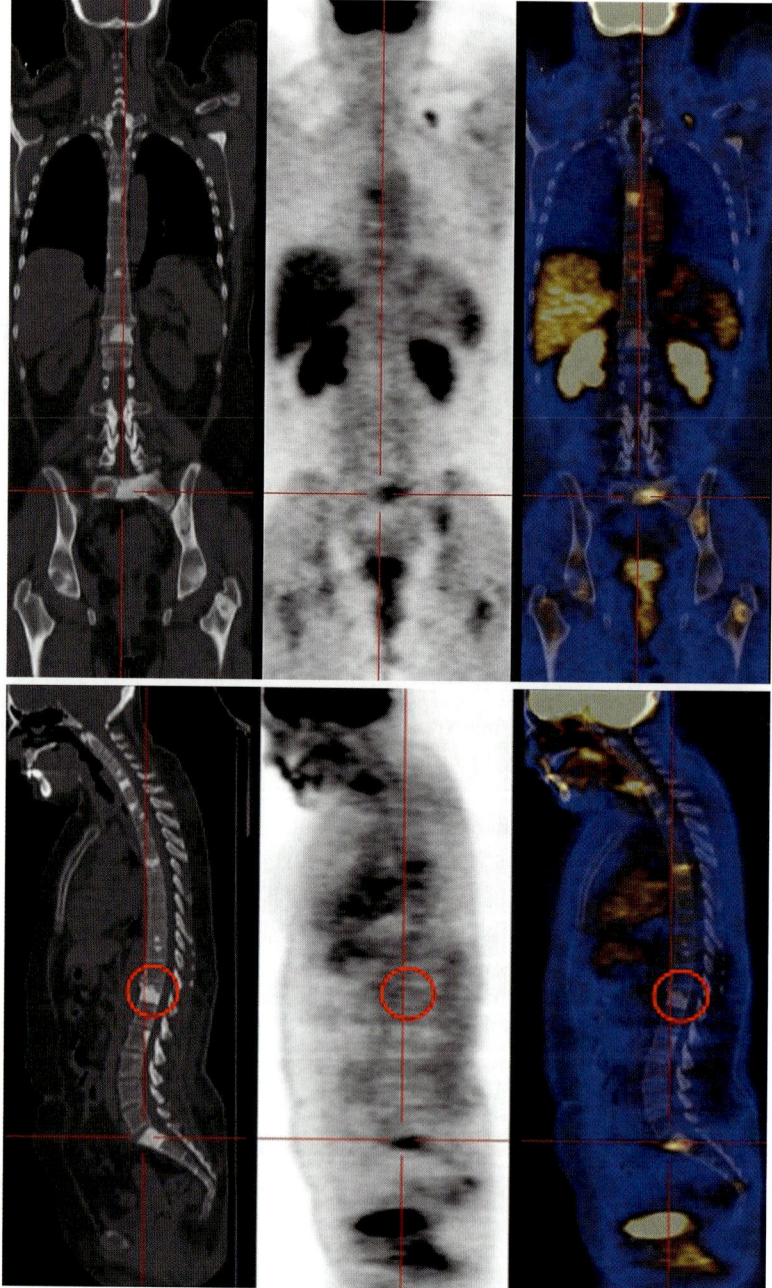

Fig. 51.2 The PET-CT scan shows a hypodense lymph node in the left clavicular fossa, with volumetric and metabolic activity progression over time. The follow up at two years shows the appearance of a new dorsal—retroscapular node. In a similar way, it detects progression of the bone disease

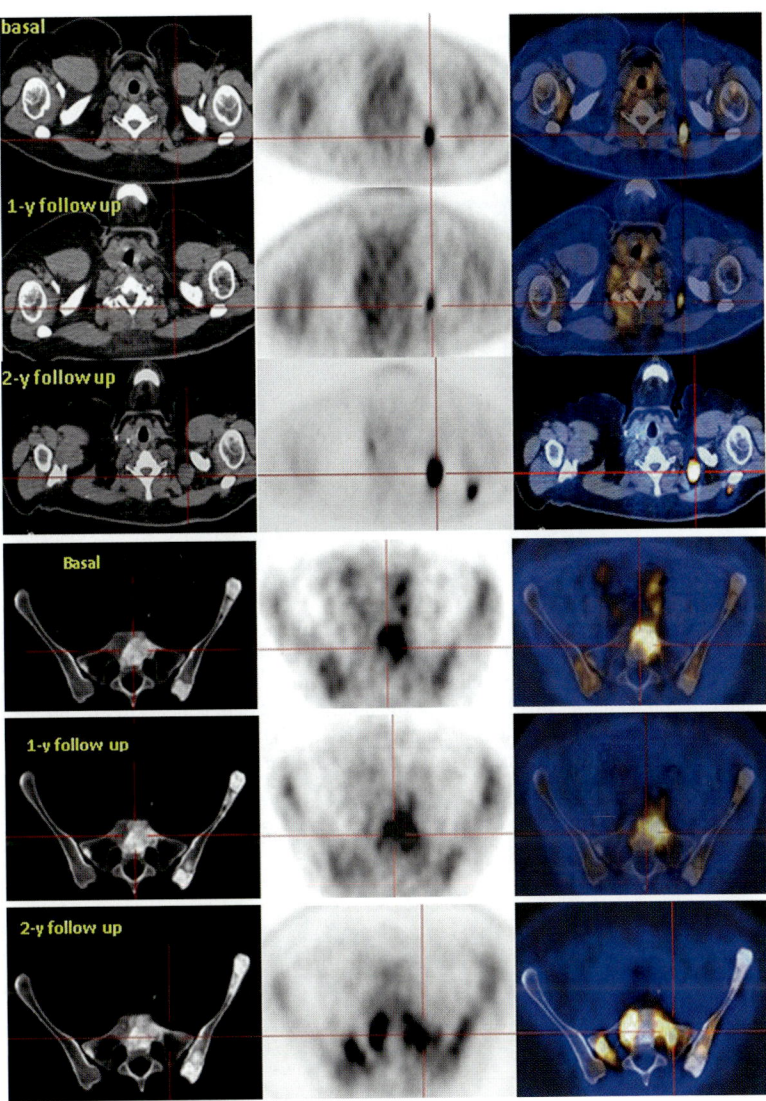

- In the presence of the secondary bone dissemination, the nuclear medicine physician must always report the skeletal sites that are at risk of fracture, with the aid of CT images.

- The radiation therapy may be recommended to relieve pain or when the risk of pathologic fracture is high.

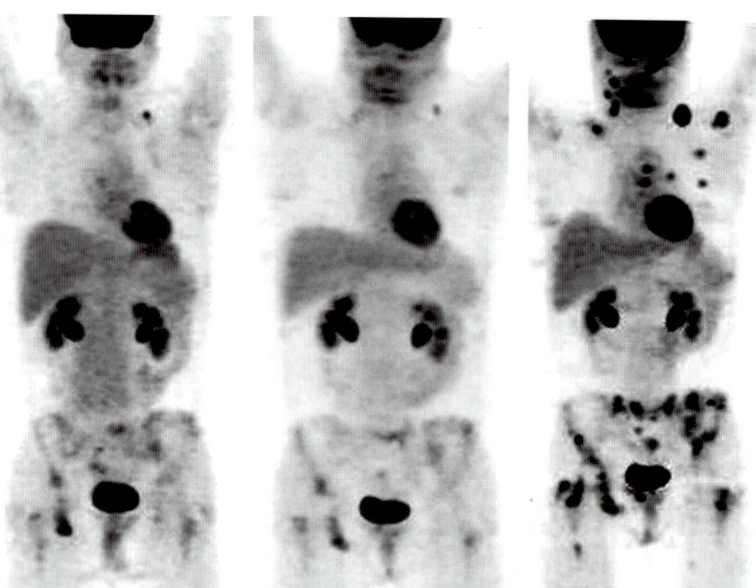

Fig. 51.3 The MIP images provide a global view, an overview the metabolic state of the disease and its progression over time. The baseline PET scan demonstrates the predominant involvement of the bones of the pelvis. The scan after a year documents the partial response to therapy, while two years after it shows a clear progression. The retroclavear lymph node has a biological behavior similar to that of bone metastases: the follow up after one year showed partial response to treatment, follow up after two years shows the progression of the metabolic activity

Bone Metastases from Breast Cancer: Progression of Disease and Subsequent Response to Radiotherapy

52

52.1 Clinical History

37-year-old woman who underwent left quadrantectomy for DIC. Subsequently adjuvant chemotherapy was performed.

Follow-up after four years:

- PET-FDG: absence of focal lesions with a high metabolism of glucose.
- Chest, abdomen with contrast medium CT scan: the absence of focal lesions.

Follow-up after four years and six months:

- PET-FDG: pathological consumption of glucose in the medium-proximal segment of the sternum (SUV max 6).
- Chest, abdomen, with contrast medium CT scan: presence of retrosternal hypodense tissue of lymphoid type (measuring 2 cm) in the anterior mediastinum. Structural rearrangement of the sternum with a substantially thickened and sclerotic appearance in the middle third of the body on the median—right paramedian area, compatible with focal skeletal lesion. Left mammary resection.

Re-evaluation after three months of therapy with "Herceptin, Femara, Decapeptyl."

- PET-FDG: progression of disease with high consumption of glucose in the sternum (SUV max 8.4).

Re-evaluation after 6 months of therapy with "Herceptin, Femara, Decapeptyl."

- PET-FDG: intense consumption of glucose in the body of the sternum (SUV max 10) with modest progression of disease compared to the previous control.

Sternal lesion to be radio-treated.

52.2 Diagnostic Question

Patient with a history of left breast cancer and sternal metastasis in the radiotreated sternum, performs today's control for the recent emergence of low back pain. Disease is being treated with Herceptin, Femara and Decapeptyl.

52.3 Report

Consumption of glucose in the body of the sternum of reduced intensity compared to previous scans reported in medical history, SUV max 4; this finding is to be referred to postactinic rearrangement.

Modest alteration of glucose metabolism in the sacrum and the right sacral wing, SUV max 2.3, not seen on CT and therefore attributed to secondary spinal cord injury.

In the left clavicular fossa there is a centimetric lymph node, characterized by modest increase in carbohydrate consumption, considered reactive in nature, SUV max 2.4. It will be useful, however, to perform an ultrasound evaluation.

Absence of focal lesions with a high metabolism in other parts of the body examined.

P. F. Rambaldi, *Whole-Body FDG PET Imaging in Oncology*,
DOI: 10.1007/978-88-470-5295-6_52, © Springer-Verlag Italia 2014

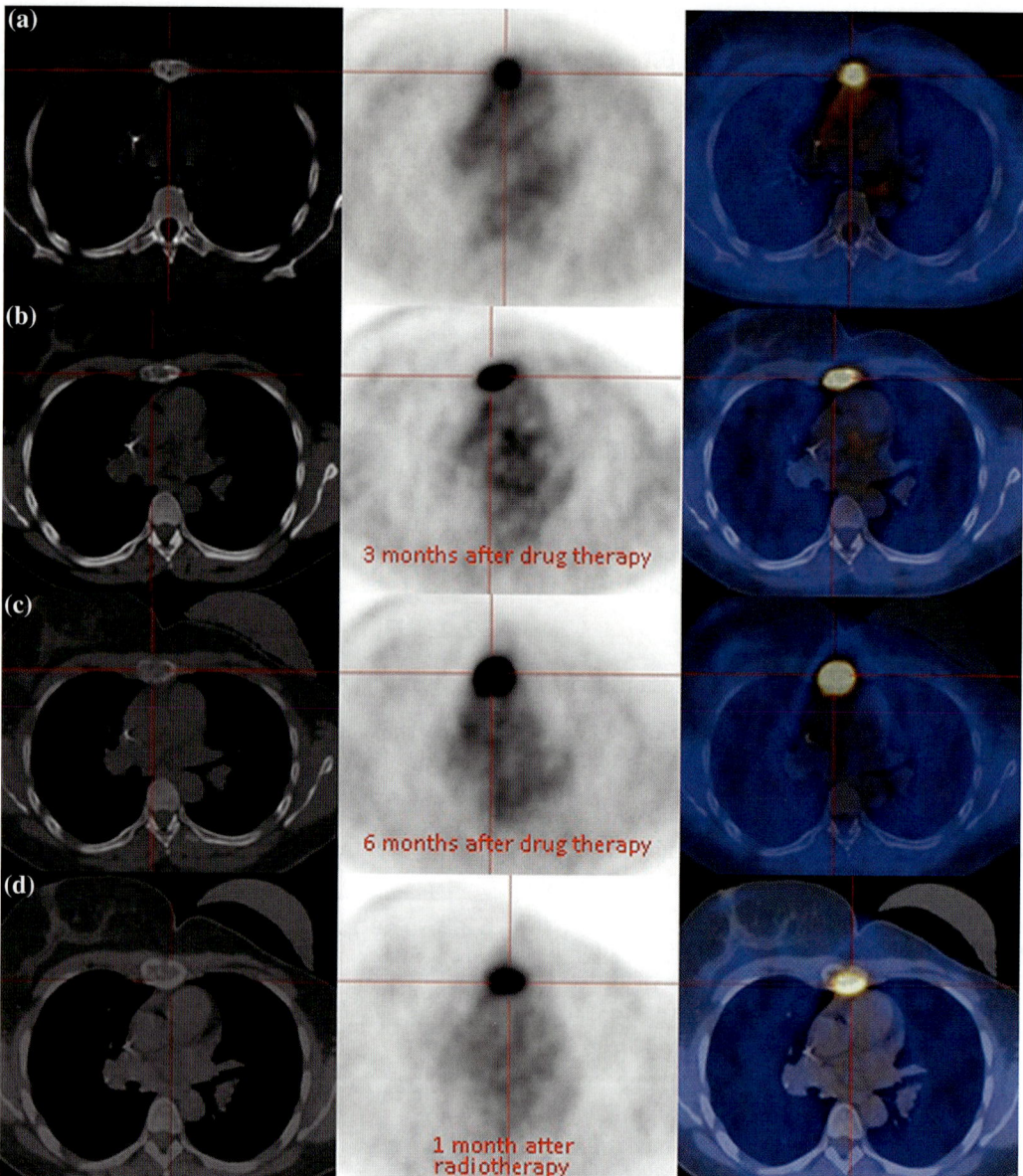

Fig. 52.1 The PET-CT axial and MIP images **a–c** show the progression of the metastasis to the sternum during follow-up and the absent response to medical therapy. The CT shows the volumetric expansion of the lytic lesion with cortical interruption in the scan performed six months later (**c**), better seen in the sagittal reconstruction. After radiotherapy (**d**) reduction of the metabolic activity of the lesion showing sclerotic margins and low carbohydrate deposition due to actinic reaction are observed

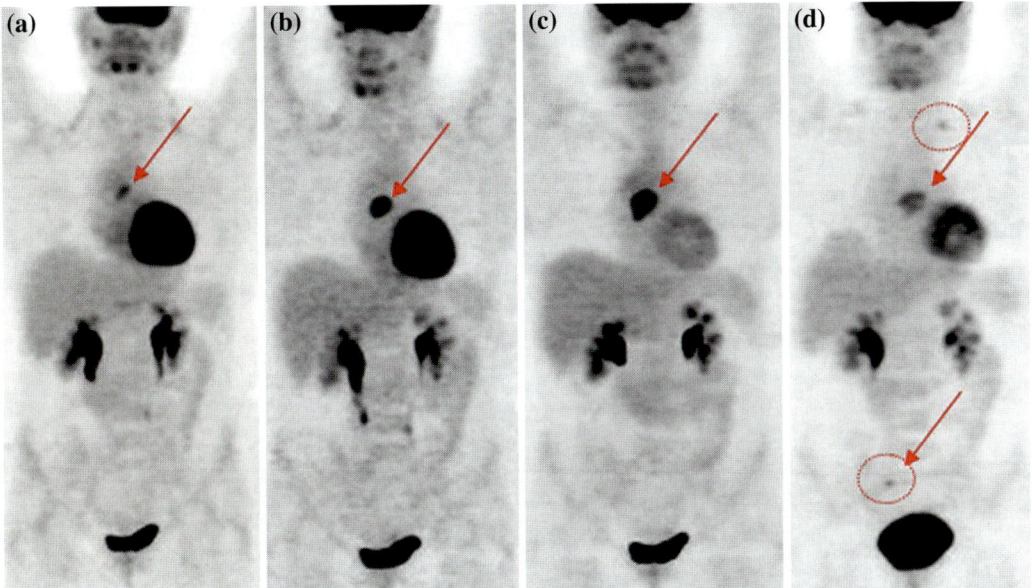

Fig. 52.2 The PET image shows two areas of modest increase in glucose consumption at the sacroiliac joint, on the right sacral side (Fig. 52.3). On CT scans, morphostructural bone changes are notobserved, although there is a scarcity of trabeculae in the sacrum right, without interruption of cortical rhyme. CT-PET suggests though a metastatic replacement of the bone marrow, that has not yet determined osteolysis on CT, an event generally is seen lately

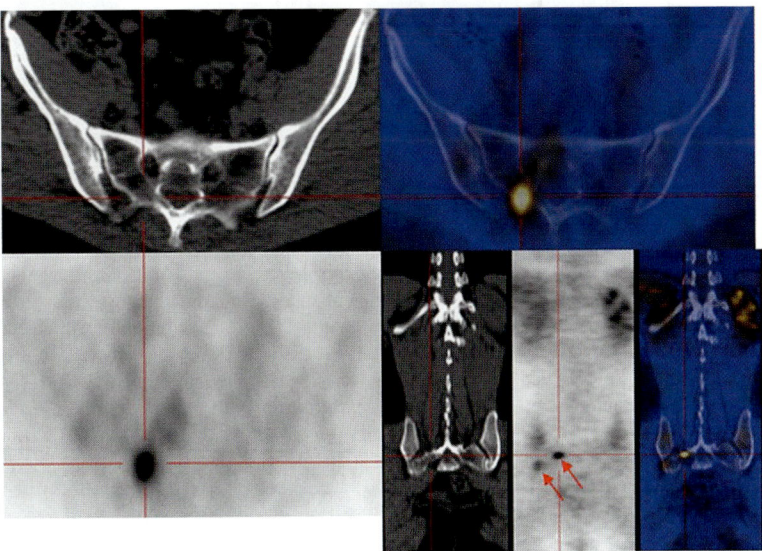

Fig. 52.3

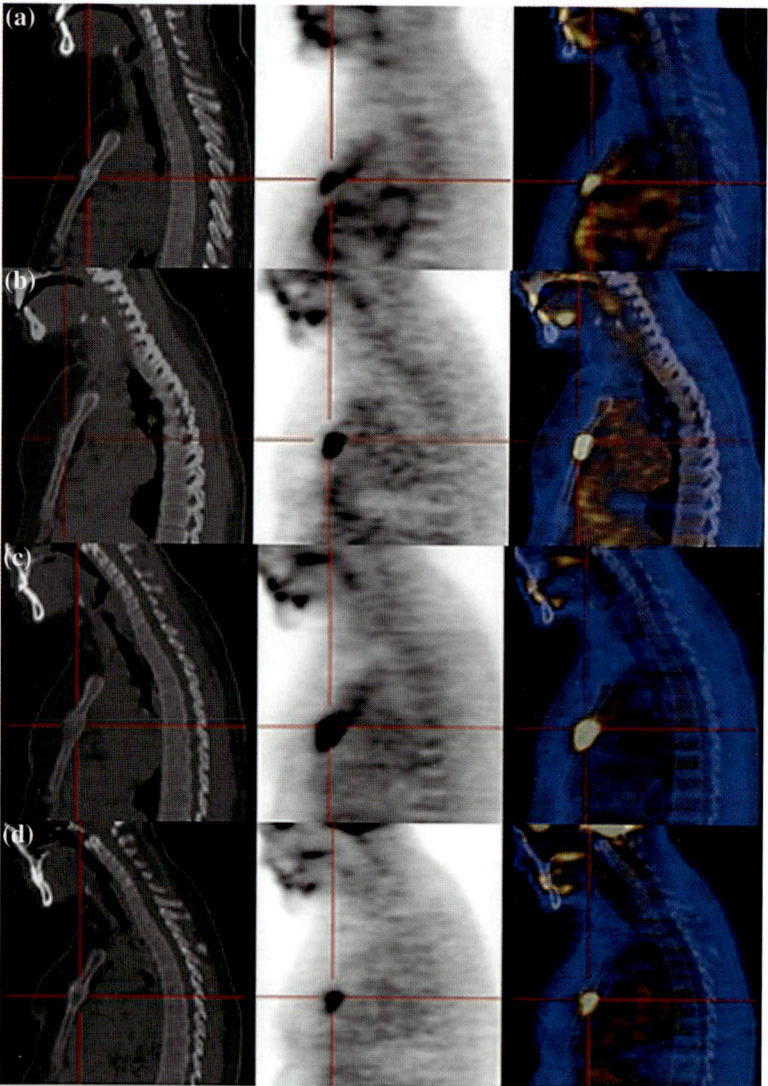

Fig. 52.4 The PET-CT sagittal reconstructions show a structural, essentially destructive, rearrangement of the sternum, with cortical interruption of the rhyme. The PET scans (**a–c**) how progression in time of the accumulation of glucose due to low response to medical therapy. After radiotherapy (**d**) metastatic bone disease tends to look thickened and sclerotic, with relative reduction in metabolic activity. You do not appreciate interruption of the cortical bone. The persistence of the lesional carbohydrate consumption is determined by actinic inflammation

52.4 Conclusions

Progression of bone marrow disease, due to impairment of the sacrum and the right sacral wing. Post-actinic remodeling of the sternal lesion with clavear reactive adenitis to be checked again over time.

At the same time new metastases appear in the sacrum and the right sacral wing, which are characterized by abnormal glucose consumption.

The clavicular fossa lymph node detected in the left shows a limited increase of FDG metabolism and is therefore reactive in nature and benign: radiation therapy at the level of sternal metastases may lead to inflammation of the region with satellite adenitis (MIP image in Figs. 52.1d, 52.2d) (See also Figs. 52.3, 52.4).

52.5 Key Points

- During follow-up of cancer patients, CT-PET may be repeated when properly justified by the appearance of new symptoms. In this woman, the scan was performed several times to document the progression of hematogenous metastasis to the sternum, the therapeutic response and the subsequent appearance of the lesion to the sacrum that determines low back pain: the "principle of justification of dose" is respected.
- When it is clear that a solitary metastatic bone lesion infiltrated by contiguity, the disease can still be considered locoregional.

- Even though the extent of the disease is limited, the patient has a high risk of progression in other districts, especially when the patient is nonresponsive to treatments with Herceptin, Femara, and Decapeptyl.
- When a solitary metastatic bone lesion is of hematogenous origin, the disease is systemic. The probability of appearance of new bone lesions (sometimes multiple) during follow-up is greater; therefore, clinical and diagnostic follow up should be more intense.
- In this patient, the risk of disease progression is very high because it is a hematogenous metastasis to the sternum, which did not respond to treatment with Herceptin, Femara, and Decapeptyl and subsequently developed chemoresistance.

Radiation therapy is palliative because it reduces the chest pain symptoms and spread of locoregional metastatic lesions. It does not affect the systemic progression of the disease though.

Axillary Lymphadenopathy of Nature to be Determined

53.1 Clinical History

83-year-old woman with left axillary lesion measuring 5 cms, mobile on the superficial and deep layers, slightly painful on palpation.

53.2 Diagnostic Question

Search of focal lesions with high metabolism of glucose in a patient with axillary lymphadenopathy of nature to be determined.

53.3 Report

The gross lesion clinically appreciable in the left axillary area shows intensive glucose metabolism, SUVmax 13 (Fig. 53.1). No significant areas of pathological glucose consumption in the remaining parts of the body examined.

53.4 Conclusions

The PET scan shows pathological glucose consumption in the left axillary area to be determined histologically (Fig. 53.2).

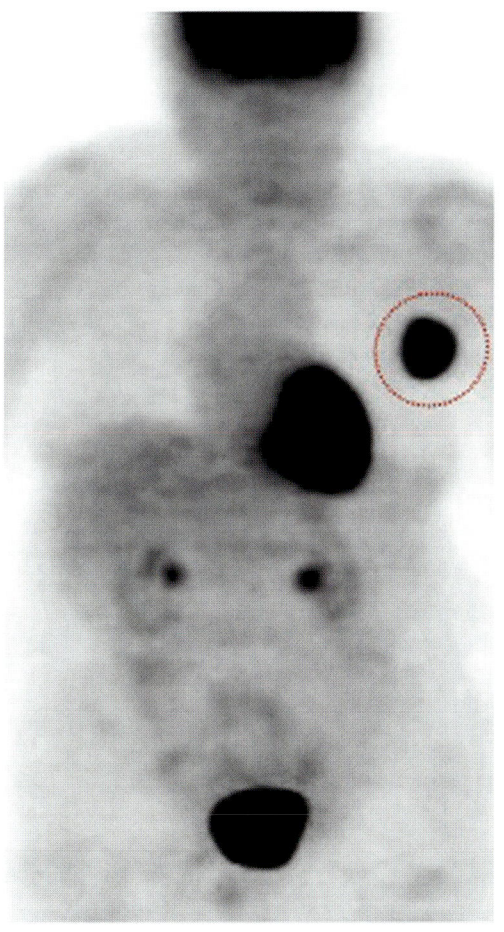

Fig. 53.1 Gross lesion clinically appreciable in the *left* axillary area

P. F. Rambaldi, *Whole-Body FDG PET Imaging in Oncology*,
DOI: 10.1007/978-88-470-5295-6_53, © Springer-Verlag Italia 2014

Fig. 53.2 The PET scan shows pathological glucose consumption in the left axillary area

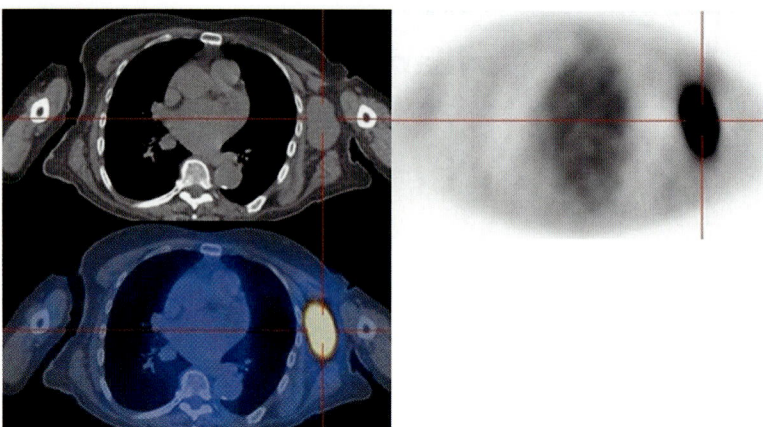

53.5   Key Points

Axillary lymphadenopathy characterized by high metabolism, requires a differential diagnosis of breast cancer, lymphoma, melanoma, or other occult disease.

The FDG-PET has a low sensitivity in the definition of mammary nodules measuring less than a centimeter.

In women, a mammogram must always be performed, even when the clinical examination of the breast is negative. In the event of a negative mammogram, it is useful to have an MRI to look for a hidden injury. When the primary tumor is not detected, a node biopsy is needed.

In this patient, an occult DIC was diagnosed in the left breast.

Brachial Plexopathy Secondary to Axillary Recurrence of Breast Cancer: Response to Chemoradiotherapy

54

54.1 Clinical History

67-year-old woman who underwent left radical mastectomy and lymphadenectomy for a moderately differentiated DIC, pT2, pN1, PM0.

Ten years after, plexopathy appears in the left upper limb.

- Echography: solid hypoechoic neoformation measuring 5 cm, in the left axillary region, with lymphadenopathy in the supraclavicular area.
- CT: in the axillary left region, adjacent to the muscular structures, a significant proportion of solid tissue (45 × 40 mm) is detected, with intense impregnation after contrast enhancement.
- Bone scan: absence of focal lesions.
- PET: left brachial plexopathy due to lymph node recurrence (SUV max 12).
  Radio-chemotherapy were then performed.

54.2 Diagnostic Question

Patient with left axillary recurrence from breast cancer (Fig. 54.1a): study of the metabolic response three months after the end of chemoradiotherapy (Fig. 54.1b).

54.3 Report

Good response to treatment performed in the left axillary region, where, today, pathological glucose consumption is not detected, except for a small lymph node in the ipsilateral clavicular fossa, SUV max 2.8.

54.4 Conclusions

The PET scan shows good response to radio-chemotherapy, even though modest metabolic activity can still be found, due to post-actinic inflammation (See Figs. 54.2, 54.3).

54.5 Key Points

In the presence of axillary recurrence, the surgical approach is to be preferred to radiotherapy for the lower incidence of acute and chronic side effects, while the radiation treatment is to be reserved for inoperable cases.

After radiotherapy is always a fair share of post-actinic phenomena mediated by immunocompetent cells according to the scheme → → →

P. F. Rambaldi, *Whole-Body FDG PET Imaging in Oncology*,
DOI: 10.1007/978-88-470-5295-6_54, © Springer-Verlag Italia 2014

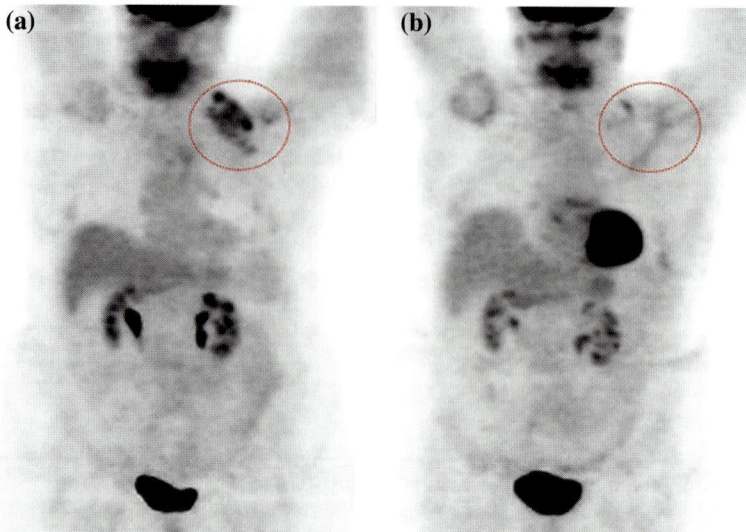

Fig. 54.1 PET scans, before (*left*, SUV max 12) and after (*right*, SUV max 2.8) chemotherapy

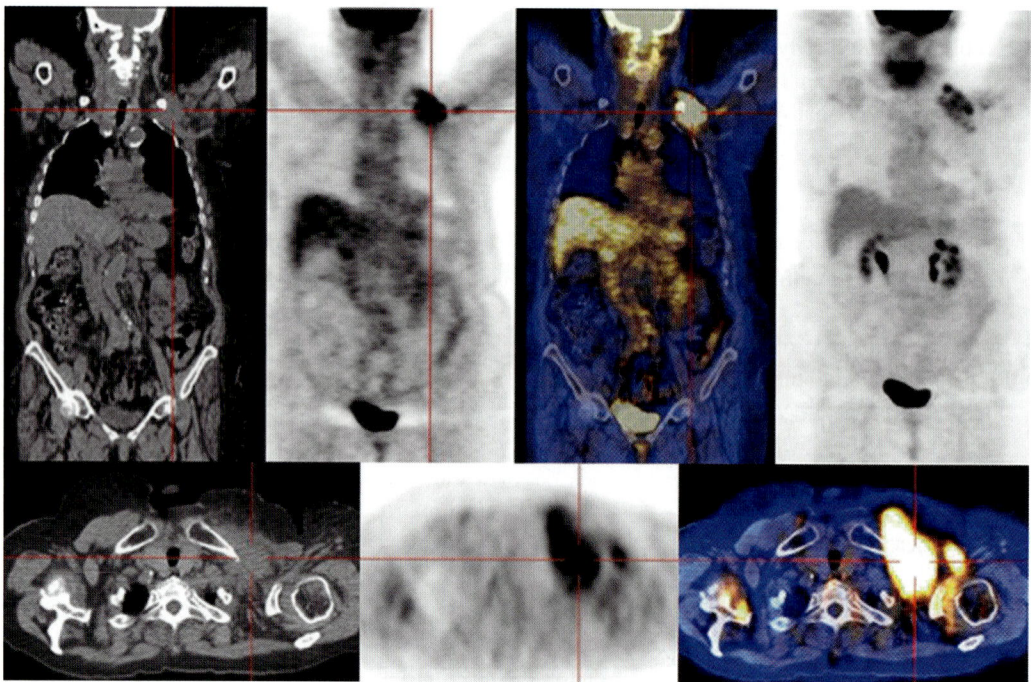

Fig. 54.2 PET-CT images and MIP reconstructions performed prior to radio-chemotherapy showed a coarse, uneven, solid lesion with irregular margins, involving the three levels of the left axillary lymph nodes, confluent with each other. More modest adenopathies could be found in the clavicular and lower ipsilateral lateral cervical region. At the PET scan these districts have a pathological glucose consumption

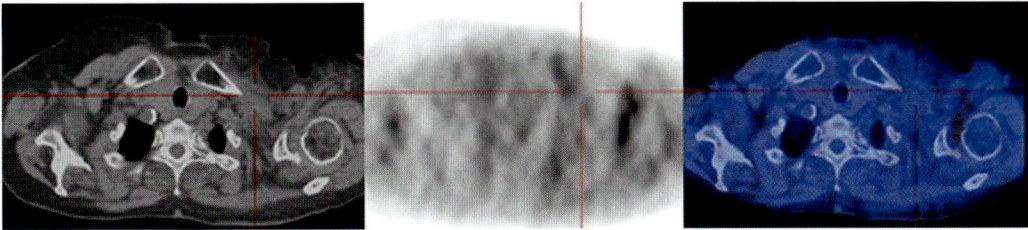

Fig. 54.3 The PET-CT scan performed 3 months after the radio-chemotherapy shows inhomogeneous tissue thickening in the left armpit due to actinic outcomes (*B*). It is associated with lymphadenopathy in the ipsilateral clavicular fossa characterized by restricted carbohydrate consumption, of nonspecific reactive nature

inflammation → → → necrosis → → → fibrosis. This process is always characterized by low metabolic activity, then by glucose consumption demonstrated by PET.

It is important to remember that the prognosis of patients with locoregional recurrence or nodal involvement is not good, about 80 % of the cases develop hematogenous metastases during the subsequent follow-up.

Malignant Melanoma

55

55.1 Clinical History

Excision of malignant melanoma in the middle third of the anterior-distal left leg in a man of 43 years.

Radicalization after a month with negative sentinel lymph node.

After 1 year: reoperation for loco-regional recurrence.

After 2 months: two surgical excisions of metastatic subcutaneous nodules, respectively on the lateral side of the left knee and the ipsi-lateral anterior distal third thigh.

- TC: presence of multiple hepatic cysts, the largest measuring 15×10 mm in segment VI. In the seventh segment a nodular lesion compatible with the diagnosis of angioma, due to the peculiar enhancement is detected.

A month later: surgical excision of some metastatic skin nodules in the middle third of the left thigh on the medial side.

Two months later: left inguinal lymphade-nectomy and surgical excision of some meta-static nodules in the ipsilateral knee and thigh. Postoperatively, a left inguinal lymphocele is created, which is afterwards aspirated.

55.2 Diagnostic Question

Search for focal lesions with high glucose metabolism in patient with metastatic melanoma.

55.3 Report

Pathological glucose consumption in two milli-metric subcutaneous nodules in the left leg in correspondence of the proximal and distal thirds, respectively with SUV max of 1.3 and 2. These lesions have hard-wood consistency on palpation.

Weak and diffuse FDG accumulation on the lateral side of the left knee, thigh and groin, due to post-surgical adaptation, SUV max 1.9.

Presence of left inguinal lymphocele that looks cool in its liquid component, while the capsule ha modest and uneven increase in met-abolic activity, of non-specific meaning, SUV max 2.4.

Glucose consumption at the right tibio-tarsic joint is secondary to a load disfunction. Absence of focal lesions with a high metabolism in the remaining body segments examined.

55.4 Conclusions

The PET scan shows progression of disease for the presence of two metastatic small lumps under the skin, clinically appreciable in the left leg (Fig. 55.1).

The deposition of glucose described in the left knee, thigh and groin has not the appearance of a focal lesion, so it is determined by non-specific post-surgical reshaping (See also Figs. 55.2, 55.3, 55.4).

P. F. Rambaldi, *Whole-Body FDG PET Imaging in Oncology*,
DOI: 10.1007/978-88-470-5295-6_55, © Springer-Verlag Italia 2014

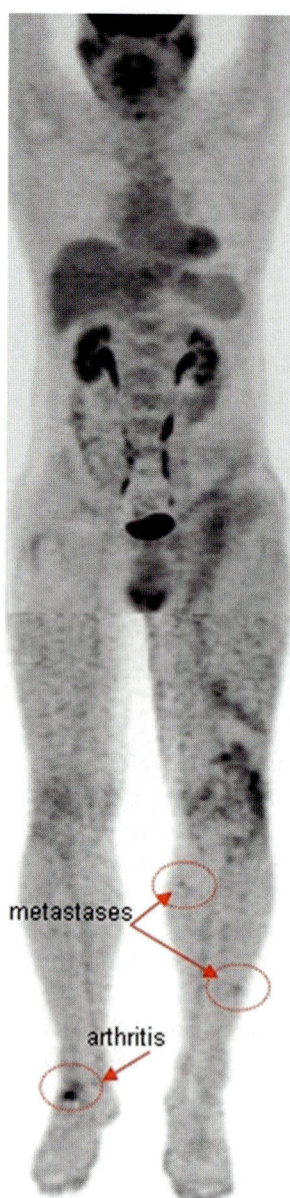

55.4.1 Methodological Note

- After surgery, there is a modest deposition of glucose determined by metabolic healing phenomena at the surgical scars.
- In some cases the PET-CT may be dubious or indeterminate because the SUV max of benign lesions characterized by nonspecific modest activity is higher than that of metastatic foci measuring less than a centimeter and that are below the limits of resolutive technique.
- The follow-up over time demonstrates a reduction in metabolism linked to the phenomena of scar remodeling and neoplastic foci have a progressive increase in the concentration of glucose.

55.5 Key Points

- The standard CT-PET does not include the upper and lower limbs. A scan addiction must always be programmed, if the underlying disease suggests a possible involvement of these districts:
- Melanomas often determine subcutaneous metastases.
- The millimeter subcutaneous nodules site of metastases may be missed on CT-PET.
- The clinical symptomatology is essential to clarify doubts, especially when the nodular uptake of glucose is limited as it is in this case.

Fig. 55.1 The PET scan shows progression of disease for the presence of two metastatic small lumps under the skin, clinically appreciable in the left leg

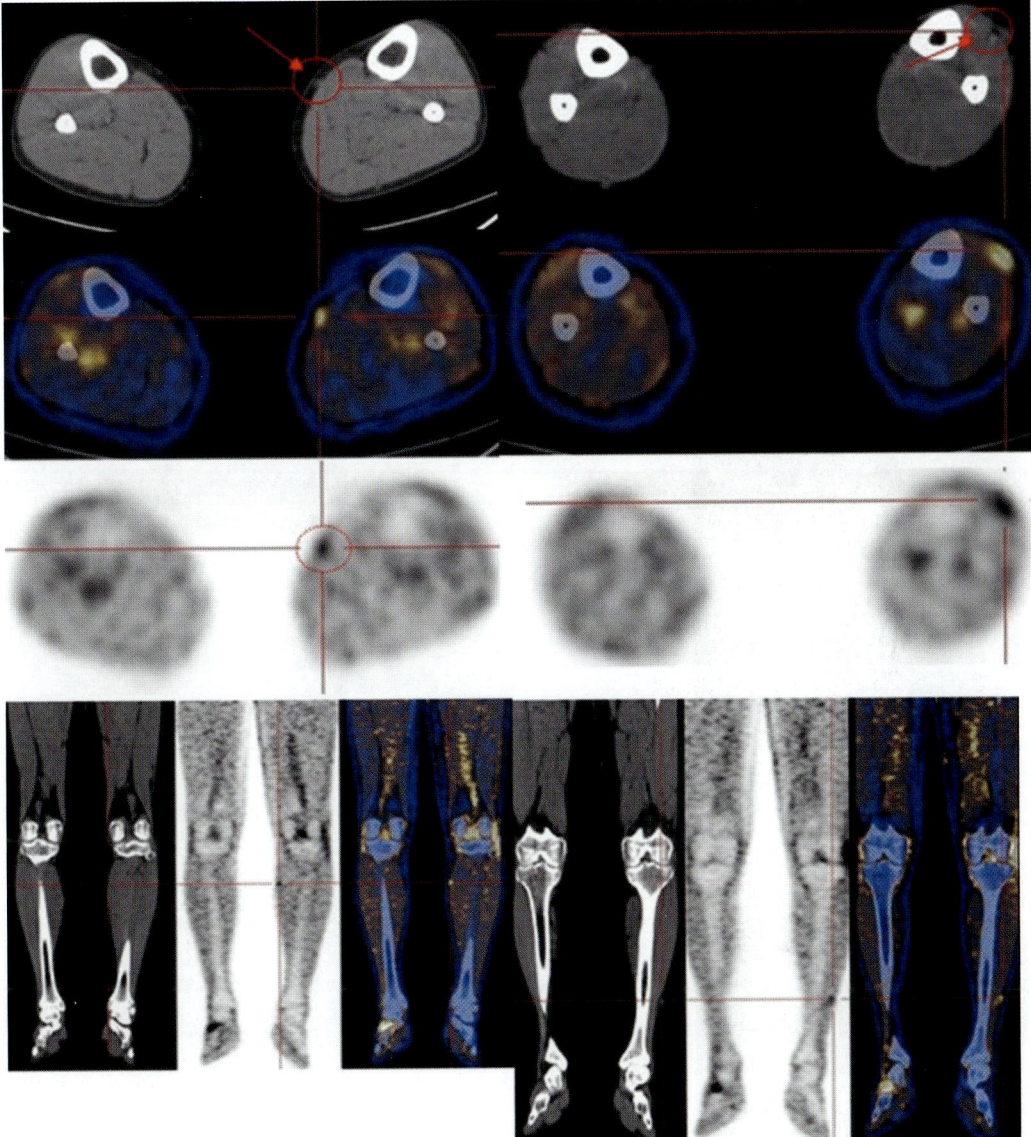

Fig. 55.2 The program that allows the calculation of the SUV max has significant limitations in the determination of the consumption of glucose in millimetric lesions because this is a limit of the resolutive technique and a relative under-estimation follows. The SUV max of the estimated subcutaneous nodules is proportional to their volume: it is higher at the bigger distal lesion and it seems lower in the proximal smaller one. Actually though, both nodules have high biological activity and metabolism

- The subcutaneous lesions have elevated glucose metabolism, the SUV max <2 does not reflect the actual metabolic activity of subcutaneous metastatic formations.

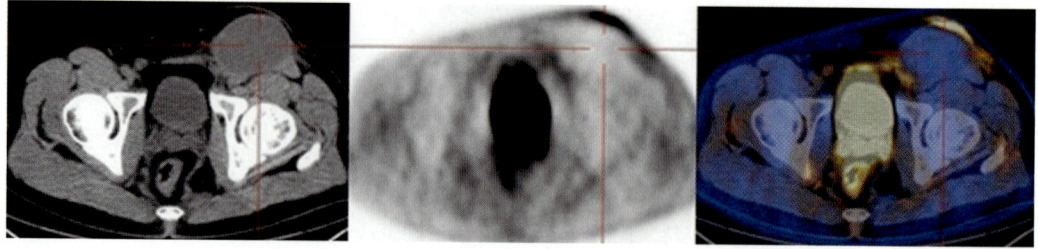

Fig. 55.3 Axial CT-PET images show the absent metabolism of the massive left inguinal lymphocele

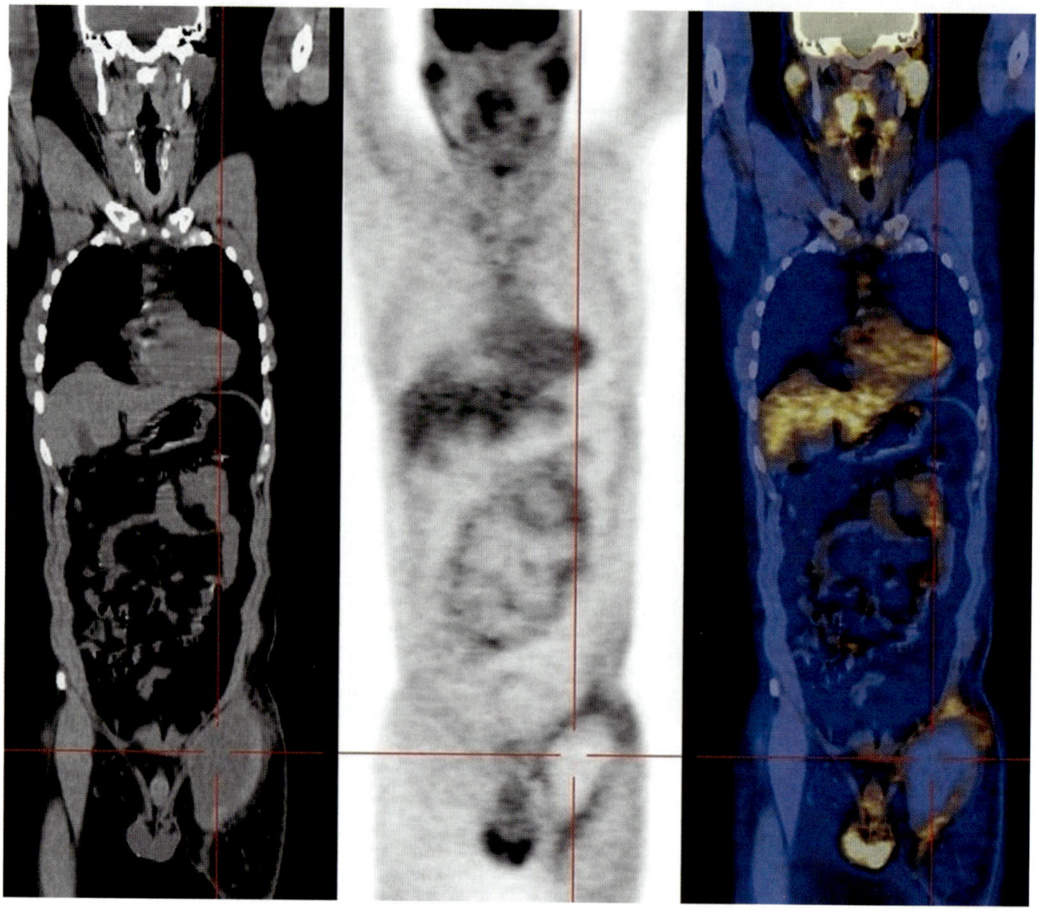

Fig. 55.4 The coronal reconstruction shows the extent and anatomical relationships of the left groin mass that is hypodense and fluid-filled (lymphocele). This lesion appears photopenic at the PET scan in its fluid component and the capsule has modest FDG metabolism, related to reactive nonspecific macrophage and fibroblast presence

- These 2 mm lesions in reality are below the limits of PET equipment. The seat and the high biological activity of metastatic nodules help to overcome the "limits of technology." The clinical symptomatology allows a correct interpretation of nuclear medicine images.

Axillary Metastases in Patient with Melanoma: Post-surgery Evaluation

56

56.1 Clinical History

79-year-old man who underwent surgery for a nodular ulcerated malignant melanoma in the left scapular region. Pathological stage: pT4b, pN0, PM0.

Immunotherapy was then performed.

Follow-up after 1 year:

- PET-FDG: multiple nodules characterized by abnormal glucose consumption in the left axilla (SUV max 9) due to extensive lymphadenopathy.

Emptying of the left axillary region: 14 lymph nodes out of 27 were found site of metastases from melanoma.

56.2 Diagnostic Question

Search for focal lesions with high glucose metabolism in patient with malignant melanoma who underwent axillary lymphadenectomy for massive recurrence (14/27 positive lymph nodes): restaging after surgery.

56.3 Report

No areas of abnormal glucose consumption in the parts of the body examined.

The coarse appreciable formation in left armpit appears to have low metabolism, SUV max 4.7 and it's probably due to nonspecific reactivity (seroma).

56.4 Conclusions

The PET scan does not show biological activity that would indicate a recurrence of pathology (See Figs. 56.1, 56.2, 56.3).

P. F. Rambaldi, *Whole-Body FDG PET Imaging in Oncology*,
DOI: 10.1007/978-88-470-5295-6_56, © Springer-Verlag Italia 2014

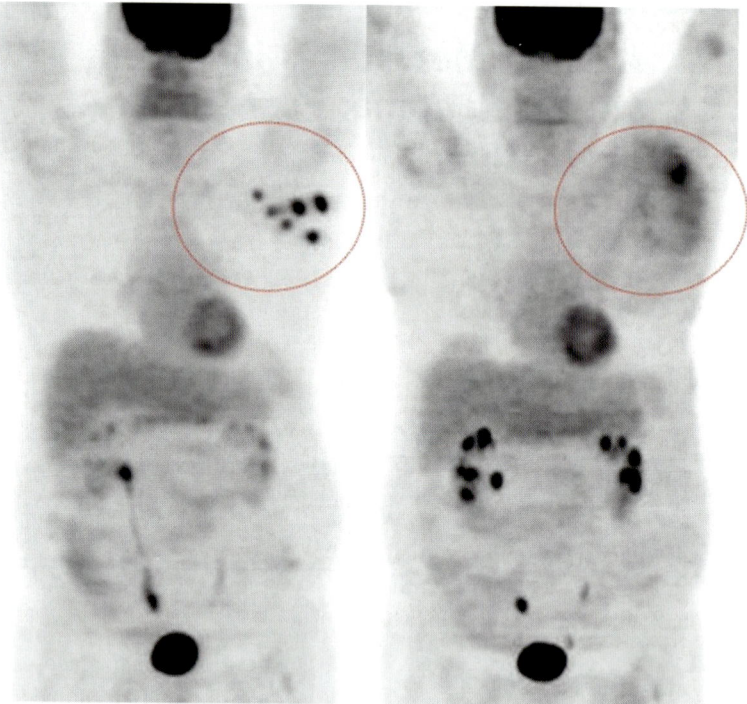

Fig. 56.1 MIP images before and after the axillary lymphadenectomy

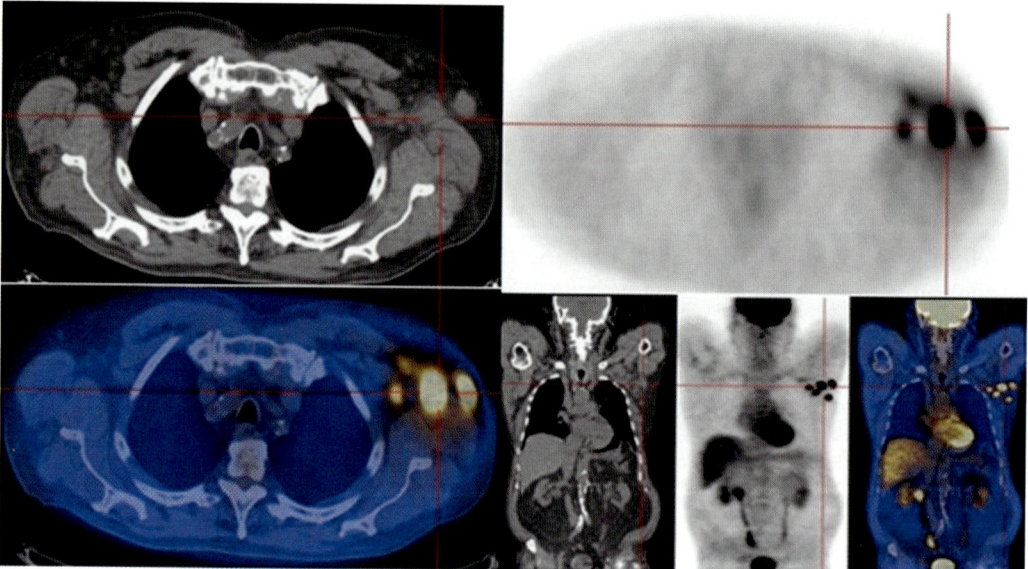

Fig. 56.2 CT-PET performed before surgery: multiple solid nodules in the left arm due to high metabolism metastatic involvement of the three lymph nodal levels

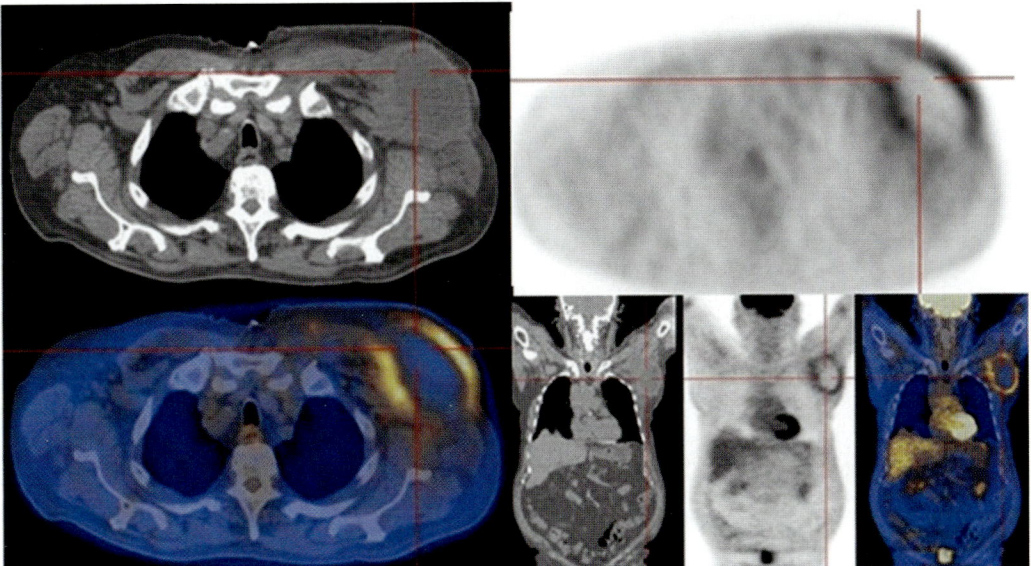

Fig. 56.3 CT-PET performed after axillary dissection: gross hypodense mass in left armpit due to a seroma, showingmodest consumption of glucose, caused by nonspecific metabolic activation

56.5 Key Points

- After surgery, the CT-PET is performed to evaluate the therapeutic efficacy, for a complete restaging and subsequent treatment planning.
- Patients with thin lesions have a survival rate of 98 %.
- Advanced melanoma survival rate is 10 %.

Ductal and Mucinous Pancreatic Adenocarcinoma: Recurrence after Surgery

57

57.1 Clinical History

66-year-old man who underwent spleno-pancreatectomy for pancreatic adenocarcinoma of mucinous and ductal type. He has not undergone radio-chemotherapy.

57.1.1 Follow-up at 6 Months

- PET: lymphadenopathy characterized by moderate increased uptake of the tracer (SUV max 3.1) in the left axillary and right inguinal regions.
- Ultrasound of the left axillary and right inguinal regions: lymphadenopathy with inflammatory-reactive appearance.

57.1.2 Follow-up at 18 Months

- CT: presence of hypodense tissue that surrounds some metal clips in the celiac-mesenteric region suspicious for recurrence. Centimetric subglissonian hypodense hepatic nodule between the V and VI segment, with moderate impregnation after contrast medium injection. Another millimetric hypodense nodule in segment IV. Both are compatible with secondary localizations.

57.2 Diagnostic Question

Restaging of mucinous adenocarcinoma of the pancreas after surgery for suspicious metastatic liver lesions: research foci of high glucose metabolism.

57.3 Report

The centimetric lump in the VI hepatic segment reported by CT in the clinical history shows moderate carbohydrate consumption; on the other hand the millimetric nodule in the fourth segment is not displayed, due to resolution limits.

The lesion lying adjacent to the metal clips in the celiac region, described in the CT scan reported in history, has a modest consumption of glucose, SUV max 2.9, so it is questionable for recurrence. RM integration and controls over time could be useful. Modest FDG metabolism in the left axillary and right inguinal regions is due to reactive nonspecific lymphadenopathy, SUV max 2.2. Uptake in the left latero-cervical region is due to the activation of the sternocleidomastoid (See Figs. 57.1, 57.2).

P. F. Rambaldi, *Whole-Body FDG PET Imaging in Oncology*,
DOI: 10.1007/978-88-470-5295-6_57, © Springer-Verlag Italia 2014

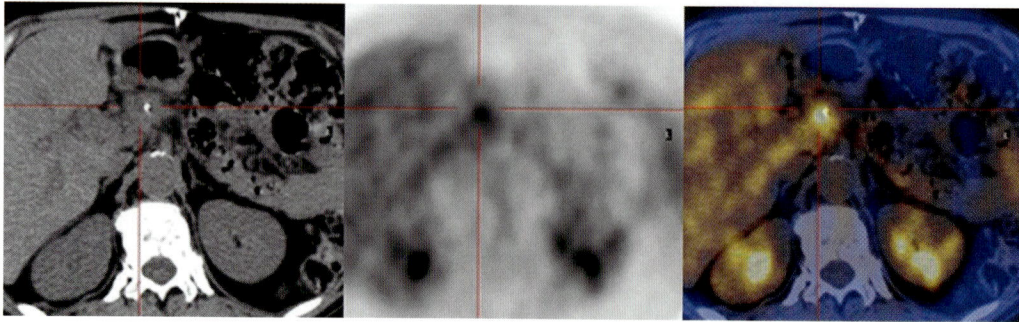

Fig. 57.1 In the celiac region adjacent to the portal trunk, at the level of the surgical area, CT-PET shows the presence of solid inhomogeneous tissue, which surrounds some metal clips, characterized by modest increase in the metabolism of glucose. This element is doubtful for locoregional recurrence of disease; nonspecific activation scar (*granuloma*) cannot be ruled out, though

Fig. 57.2 The patient comes with a CT diagnosis of liver metastases but CT-PET shows only a slight increase in the metabolic activity of the nodule in segment VI. We can say that this tumor is characterized with limited metabolism of FDG

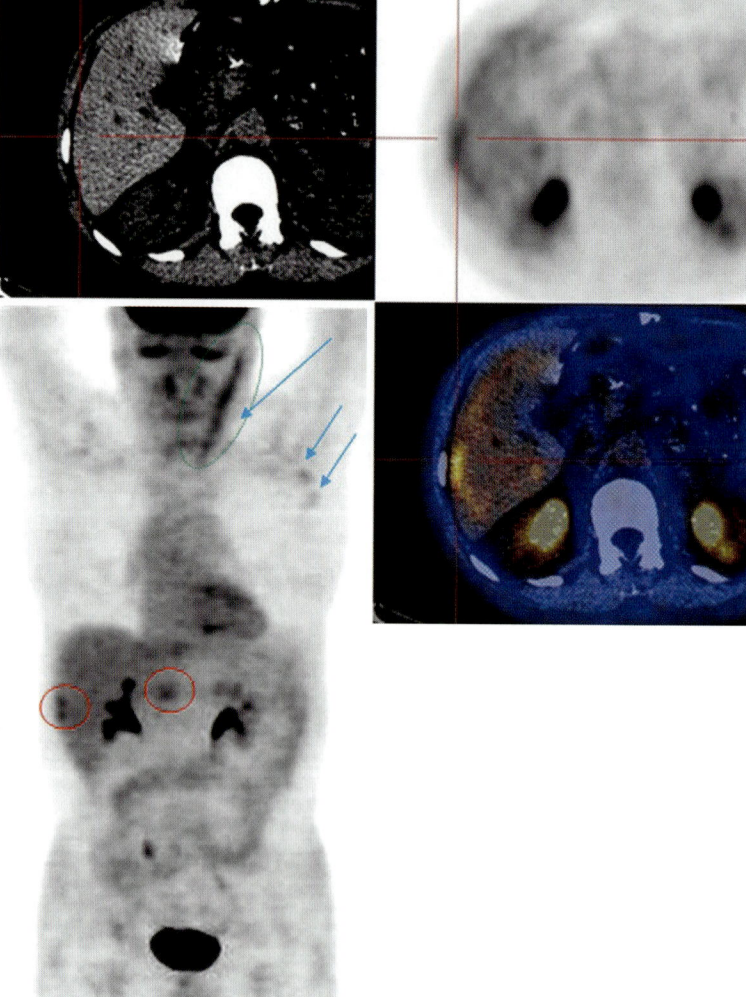

57.4 Conclusions

The PET scan shows limited metabolism of the hepatic nodules reported in the previous contrast-enhanced CT. This element is compatible with secondary lesions from mucinous adenocarcinoma of the pancreas. Biopsy confirmation has to be done (Fig. 57.2).

57.5 Key Points

The FDG-PET has limited sensitivity in the study of mucinous neoplasms because of the low consumption of glucose, but a lesion that accumulates FDG is suspicious for recurrent disease.

In this patient, the contrast-enhanced CT previously performed identified two metastatic liver lesions; therefore, the duty of the nuclear physician is to define the lesional metabolism.

In the surgically treated patients, the surgical area should always be identified anatomically by CT. This locates the metal clips used while the PET determines the presence of metabolic activity in the area.

Similarly, the analysis of CT and CT-PET images helps to better identify metastatic lesions anatomically.

58.1 Clinical History

62-year-old man, who underwent gastroresection for peptic ulcer at age 41, performs clinical and instrumental evaluation for recurrent abdominal colic.

- Gastroscopy: presence of diverticula of the duodenum in gastro-resected patient.
- Tumor markers: CEA = 5.2 (NV < 4.5), CA19-9 = 57.8 (NV < 37).

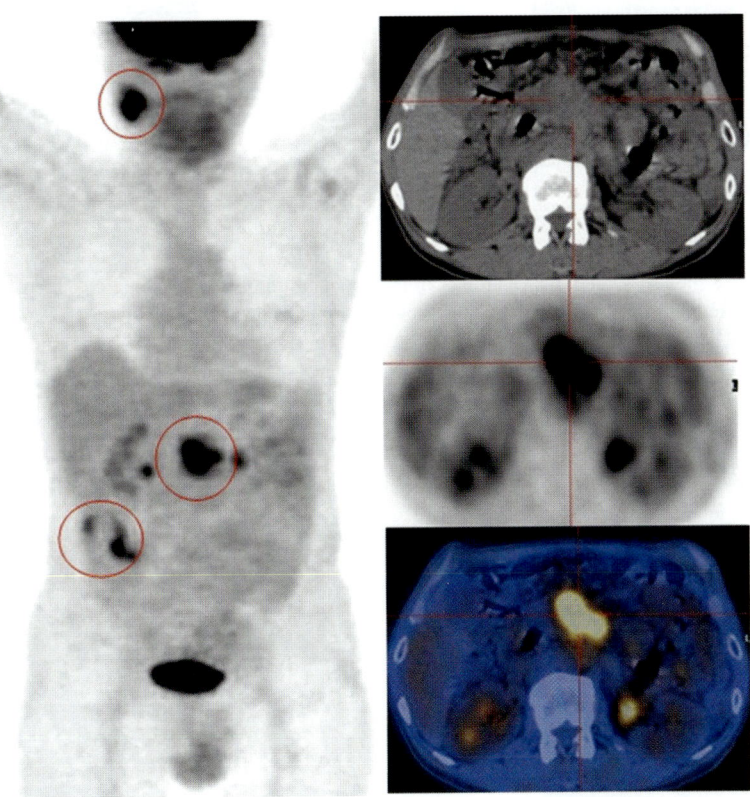

Fig. 58.1 The PET scan showed a focal lesion of the pancreas with a high metabolism

P. F. Rambaldi, *Whole-Body FDG PET Imaging in Oncology*,
DOI: 10.1007/978-88-470-5295-6_58, © Springer-Verlag Italia 2014

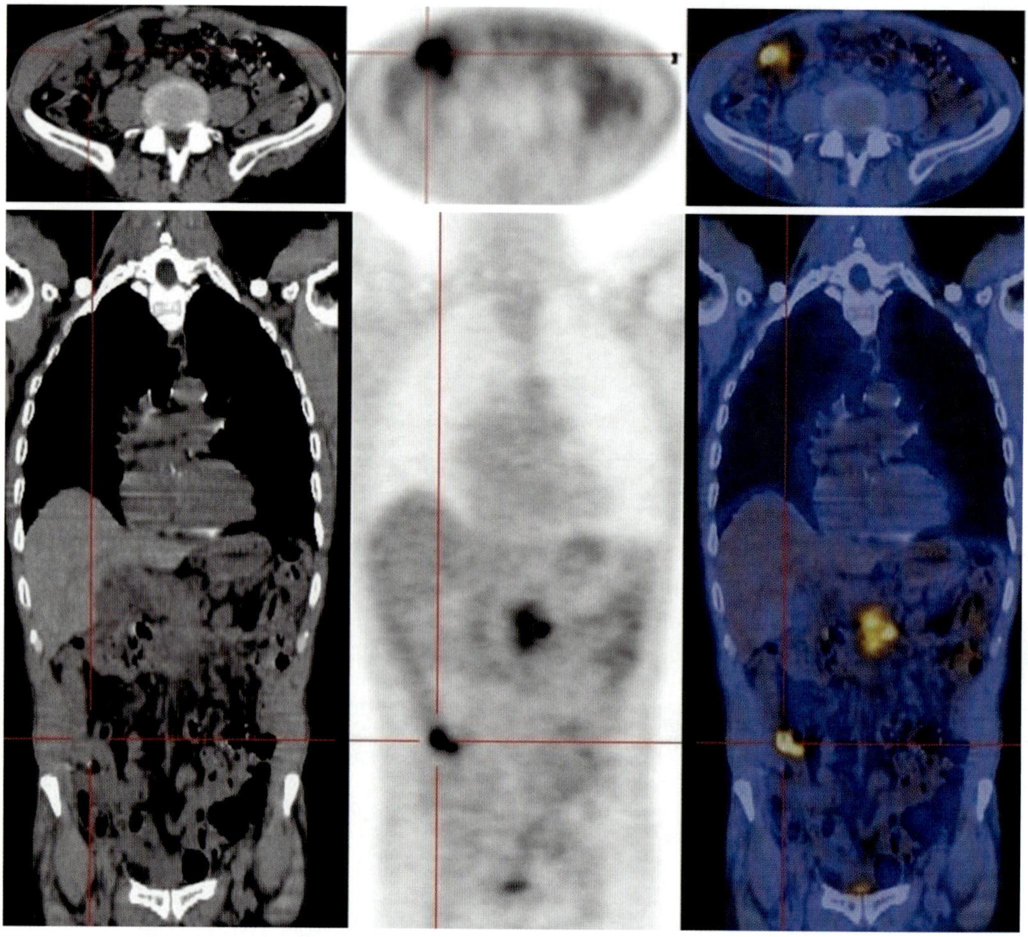

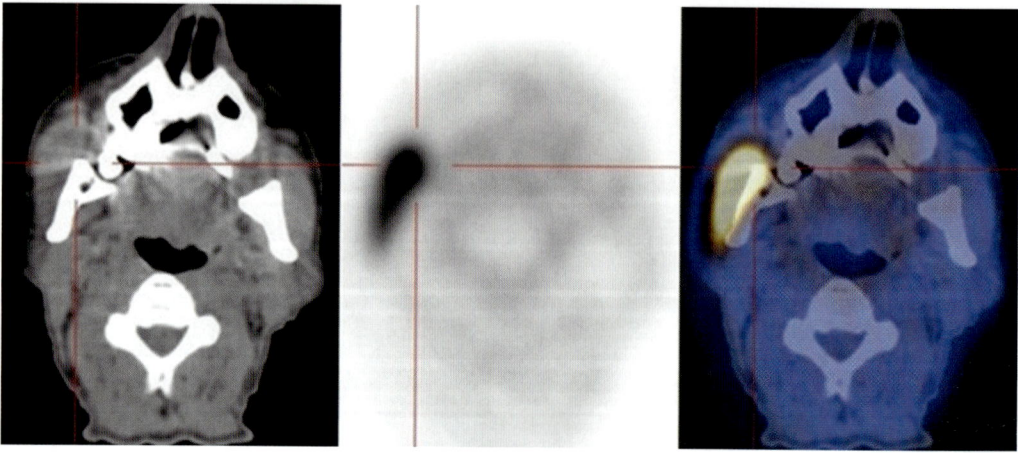

Fig. 58.2 CT-PET showed a solid, uneven tumor in the middle third of the ascending colon, characterized by high carbohydrate consumption. The subsequent colonoscopy showed an adenomatous polyp

Fig. 58.3 Presence of metal synthesis at the right ramus of the jaw, which at the PET scan is shown as a hot spot due to anomalous correction

58.2 Diagnostic Question

Search for focal lesions with high glucose metabolism in patient with recurrent abdominal colic and alteration of tumor markers' levels.

58.3 Report

In correspondence of the body of the pancreas a mass is detected, indissociable from the surrounding tissues, presenting intense consumption of FDG, SUV max 8.7.

Focal modest increase in glucose metabolism in the ascending colon, SUV max 6.5. Endoscopic control could be useful.

58.4 Conclusions

The PET scan showed a focal lesion of the pancreas with a high metabolism (Fig. 58.1). See also Figs. 58.2, 58.3.

58.5 Key Points

Unexplained elevation of tumor markers suggests a PET study. The MIP reconstruction shows three areas of altered metabolism of glucose, respectively, in the pancreas, ascending colon, and the jaw.

To reduce the rate of "false positives," PET images must be interpreted in light of the history and the CT scan:
- The lesion responsible for the alteration of tumor markers is pancreatic.
- The other two accumulations are determined by an intestinal polyp and from an artifact from abnormal attenuation caused by the presence of a metallic means of synthesis.

Diffuse Peritoneal Carcinosis Due to Pancreatic Adenocarcinoma

59

59.1 Clinical History

77-year-old man who already underwent gastroresection for peptic ulcer.

Recent surgically treated fracture of the left femur. After surgery, there has been a deterioration of general condition, jaundice and a marked alteration of laboratory data, especially liver function markers.

- CT: solid lump between the body and tail of the pancreas measuring 28 × 29 mm, with dilatation of the bile ducts inside and outside the liver, incarceration of the vessels of the celiac trunk and its branches.
- Extended commitment of the retroperitoneal and celiac-mesenteric lymph node chains. Free fluid in the abdomen and pelvis with detachment of the higher parenchymal splanchnic organs; jumble of bowel loops with thickened omentum and mesentery. Thrombosis of the inferior mesenteric artery.
- Cancer markers: CA15-3 = 26.88 U/mL (nv < 25); CA125 = 201.2 U/mL (nv < 40), CA 19-9 = 9257 U/mL (nv < 39).

59.2 Diagnostic Question

Search for focal lesions with high glucose metabolism in patient with suspected cancer of the pancreas.

59.3 Report

Mass with high glucose metabolism which occupies the body and tail of the pancreas, SUV max 8.8.

Mesenteric and retroperitoneal celiac lymphadenopathy, SUV max 7.5.

Multiple solid nodules in the abdomen and pelvis characterized by high glucose metabolism, suggesting a diffuse peritoneal carcinomatosis, SUV max 8.1 (See Figs. 59.1, 59.2, 59.3).

59.4 Key Points

When the primary tumor causes a diffuse peritoneal carcinomatosis, prognosis worsens dramatically.

In advanced stages of the disease, a condition characterized by worsening ascites and cholestatic jaundice from obstructive neoplastic infiltration may appear. It is sometimes associated with other nonspecific symptoms such as feeling of abdominal distension and pain.

The presence of peritoneal lesions that infiltrate the ureter determines hydronephrosis, while the intestinal involvement is associated with alvus disorders and abdominal pain.

Not all peritoneal carcinomatosis are characterized by a high consumption of glucose.

P. F. Rambaldi, *Whole-Body FDG PET Imaging in Oncology*,
DOI: 10.1007/978-88-470-5295-6_59, © Springer-Verlag Italia 2014

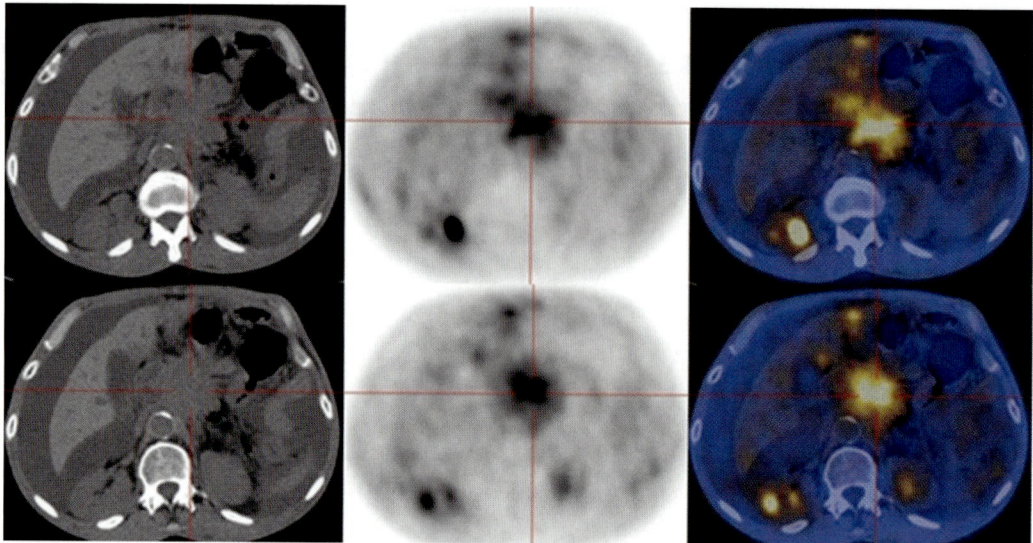

Fig. 59.1 In correspondence of the body and tail of the pancreas CT-PET shows a coarse expansive, diffusely inhomogeneous solid mass, which infiltrates locoregional tissues, in particular lymph nodes, especially celiac-mesenteric and retroperitoneal ones. This mass has a high FDG metabolism. There are multiple peritoneal nodules characterized by abnormal glucose consumption. Conspicuous neoplastic ascites. Obstructive expansion of intra- and extra-hepatic biliary ducts

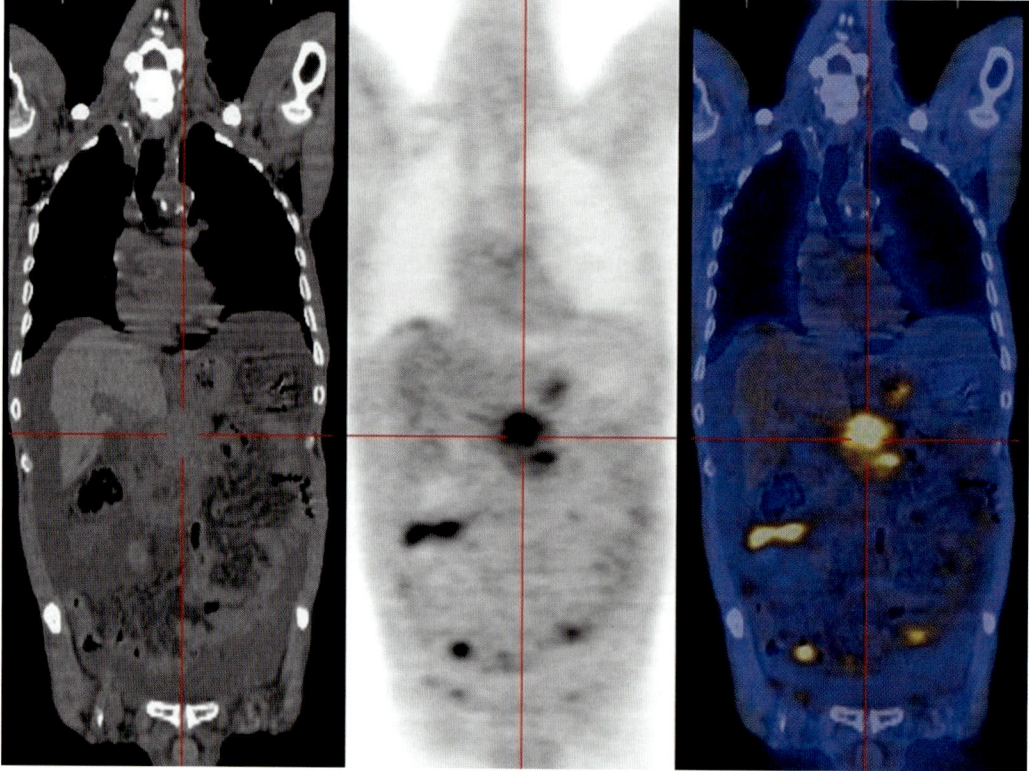

Fig. 59.2 The PET scan shows a tumor of the pancreas with a high metabolism with nodal metastases, peritoneal carcinomatosis and secondary ascites. Moderate obstructive dilatation of the biliary tract

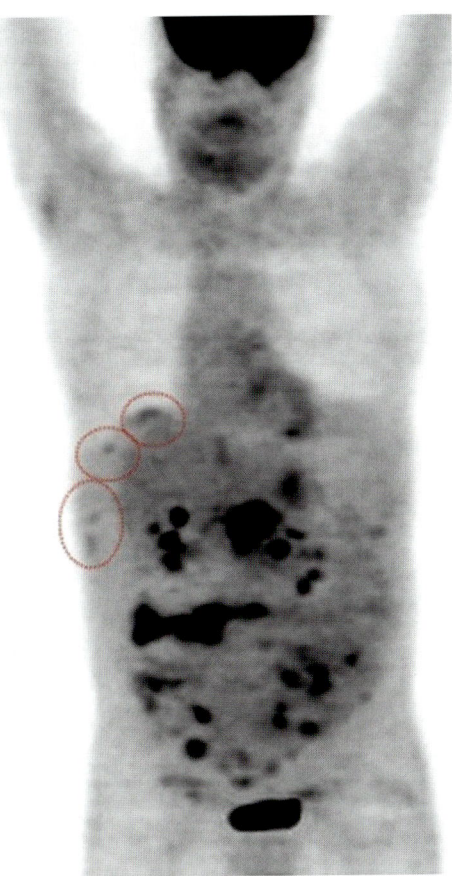

With the help of clinical, laboratory, and CT data, the nuclear physician must always seek out and report those carcinomatosis characterized by low FDG metabolism which, in any case, require a different management of the patient and have a worse prognosis.

This piece of information is essential to define the treatment protocol and subsequent supportive care.

Fig. 59.3 MIP image allows to appreciate the extent of the disease, in particular the severity of peritoneal carcinomatosis

Pulmonary Nodule in Patient with Severe Interstitial Fibrosis

60

60.1 Clinical History

79-year-old man with pulmonary fibrosis, in oxygen therapy for dyspnea:

- Chest CT: postero-basal para-hilar right pulmonary condensation not separable from the ipsilateral bronchus.
- Chest CT (performed after 3 months) in the basal right region, parenchymal consolidation with air bronchograms by inflammatory phenomena can be seen. Multiple areas of thickening and bilateral ground-glass appearance due to severe nodular interstitial fibrosis. Moderate pleural effusion on the right. Apical ipsilateral fibro-calcific remnants.

60.2 Diagnostic Question

Search for focal lesions with high glucose metabolism in patient with severe pulmonary fibrosis and pulmonary nodule, of nature to be determined.

60.3 Report

The PET shows widespread alteration of the carbohydrate consumption of the lung parenchyma bilaterally, with more severe metabolic disorder in the right, due to interstitial disease of modest activity, SUV max 2.8.

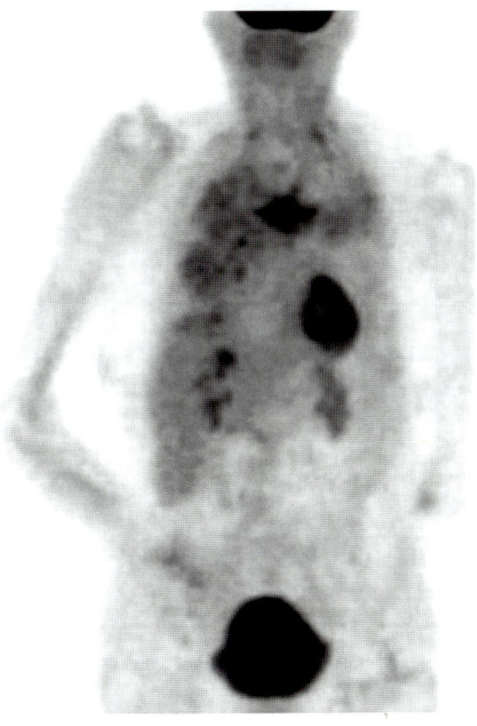

Fig. 60.1 MIP image: The high lung deposition of FDG is determined by the condition of chronic inflammation of the interstitium and by the presence of lymphocytic alveolitis

Pulmonary nodule in the posterior—basal right segment of the lower lobe, para-hilar with SUV max 3.6. Increased glucose consumption to the sternum, of nonspecific type due to regressive, degenerative phenomena, with osteoblastic remodeling, SUV max 6.9.

P. F. Rambaldi, *Whole-Body FDG PET Imaging in Oncology*,
DOI: 10.1007/978-88-470-5295-6_60, © Springer-Verlag Italia 2014

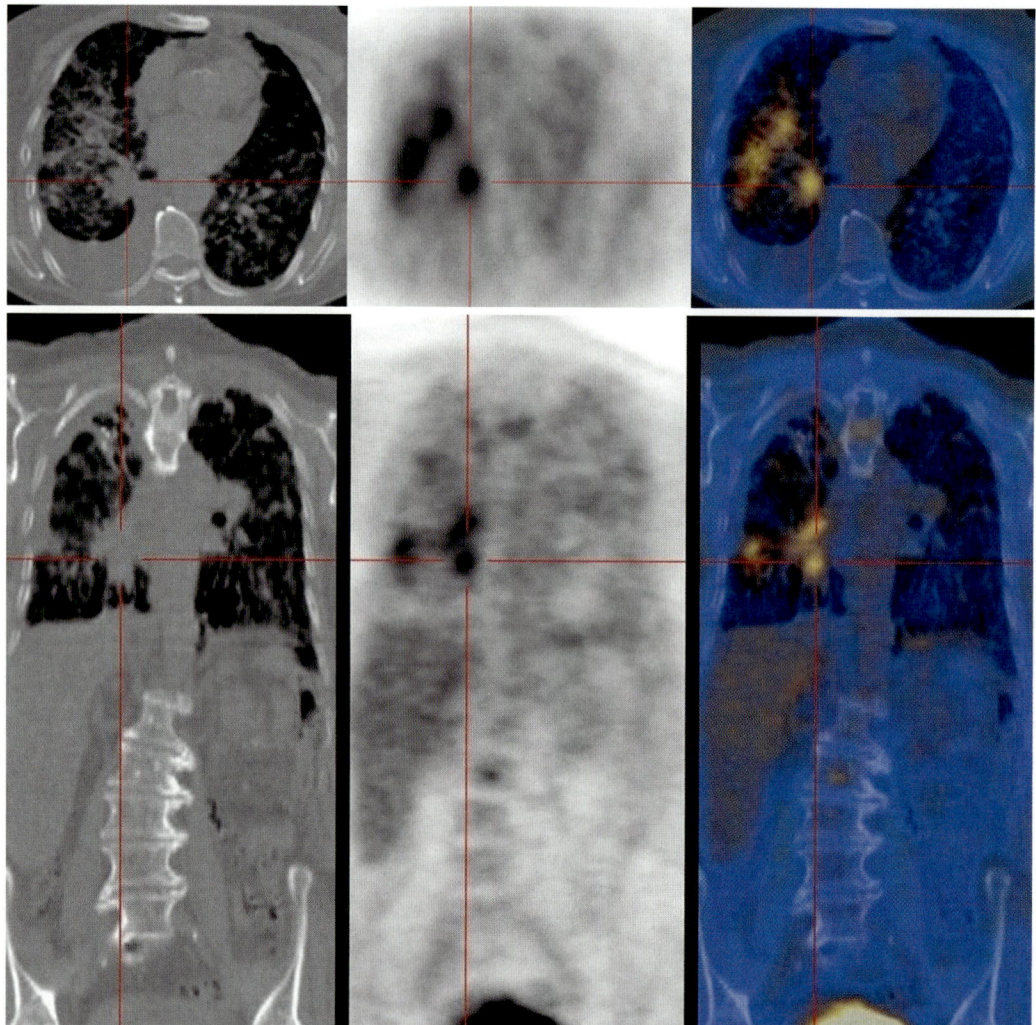

Fig. 60.2 At CT, a marked reticular thickening of the interstitium, diffusely involving the parenchyma of both lungs, can be seen. At the inferior bronchus of the *right* lung, a ground-glass nodule is seen, characterized by ill-defined margins and satellite areas of parenchymal consolidation. The FDG-PET demonstrates limited consumption of glucose in the lesion

60.4 Conclusions

The PET shows activation with severe interstitial lung disease, with more marked impairment on the right.

The lump in the posterior basal segment of the right lower lobe shows low metabolic activity, so it must be checked over time at CT. The intense deposition of glucose to the sternum is degenerative in nature.

60.5 MIP Picture

See Figs. 60.1, 60.2, 60.3.

The extent of the interstitial disease in this patient seems remarkable: the pulmonary uptake exceeds that of the mediastinum and liver.

As the gallium scintigraphy, PET-FDG allows us to evaluate the biological activity of the disease, while the CT shows the morphology of the fibrotic damage.

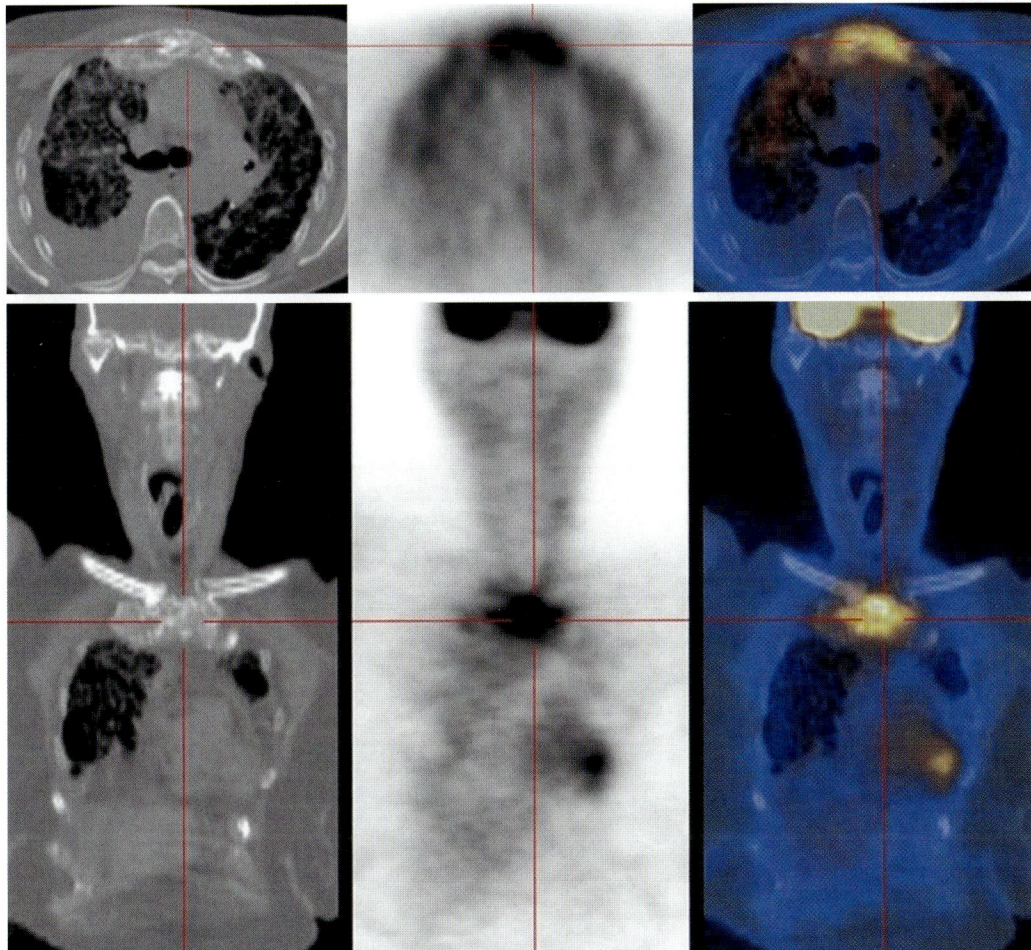

Fig. 60.3 The CT scan shows a gross structural alteration of the manubrium, with areolas of sclerotic bone reabsorbing and arthritic remodeling. No interruption of the cortex detected. PET shows that the increase in glucose consumption is widespread and does not show the focal characteristics typical of metastatic lesions. In axial sections, right pleural effusion is seen, responsible, at least in part, of the progression of dyspnea

60.6 Key Points

The patient is on oxygen therapy for severe interstitial disease. The poor clinical conditions discourage aggressive diagnostic and therapeutic approaches.

- The interstitial diseases recognize a variety of etiologies and the current classification is quite complex.
- The pulmonary nodule is probably benign, because the two CT scans reported in medical history showed no progression of the lesion volume; the PET also documented only a limited increase in the metabolism.
- The lump is located at the inferior bronchus of the right lung; therefore, bronchoscopy and BAL possibly can exclude the presence of carcinoma and certify the etiological of the interstitial disease, which is essential to define the therapeutic approach.

PS: In this patient, the subsequent bronchoscopy and BAL showed no malignant disease. The presence of alveolitis suggested therapy with corticosteroids.

After Surgery Follow-Up in Patient with NSCLC: Muscular Metastases

61

61.1 Clinical History

73-year-old patient with surgically treated right NSCLC.

Revaluation 3 months after surgery.

- PET-FDG: Focal pathological glucose consumption at the right lateral chest wall, SUV max 8.3. Nodular mass in the left iliac muscle with high metabolism, SUV max 7.2.
- Bone scan: absence of focal lesions.

Excision of the lesion involving the subcutaneous muscles of the right lateral chest wall, positive for metastases from lung cancer.

Chemotherapy and subsequent re-evaluation in 6 months.

- CT: lung fields with asymmetric right hypo-expansion due to surgical outcomes and calcified pleural thickening in the lower ipsilateral regions. Millimetric ilo-mediastinal lymph node stations. Nodular mass in the left iliac muscle, smaller than in the previous scan (max 18 mm). Morpho-structural alteration of the right iliac wing, as already seen at the previous CT scan.

The patient complains of low back-sciatic and left hip pain.

61.2 Diagnostic Question

Surgically treated NSCLC with subsequent chest muscle relapse, treated with surgery and adjuvant chemotherapy: search for focal lesions with high glucose metabolism, "restaging".

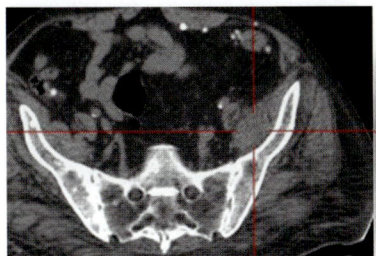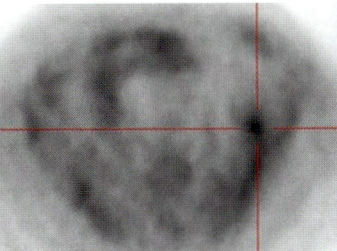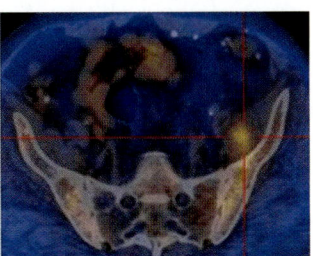

Fig. 61.1 CT-PET shows a solid, patchy nodule with irregular margins, contained within a marked thickening of the left iliac muscle, showing focal glucose consumption. There is no locoregional bone infiltration. At CT, the right iliac wing has osteosclerotic alterations that do not have typical characteristics of a recurrent injury, the absent carbohydrate consumption supporting the hypothesis of a dystrophic condition, or involution, in a patient with bilateral hip prostheses

P. F. Rambaldi, *Whole-Body FDG PET Imaging in Oncology*,
DOI: 10.1007/978-88-470-5295-6_61, © Springer-Verlag Italia 2014

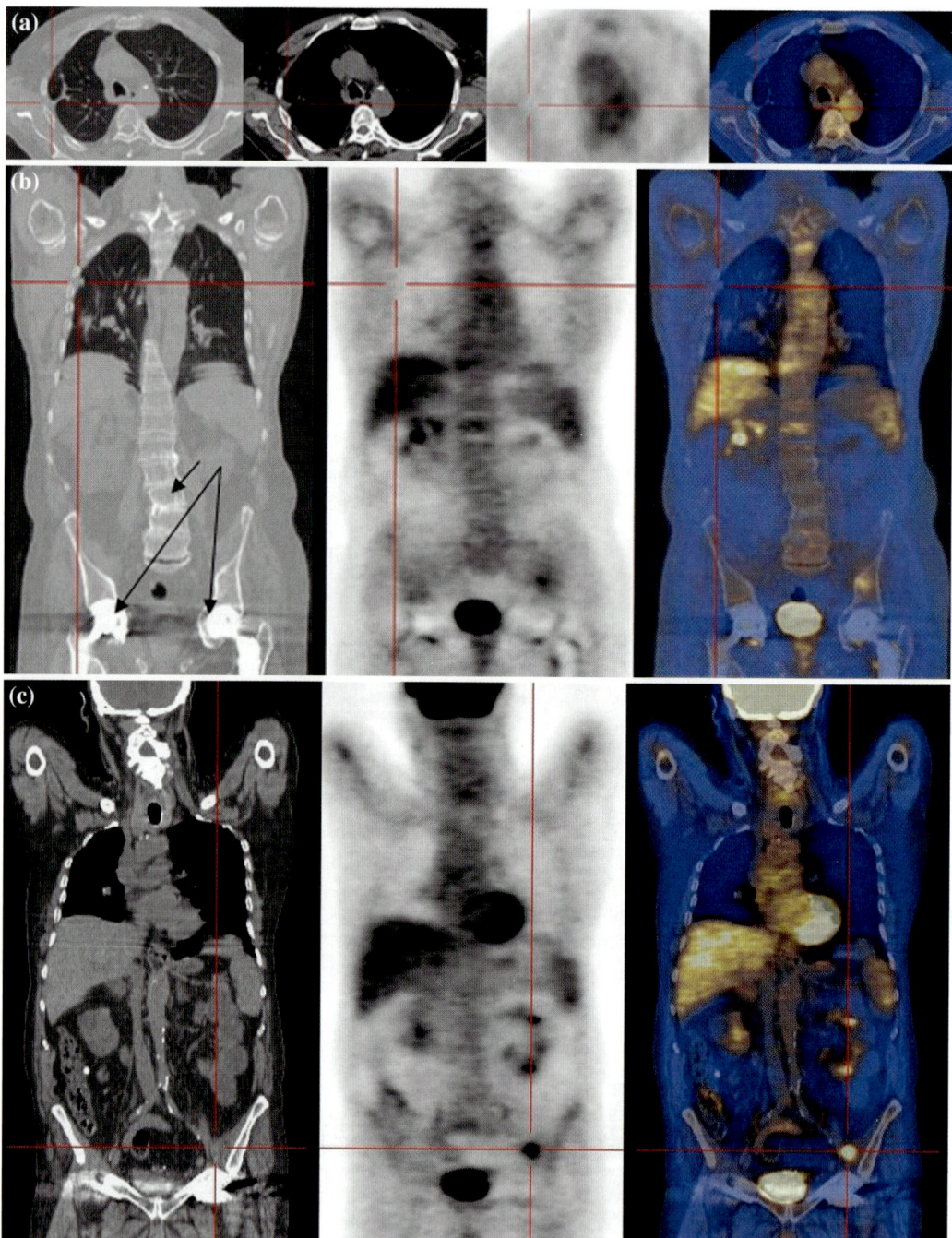

Fig. 61.2 The PET-CT scan shows asymmetric lung fields with right hypoexpansion due to surgical outcomes ad alteration of the chest wall; it does not detect pathological glucose consumption indicating a loco-regional recurrence (**a**). The coronal CT reconstruction shows the patient's scoliosis and the presence of bilateral hip replacement, elements that justify dystrophic - degenerative bone changes (**b, c**)

61.3 Report

Presence of nodule in the left iliac muscle, characterized by increased glucose consumption, SUV max 5.2.

Absence of lesions with intense FDG deposition in the remaining parts of the body. See Fig. 61.1.

61.4 Conclusions

The PET scan shows incomplete response of muscular metastases to chemotherapy. See Fig. 61.2.

61.5 Key Points

- Skeletal muscle is a rare site of hematogenous and lymphatic spread metastases of lung cancer, although their incidence is underestimated in relation to the lack of systematic evaluation during post-mortem examinations.
- The metastases follow the laws of hydrodynamics, the quality of the surrounding tissue, and the quality of the filters, for which the muscle is an unfavorable seat for them to invade.
- The contractile activity, local variations of pH, the accumulation of lactic acid and other metabolites, the local temperature, and intramuscular blood pressure are probably the basis of this refractoriness.
- In this patient, the presence of two muscle lesions and absent impairment of other organ systems suggest the particular tropism of this cancer for the muscular system; therefore, in the ongoing follow-up, muscles are to be evaluated much more carefully.

Anaplastic Metastatic Pulmonary Cancer: Follow-Up After Radiotherapy

62

62.1 Clinical History

80-year-old patient with left lung anaplastic cancer.

COMORBIDITY: previous malignant right clear cell renal cancer, in remission.

- CT: At the posterior segment of the upper lobe of the left lung, there is a massive solid focal lesion, with axial diameter of 62 × 53 mm showing marked and heterogeneous enhancement after contrast medium. Adenopathy in the aorto-pulmonary and right hilar regions. Solid secondary hypodense lesion at the anterior pole of the spleen. Small nodal centimetric swellings at the splenic hilum and in the peripancreatic region. The lower pole of the right kidney shows an irregular solid formation measuring 37 × 46 mm, that has no enhancement after contrast medium. Small nodes can be seen in the intercavo—para-aortic and left aortic regions.

- PET-FDG: pathological glucose consumption of the left upper lobe lung mass at the dorsal segment in the sub-pleural posterior region, SUVmax 23. Lymphadenopathy with increased metabolic activity in the aorto-pulmonary window and right hilum (SUVmax 9). Presence of some lymph nodes with intense metabolism of glucose in the abdomen, respectively at splenic hilum, in the peripancreatic region (SUVmax 7) and in the left para-aortic region (SUVmax 10). Non-pathological FDG metabolism of kidney lower right polar mass, already treated with radiotherapy in the past.

Stereotactic radiotherapy (SRT) of the left lung lesion associated with chemotherapy.

62.2 Diagnostic Question

Search for focal lesions with high metabolism of glucose in a patient with double cancer: restaging 3 months after the radio-chemotherapy treatment.

62.3 Report

Compared to the previous PET study, the lung mass seen at the dorsal segment of the left upper lobe shows marked reduction of carbohydrate consumption, SUVmax 2.4.

Lymphadenopathy with high deposition of FDG at the aorto-pulmonary window, right pulmonary hilum, SUVmax 16, in the left lateral cervical region and more intense in the ipsilateral clavicular fossa, SUVmax 14.

Lymph nodes with increased metabolism of glucose at the anterior pole of the spleen, splenic hilum and in the peripancreatic region, SUVmax 19.

Slight increase in the deposition of the tracer in a right costal arch.

No substantial accumulation of the previously radiotreated renal cancer.

P. F. Rambaldi, *Whole-Body FDG PET Imaging in Oncology*,
DOI: 10.1007/978-88-470-5295-6_62, © Springer-Verlag Italia 2014

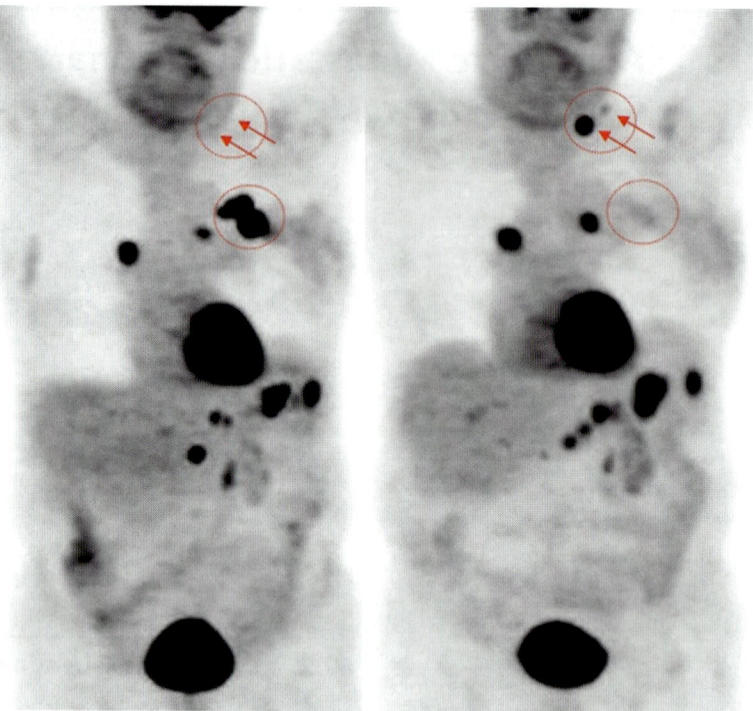

Fig. 62.1 The MIP image shows metabolic response of the left lung mass but there is a clear progression of disease in all mediastinal and abdominal injuries. Moreover, we find the appearance of new metastatic lymph nodes in the left clavicular fossa and in the ipsilateral region 81 lateral cervical

62.4   Conclusions

The PET study shows a net reduction of glucose metabolism at the left lung mass due to response to radiation therapy.

Progression of disease in the remaining districts is reported as poor response to chemotherapy. See Figs. 62.1, 62.2, 62.3, 62.4, 62.5.

62.5   Key Points

- The double primary tumors are not uncommon in the elderly. They are divided into synchronous and metachronous: Synchronous are those that arise simultaneously, metachronous are those that are detected after a certain time interval. The metachronous primary lung cancers are the most common class of multiple primary lung cancers, accounting for 50–70 % of metachronous tumors.
- The high carbohydrate consumption supports the biological aggressiveness of lung cancer both before and after treatment.
- In the presence of multiple metastases, an aggressive chemoradiotherapy approach rarely substantially alters the natural history of the disease.
- In this patient, both primary tumors responded to radiation therapy, but the progression of metastases at follow-up shows the chemoresistance of the disease.

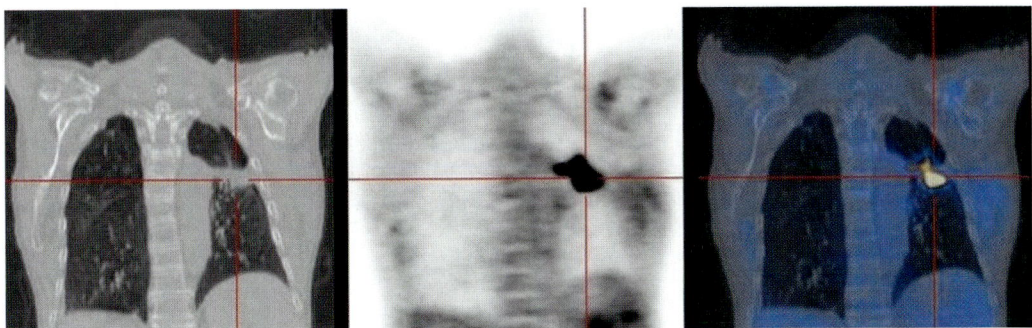

Fig. 62.2 The coronal reconstruction of CT-PET performed before radiation therapy shows the metabolism of the left lung neoplasm, presenting with dendritic branches in connection with the parietal pleura and mediastinum

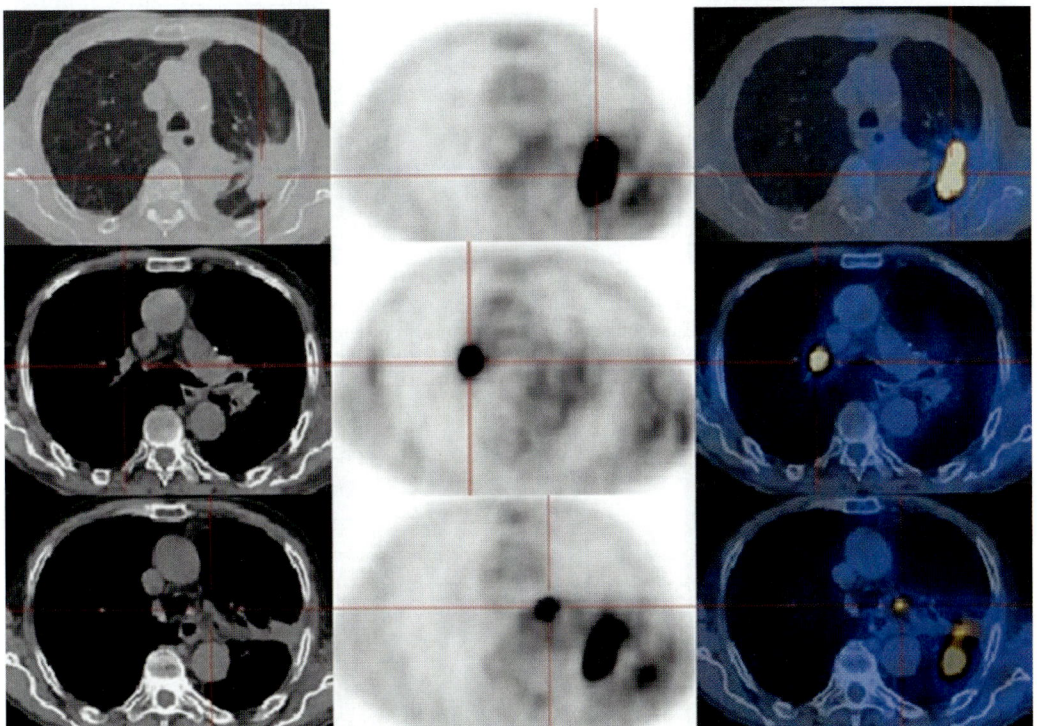

Fig. 62.3 Before the radio-chemotherapy, CT-PET shows the dorsal segment of the upper lobe of the left lung in close contact with the posterior parietal pleura, a solid speculated mass with irregular margins, which has extensive metabolism. Lymphadenopathy is associated with increased deposition of FDG at the level of the aorto-pulmonary window and right hilum

Radiation therapy in these cases only has a palliative role, and the evolution of the disease does not change.

In patients with two tumors, it is not always possible to understand the exact origin of each metastasis.

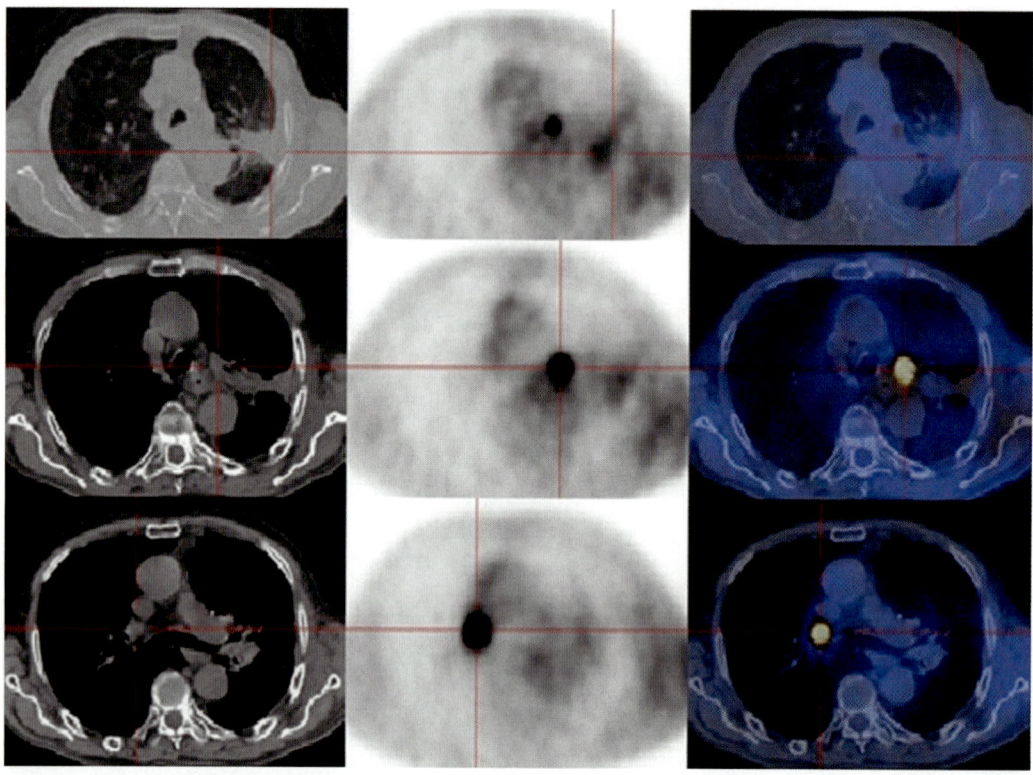

Fig. 62.4 After radio-chemotherapy, CT-PET shows volume reduction and the metabolism of left lung cancer. Increased deposition of glucose in correspondence of the lymph nodes at the aorto-pulmonary window and right hilum as in progression of disease

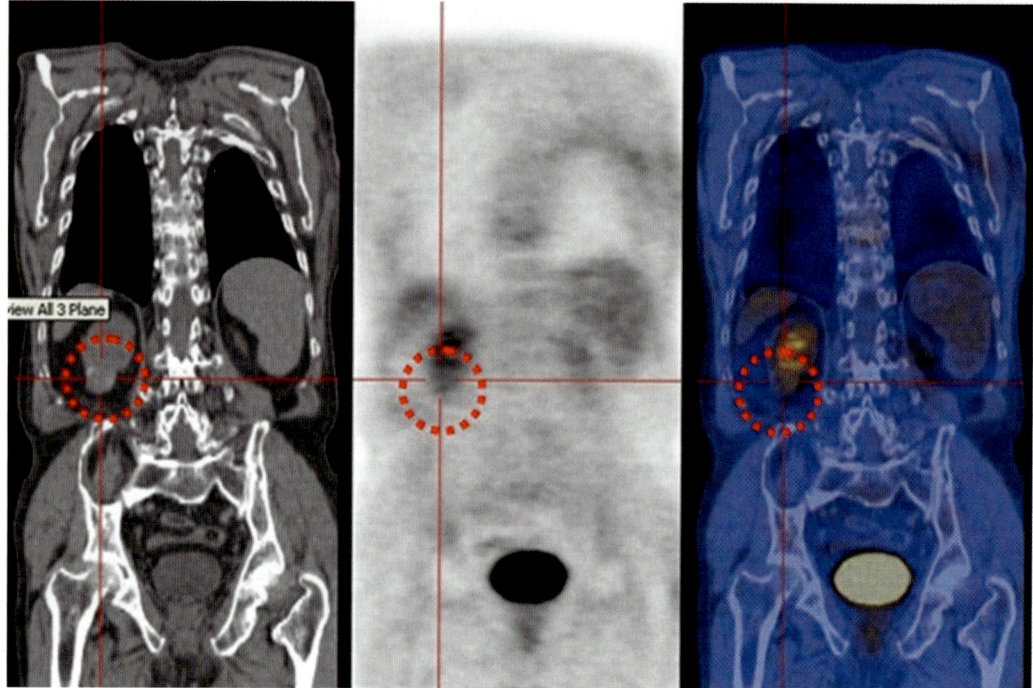

Fig. 62.5 Coronal reconstruction CT-PET detects a solid mass at the lower pole of the right kidney, with regular margins and a low consumption of glucose, due to post-actinic stabilized fibrotic outcomes

The clear-cell renal cell carcinomas usually express a low consumption of FDG and rarely determine lymph node metastases with a high metabolism.

Lung cancers are characterized by high concentration of FDG.

In this patient, the CT-PET performed before radiotherapy showed the intense deposition of glucose and lung masses and lymph nodes therefore appear to have comparable metabolic and biological behavior, so they are compatible with metastasis of lung cancer.

Lymphocytic Interstitial Pneumonia in Patient with History of Breast Cancer

63

63.1 Clinical History

47-year-old woman, who underwent left mastectomy for intraductal multifocal carcinoma, G3. Quadrantectomy was subsequently performed for a right mammary lobular in situ carcinoma.

Follow-up after 2 years:
- CT: presence of multiple pulmonary nodules on both sides.
- PET-FDG: multiple pulmonary nodules bilaterally with high accumulation, the most evident on the right, SUVmax 4.9.
- atypical resection of the dominant right pulmonary nodule and histologic diagnosis of lymphocytic interstitial pneumonia (LIP) with diffuse lymphoid hyperplasia.

63.2 Diagnostic Question

Search for focal lesions with high glucose metabolism in woman with lymphocytic interstitial pneumonia and bilateral breast cancer in clinical-instrumental remission, in the third year of follow-up.

63.3 Report

The PET scan shows multiple pulmonary nodules characterized by a pathological increase in the consumption of glucose, the most evident at the dorsal segment of the right lower lobe, SUVmax 5.3. No areas of abnormal metabolism in the remaining parts of the body examined.

63.4 Conclusions

PET framework compatible with persistence of biological activity of disease (LIP). See Figs. 63.1, 63.2.

63.5 Key Points

In the presence of multiple pulmonary nodules of dubious nature, excisional biopsy rules out metastatic disease. This should not be repeated during follow-up if the patient is stable.

A chronic, rheumatic systemic disease should be suspected when there are obvious signs and symptoms of infection. We can say that the PET in this patient allows us to:

P. F. Rambaldi, *Whole-Body FDG PET Imaging in Oncology*,
DOI: 10.1007/978-88-470-5295-6_63, © Springer-Verlag Italia 2014

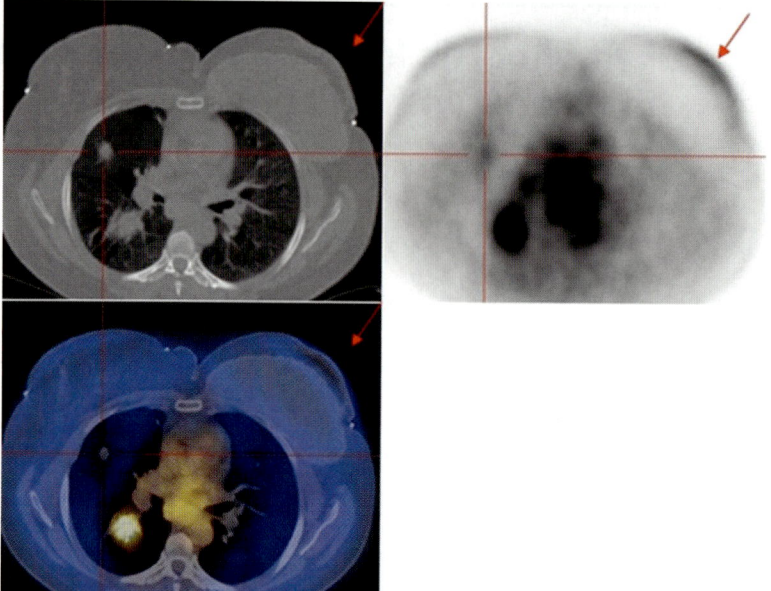

Fig. 63.1 In the same axial scan, CT-PET shows two pulmonary nodules on the right that have different sizes and carbohydrate consumption. On the left, the CT shows some millimetric pulmonary nodules, not detected by PET due to resolving limits. Presence of left breast implant with moderate carbohydrate consumption and widespread adjacent soft tissue non-specific inflammatory reaction

- exclude metastases from breast cancer with high glucose metabolism in other organs and systems,
- exclude the occurrence of a second tumor,
- evaluate the metabolic activity of the lymphocytic pneumonia as an accessory element.

In immunocompromised patients, the clinical and instrumental surveillance must be very close because there is a greater likelihood of recurrence of disease or the occurrence of a second tumor.

Fig. 63.2 a The CT scan shows the presence of multiple solid pulmonary nodules with irregular margins, which does not have the typical characteristics of metastases. The PET shows glucose consumption due to the persistence of biological activity of lymphocytic ▶ interstitial pneumonia (**b**)

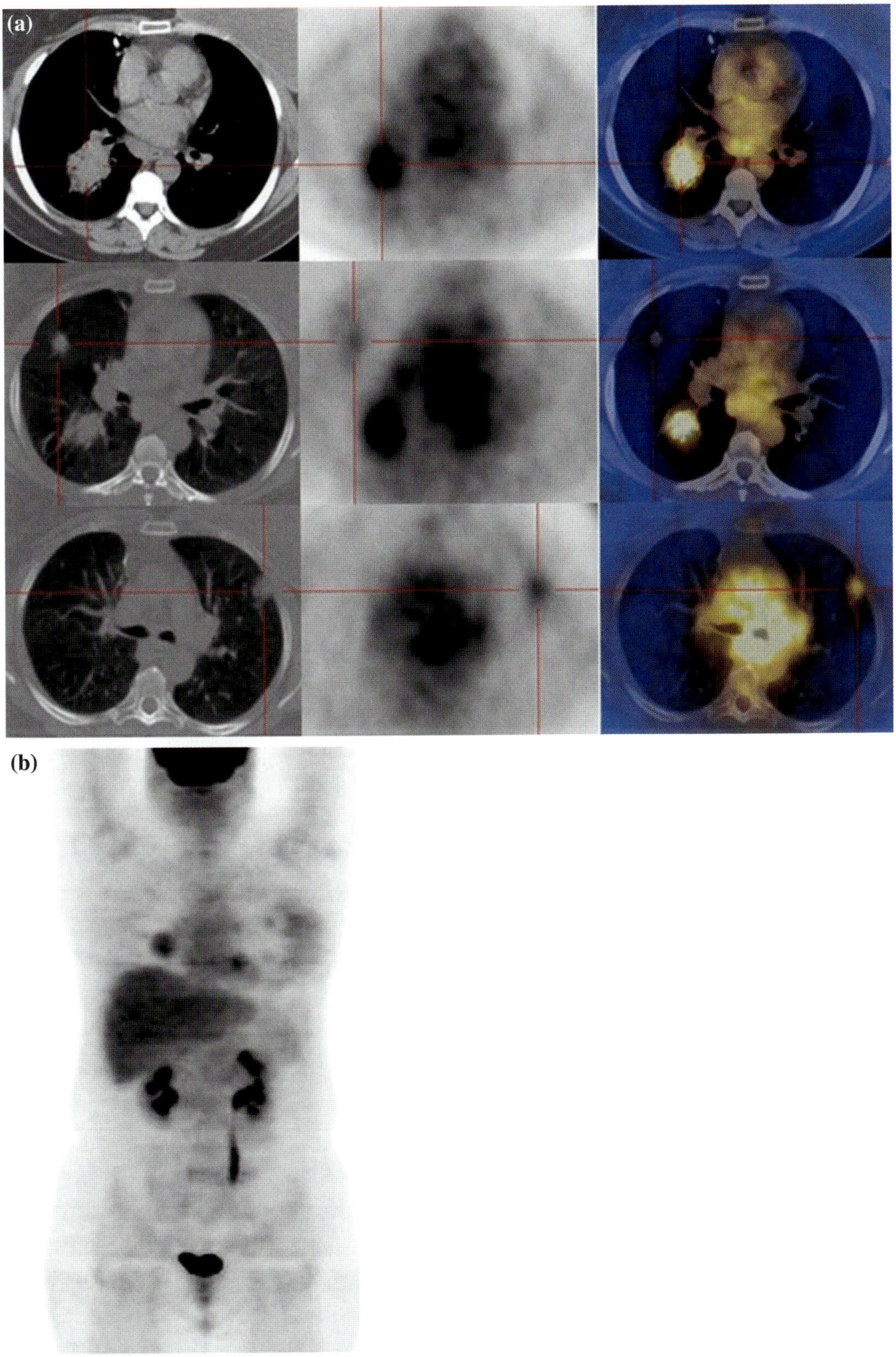

(a)

(b)

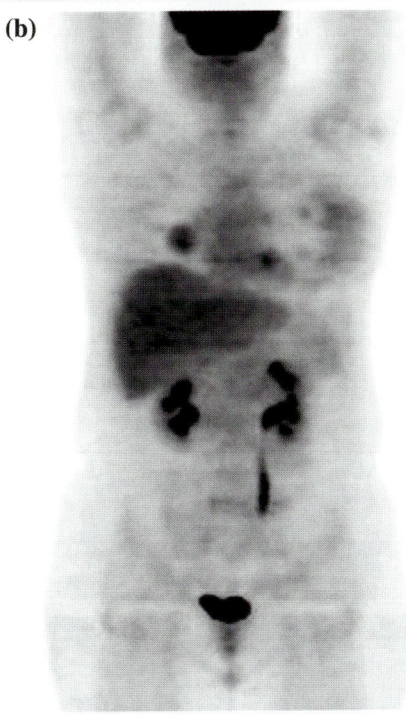

Mucinous Cancer Recurrence

64

64.1 Clinical History

Atypical pulmonary resection for adenocarcinoma with papillary and mucinous aspects, pT2, pneumothorax, PMX in 61 year-old patient, bearer of liver transplantation.

Post-surgical revaluation.

- CT: presence of adenopathy adjacent to the left pulmonary artery and ipsilateral hilar lower region, with a maximum axial diameter of 20 and 18 mm. Centimetric tissue thickening at the site of previous surgery.
- PET does not detect disease with high metabolic activity.

Follow-up at six months.

- CT: minimum volumetric increase of lymph node near the left pulmonary artery which shows now a maximum axial diameter of 25 mm and has partially necrotic appearance; slight volumetric increase of the lower left hilar adenopathy. Although both negative at a recent PET study, they are likely metastatic. Unchanged disventilatory fibrotic striae contiguous to the likely origin of the surgical scar.
- Trans-bronchial fine-needle aspiration cytology of a mediastinal lymph node: in one of the nine prepared slides there are massive atypical cells, with occasional intra-cytoplasmic inclusions related to adenocarcinoma.

64.2 Diagnostic Question

Search for lesions with high FDG metabolism in patient with recurrent pulmonary adenocarcinoma with papillary and mucinous aspects: restaging.

64.3 Report

Modest consumption of glucose in the latero-basal segment of the lower lobe of the left lung due to scarring, SUVmax 2.3.

Lymphadenopathy of low metabolic activity in the left hilar middle-lower region and at the aorto-pulmonary window, SUV max 1.7.

Modest glucose consumption of the left sixth rib, SUV max 1.6, of the right femur in the trochanteric region and cervical spine at C3—C4 level, SUV max 2.9. Useful correlation with bone scan and or MRI with contrast medium.

64.4 Conclusions

Patient with histologically documented metastases at a mediastinal lymph node, shows low carbohydrate consumption disease at PET study

P. F. Rambaldi, *Whole-Body FDG PET Imaging in Oncology*,
DOI: 10.1007/978-88-470-5295-6_64, © Springer-Verlag Italia 2014

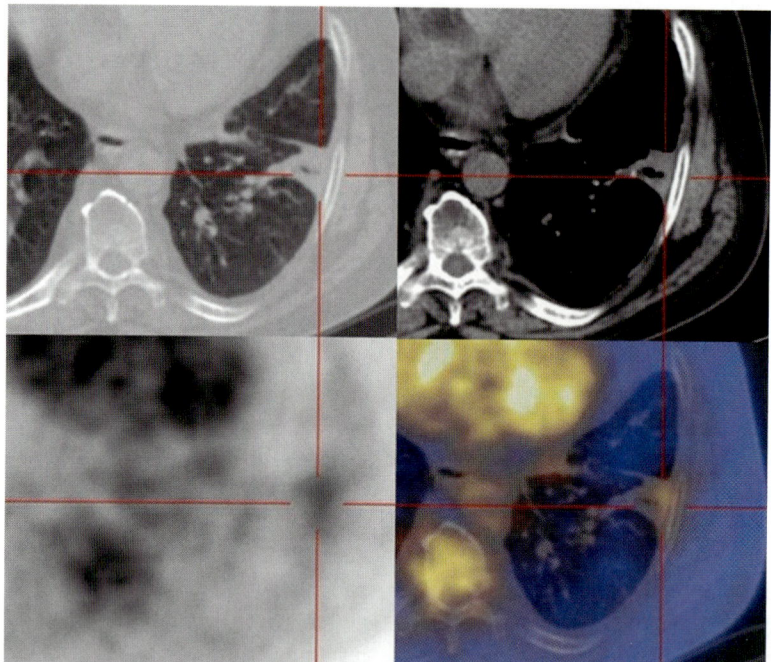

Fig. 64.1 CT-PET shows partial resection the lower left lung lobe, with centimetric contextual fibrotic tissue thickening and striae—scars that reach the hilum; mild carbohydrate consumption of the lesion

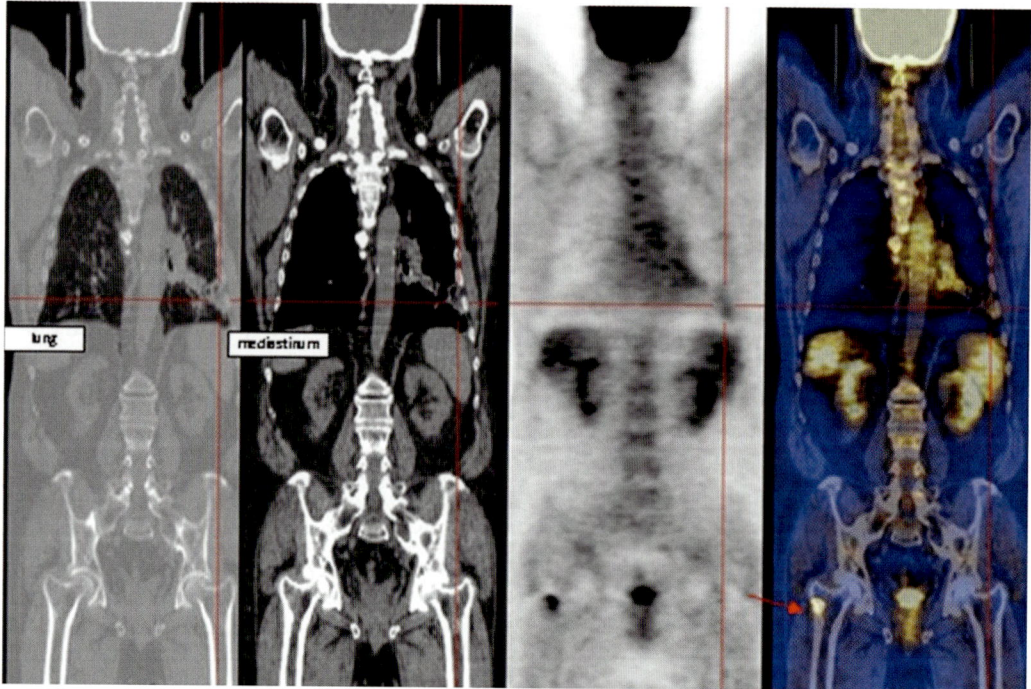

Fig. 64.2 The coronal reconstructions show a bone-producing lesion to the greater trochanter of the right femur, that has limited metabolism

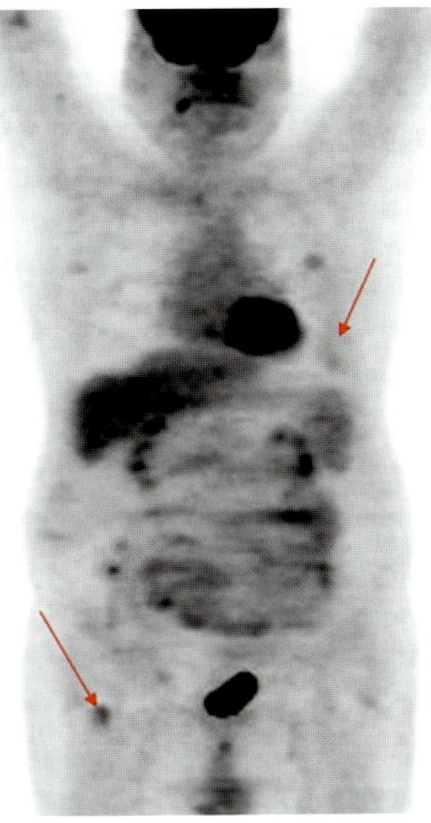

Fig. 64.3 MIP image in patients with liver transplantation, FDG-PET examination frequently shows nonspecific background high uptake due to the slow clearance of the tracer, especially in the abdomen. As immunosuppressed patients have a higher incidence of new cancers and are therefore considered a high-risk category, some authors suggest surveillance with CT-PET

today, typical of papillary and mucinous adenocarcinomas.

In subsequent follow-up after therapy, contrast-enhanced CT is suggested to evaluate the therapeutic response and the growth parameters of individual lesions. See Figs. 64.1, 64.2, 64.3.

64.5 Key Points

Mucinous tumors generally have a limited glucose metabolism.

It is also known that PET with FDG can be positive even in the presence of inflammatory phenomena.

Many experiments have shown that FDG accumulates significantly in the case of inflammation that, if determined by neoplasia (peritumoral inflammation), may also be of help in improving the localization of small lesions. This phenomenon is due to the overexpression of the glucose transporters, especially type Glut-1; it is also known that the FDG accumulates in activated granulocytes.

The lack of cellular metabolism of FDG generally correlates with a slower progression of the disease.

The potential of PET in establishing a diagnosis in mucinous neoplasms may therefore be limited by the possible impact of false positives and false negatives.

When the FDG-PET shows low-activity lesion in the post-chemotherapy follow-up, a contrast-enhanced CT should be performed.

To reduce diagnostic errors, the following are essential:

- A precise clinical history,
- An evaluation of previous diagnostic tests (CT, MRI, echo, etc.)
- re-evaluate the PET examination performed at diagnosis to define the biological activity of the primary tumor.

In the course of restaging, a meticulous comparison of PET and CT images performed during the diagnosis or staging to determine even small volumetric changes and metabolic disorders must be made.

Epidermoid Pulmonary Cancer: Follow-up After Surgery

65

65.1 Clinical History

Left superior pulmonary lobectomy and mediastinal lymphadenectomy for epidermoid carcinoma infiltrating the parietal pleura, pT3, pN0, PM0 in a 74-year-old man.

  Post-surgical revaluation.
- CT: right adrenal thickening with small focal, probably metastatic lesion measuring 15 mm.
- PET-FDG: small nodular area of hyperaccumulation in the right adrenal gland.

  Follow-up three years after.
- CT: volumetric increase of the right adrenal gland, inhomogeneous in densitometry due to the presence of a small focal lesion, which was unchanged compared to the previous controls.
- Bone scan: absence of focal lesions. Intense accumulation of the tracer in some ribs on the right, due to previous trauma.

65.2 Diagnostic Question

Left lung cancer in follow-up: look for focal lesions with a high metabolism of glucose.

65.3 Report

The PET scan shows no areas of abnormal glucose consumption in the body areas examined, therefore excluding focal lesions in place.

The right adrenal nodule reported by previous diagnostic tests has no pathological metabolism.

Modest increase in the deposition of FDG in some right ribs, due to recent trauma, SUV max 2.2.

65.4 Conclusions

The survey PET revealed no significant focal areas of pathological consumption of glucose in the body areas examined indicate a resumption of pathology within the limits solving and biological method. See Figs. 65.1, 65.2.

65.5 Key Points

The trauma may be direct or indirect: in the first case, the fracture occurs at the point of application of force, and in the second case, at a distance from the point of application.

In bone fractures caused by primary or metastatic tumors of the skeleton, the CT shows a morphostructural lytic or thickening alteration. In some cases, this can be a fair share of the newly formed tissue that exceeds the margins of the bone itself. The metabolic alteration is determined by the high biological activity of neoplastic cells that occupy the marrow space in a disorderly and irregular manner, until reaching the cortex than in the advanced stages is thinned and eroded. Under these circumstances, even small traumatic events may be critical. In the

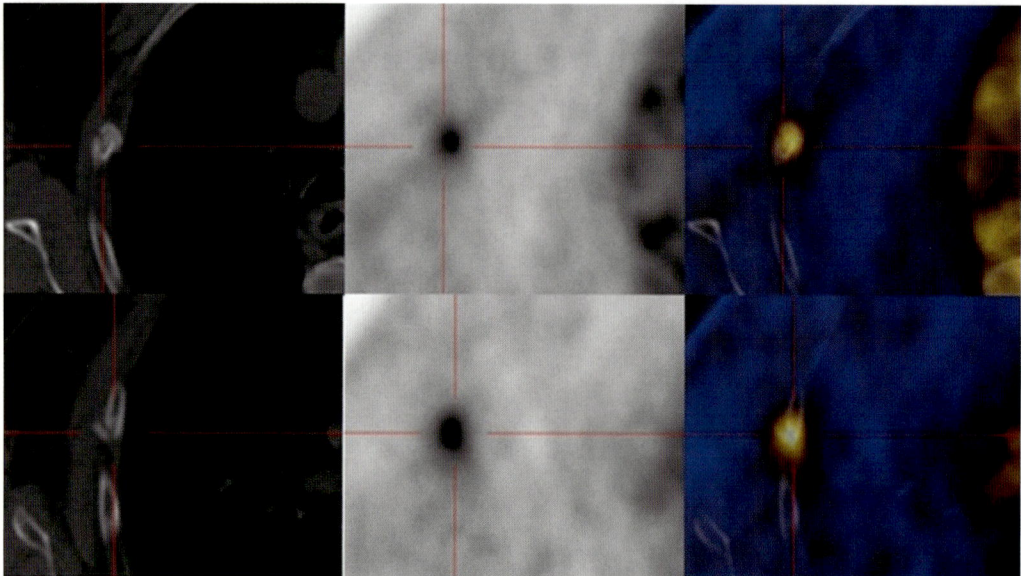

Fig. 65.1 The PET-CT scan shows apparent two broken ribs, and there is no contextual detects the newly formed tissue even if there is moderate carbohydrate consumption by activating reparative bone marrow

Fig. 65.2 CT-PET detects the volumetric expansion of the right adrenal gland that appears hypodense but is not characterized by abnormal metabolism, so it is benign In a patient who does not show signs and symptoms of endocrine disorders, an adrenal nodule that has no volumetric increase in time and does not concentrate FDG can be considered an incidentaloma

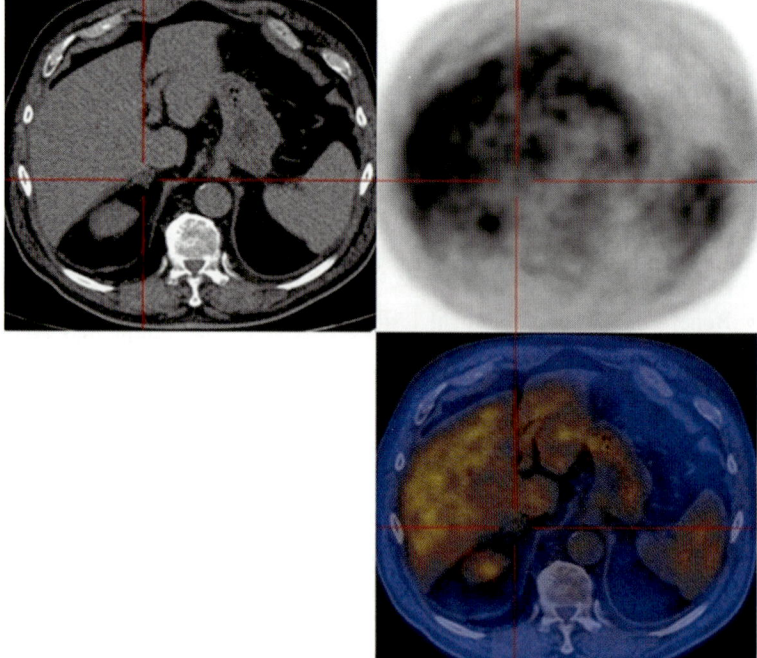

long bones, the concentration of the tracer assumes a characteristic elliptical shape for the prevailing marrow expansion of the tumor.

The "pathological fractures" may also be determined in several benign diseases of the bone, first of all osteoporosis. In these cases, it is not always a traumatic event the cause of the fracture. These fractures are characterized by an increase in carbohydrate consumption in the early stages at PET scans, the expression of moderate inflammatory reaction associated with cellular reparative bone marrow activity. Metabolism is reduced progressively returning to normal after a few months, when the healing is complete.

The post-traumatic benign bone lesions appear with rounded development of the biological activity at the edge of the fracture along the lines of direct and indirect forces that determined the skeletal and bone marrow damage.

In case of an accident, you have to suspect a post-traumatic fracture.

Pulmonary Cancer with Numerous Nodal Hilar-Mediastinic and Bone Metastases

66

66.1 Clinical History

Left quadrantectomy performed for a DIC pT1, pN0, PM0, in a 68-year-old woman.

The patient underwent chemotherapy.

Follow-up seven years after.

- Bone scan: negative for focal lesions.
- XR of dorsal-lumbar-sacral spine: absence of focal lesions.

After six months.

- Tumor markers: CEA, CA 125, CA 19-9, alpha-fetoprotein are all normal.
- MR-lumbosacral spine: signal alteration of the soma of D11 and L5 extended to pedicles, characterized by low signal on T1 and homogeneous signal on T2, as secondary localizations of the underlying disease.

The patient complains of diffuse bone pain, worst in the dorsal and lumbar spine, that prevents her from performing normal daily activities.

66.2 Diagnostic Question

Search for focal lesions with high glucose metabolism in patient with breast cancer in remission for seven years and recently diagnosed with bone metastases.

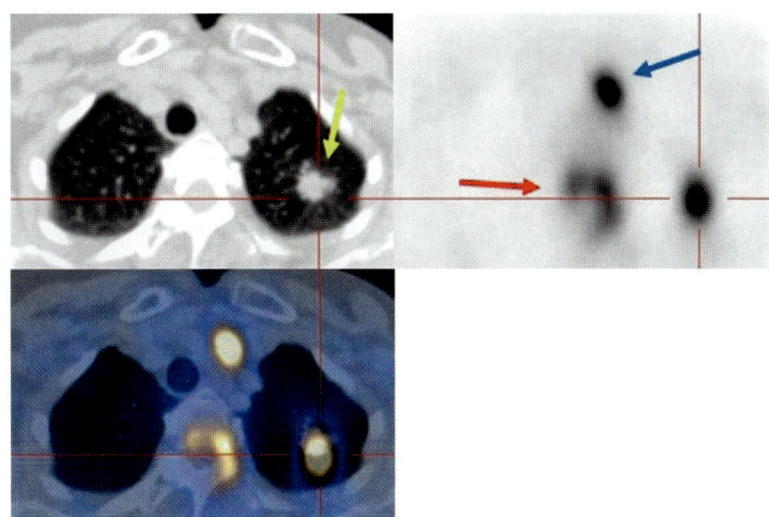

Fig. 66.1 PET-CT images with parenchymal window show a left solid, uneven, apical lung nodule, with branches infiltrating the surrounding parenchyma (*yellow arrow*). There are also multiple lymph nodes of increased size (*blue arrow*) and a metastasis at the level of a dorsal vertebra (*red arrow*). All of these lesions have high metabolism

P. F. Rambaldi, *Whole-Body FDG PET Imaging in Oncology*,
DOI: 10.1007/978-88-470-5295-6_66, © Springer-Verlag Italia 2014

66.3   Report

Left apical lung nodule characterized by abnormal glucose consumption, SUV max 16. High metabolic activity of multiple mediastinal lymph nodes at the hilar, prevascular, pretracheal, carinal, subcarinal level on both sides, internal mammary chain, Barety space and the aorto-pulmonary window, SUV max 17.

Abnormal glucose metabolism in multiple vertebrae (D3, D4, D5, D7, D10, D11, L5), left sacroiliac, the shaft of the proximal ipsilateral humerus and the right scapula to report to metastatic injuries, SUV max 12. See Fig. 66.1.

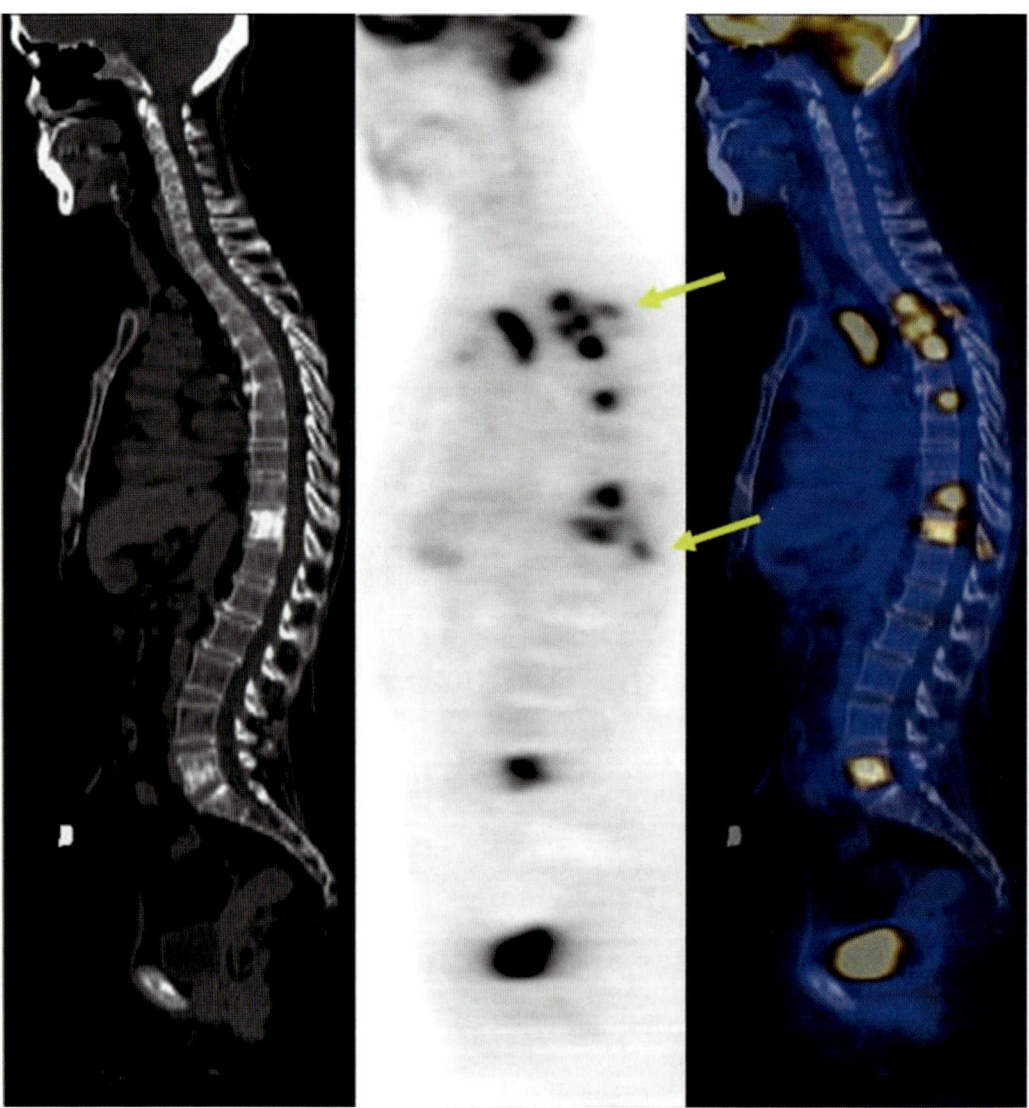

Fig. 66.2 The sagittal CT scan reconstruction of the spine shows thickening of two vertebral bodies, D11 and L5 that at the PET scan have high metabolism. There were no thickening morphostructural alterations at D3, D4, D5, D7, D10 and some spinous processes (D3, D11), which, however, are characterized by high consumption of glucose. This finding suggests the presence of bone marrow metastases that have not yet determined a bone producing skeletal alteration in, an event that is realized only belatedly

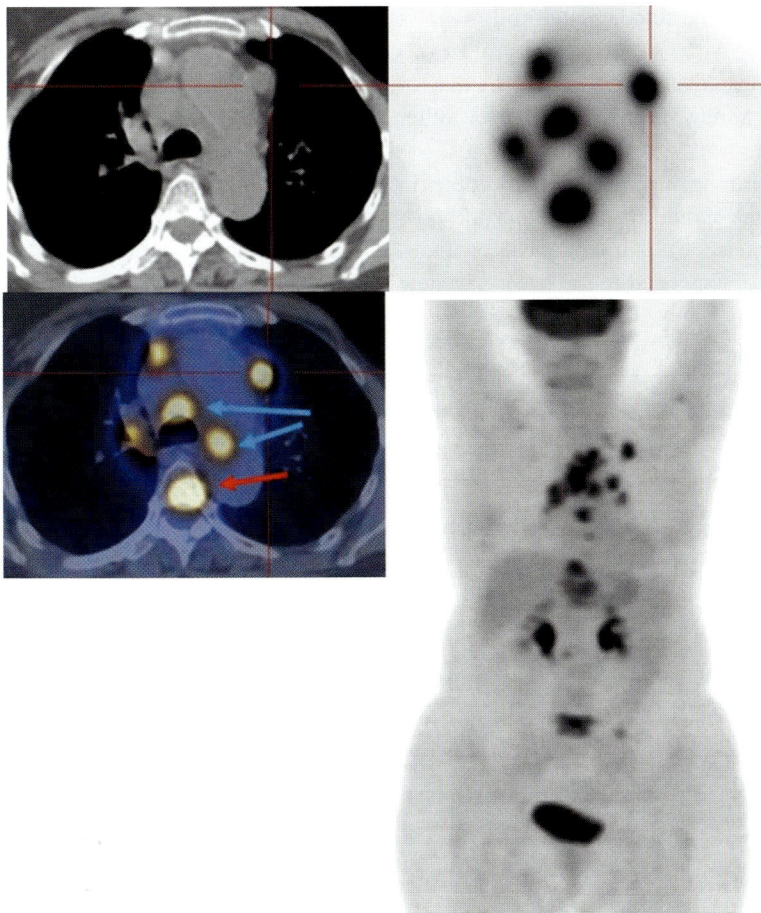

Fig. 66.3 PET-CT images with mediastinal window show multiple enlarged lymph nodes increased in size at the hilum, prevascular, pretracheal, the internal mammary chain, in the Barety space and aorto-pulmonary window (*blue arrow*). All have elevated glucose metabolism. Evidence of a vertebral dorsal metastasis (*red arrow*)

66.4 Conclusions

The PET scan suggests left lung cancer with multiple lymph node and bone metastases.

Histological definition of pulmonary nodule is suggested.

Less likely is the possibility of metastasis of breast cancer operated in 2001. See Figs. 66.2, 66.3.

66.5 Key Points

As we cannot exclude that a breast cancer (pT1, pN0, PM0) with negative follow-up for seven years is the cause of a dramatic and devastating lymph node and bone metastatic dissemination, a metachronous carcinoma should be suspected and excluded.

• Even if it depends on the location and histological type of the tumor, if the follow-up is negative for 5 years, the possibility of developing a metastatic lesion is equal to that of diagnosing a new primary cancer of other body districts.

- When performing a diagnostic procedure in oncology, one should never rule out the possible occurrence of morphological or functional alterations related to the onset of a new benign or malignant disease of other organs and systems.

- The probability that a finding can be attributed to new diagnostic pathology is as follows:
  - directly proportional to the number of years of follow-up spent in the absence of recurrence;
  - inversely proportional to the aggressiveness of the already known disease.

Follow-Up of Pulmonary Cancer After Surgery: Granulomatous Reaction on Scar

67.1 Clinical History

Atypical right upper lobe pulmonary resection for adenocarcinoma pT2, pN0, PM0 in man of 76 years.

The patient did not undergo chemotherapy and or radiotherapy.

Follow-up after one year:

- CT: lung fields are asymmetric due to outcomes for resection of the right upper lobe; residual fibrotic shoots and small subpleural parenchymal consolidation in the medium-apical and posterolateral regions. Modest thickening of the ipsilateral costal pleura. Mediastinum in axis with some subcentimetric lymph node swellings. Left adrenal gland slightly increased in size.

- Cancer markers: CEA = 4.45 ng/ml (nv < 4.5), CA19-9 = 7.52 U/ml (nv < 33) Alpha-fetoprotein = 0.90 IU/ml (nv < 10).
- PET-CT: pathological glucose consumption in the upper lobe of the right lung at the surgical site, SUV max 8. Lymphadenopathy in the Barety space with modest increase in carbohydrate consumption, SUV max 3.3.
- Bronchoscopy: absence of neoplastic cells, therefore we refer the patient to close follow-up CT.

Follow-up after two years:

- Bronchopneumonia treated with antibiotics. Presence of persistent cough and haemoptysis.
- CT: in the middle right lung field, presence of solid tissue with air bubble inside and metal clips from previous surgery. Evidence of

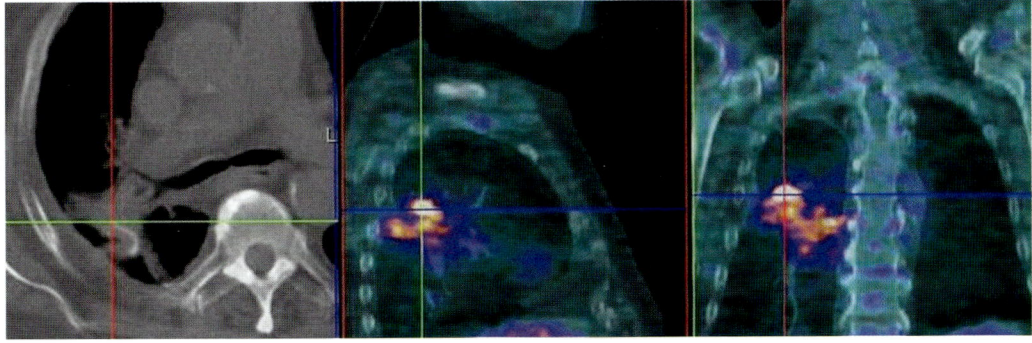

Fig. 67.1 The PET scan suggests granulomatous reaction of surgical scar to be confirmed by follow-up

P. F. Rambaldi, *Whole-Body FDG PET Imaging in Oncology*,
DOI: 10.1007/978-88-470-5295-6_67, © Springer-Verlag Italia 2014

Fig. 67.2 The CT-PET demonstrates lung fields to be asymmetric due to previous atypical pulmonary resection with some metal clips in correspondence of which seems to be a nodule with intense carbohydrate metabolism

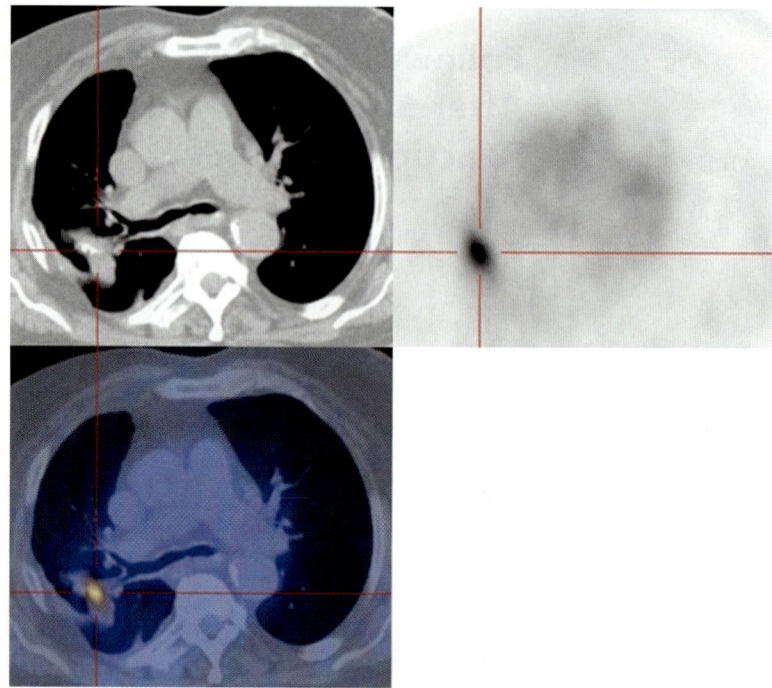

fibrotic stria continuous with the pleura. Subcentimetric node in the Barety space.

67.2　Diagnostic Question

Search for focal lesions with high glucose metabolism in patient with suspected recurrence of right lung adenocarcinoma.

67.3　Report

Nodule characterized by abnormal glucose consumption in the upper lobe of the right lung at the surgical site, intensity slightly decreased compared to the previous scan, SUV max 6.8.

No areas of abnormal metabolism in other parts of the body examined.

67.4　Conclusions

The PET scan suggests granulomatous reaction of surgical scar to be confirmed by follow-up (Fig. 67.1).

The CT-PET demonstrates lung fields to be asymmetric due to previous atypical pulmonary resection with some metal clips in correspondence of which seems to be a nodule with intense carbohydrate metabolism (Figs. 67.2, 67.3). This mass shows fibrotic branches that are

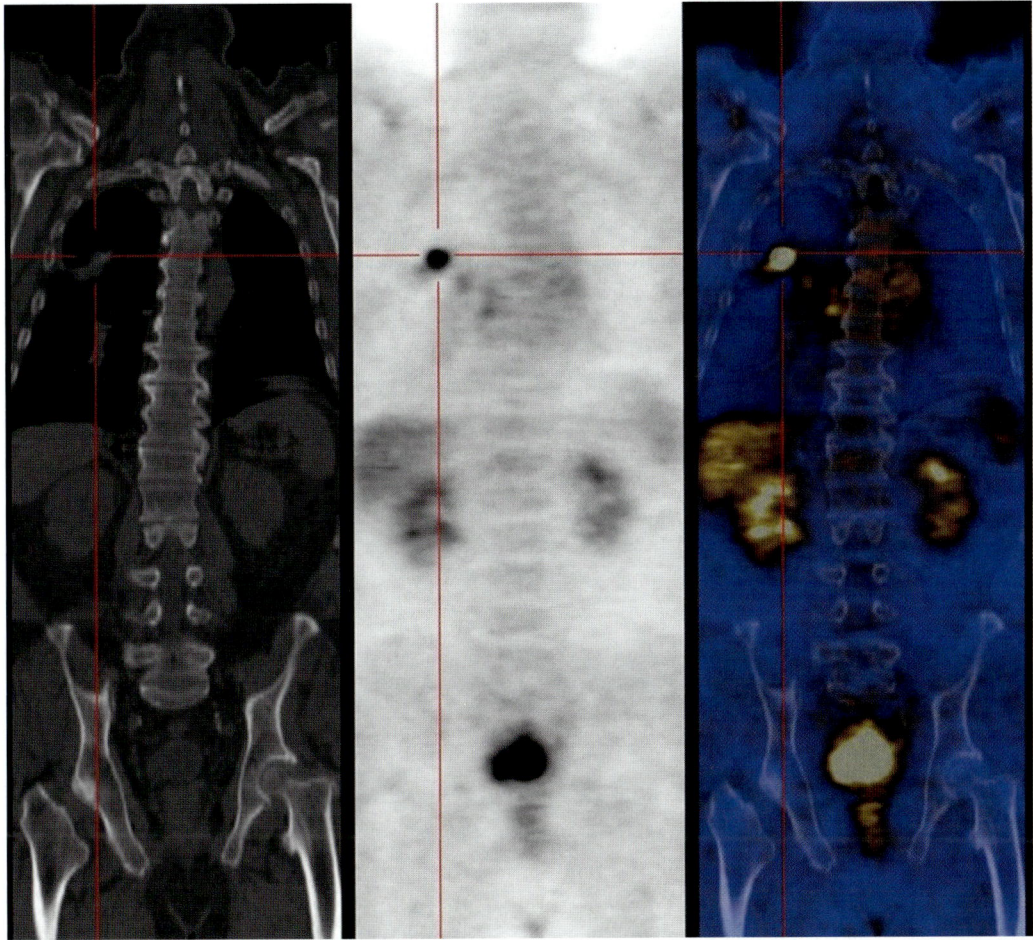

Fig. 67.3 This mass shows fibrotic branches that are related to the posterolateral pleura, which appears thickened although with no pathological metabolism.

related to the posterolateral pleura, which appears thickened although with no pathological metabolism.

In Figure 67.4, MIP image 1 year after the treatment (Fig. 67.4a) and 2 years after the treatment (Fig. 67.4b).

67.5 Key points

In patients undergoing atypical lung resection, differential diagnosis between locoregional recurrence of scar and granulomatous reaction is difficult.

- The first few months following surgery are characterized by an inflammatory reaction—reactive and later reparative—scar, sometimes intense, that later fades until it disappears almost completely at 6–12 months.
- The persistence of high metabolism suggests a chronic granulomatous reaction, especially when metabolic activity is restricted to the area adjacent to the metal clips or other devices used in resections.

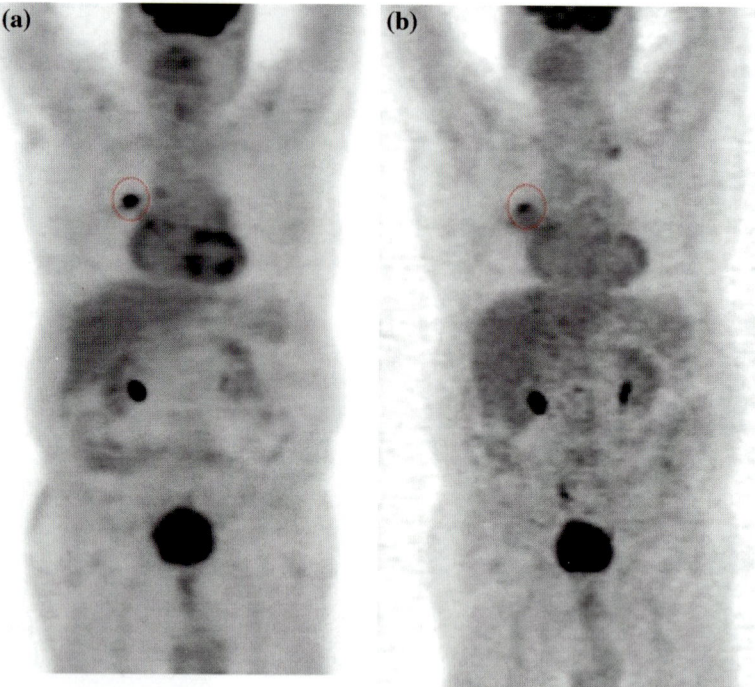

Fig. 67.4 In patients undergoing atypical lung resection, differential diagnosis between locoregional recurrence of scar and granulomatous reaction is difficult.

- In the differential diagnosis between recurrence and granulomatous reaction, the fundamental element is the critical review of previous CT and CT-PET scans to demonstrate the change in volume and metabolic activity of the nodule.

- It would be more appropriate to perform a bronchoscopy and or a FNAB. Alternatively, CT follow-up at three months is suggested following any volumetric increase of the lesion, without forgetting that these increases should be evaluated on the three-dimensional plane.

68.1 Clinical History

Left pneumonectomy for lung adenocarcinoma in a 59-year-old man.

He underwent adjuvant and neoadjuvant chemotherapy.

Follow-up after one year.

- FDG-PET: No focal lesions indicate a resumption of pathology. Area of increased uptake in the left, anterior to the heart, probably nonspecific.
- CT scan, chest, abdomen and pelvis: left pneumonectomy with a layer of residual liquid in the pleural cavity. Presence of fibrotic striae in the upper and in the basal lobe of the right lung.

Follow-up 2 years after.

- Abdominal ultrasound: negative for focal lesions.

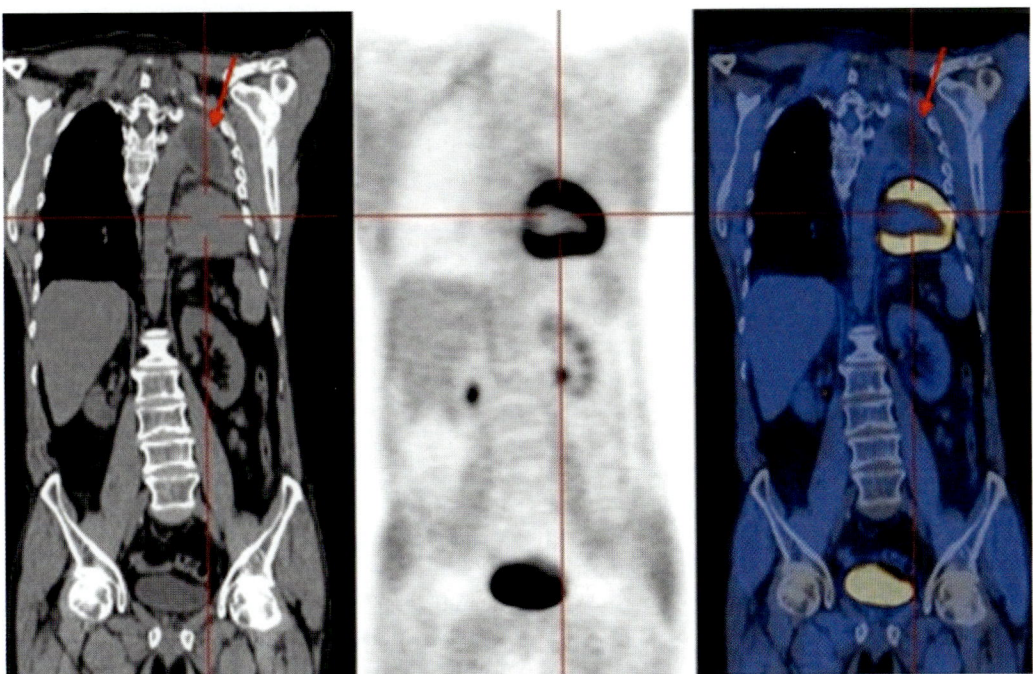

Fig. 68.1 At the CT there is evident massive opacification of the left hemithorax with marked attraction of mediastinal structures and pleural effusion

P. F. Rambaldi, *Whole-Body FDG PET Imaging in Oncology*,
DOI: 10.1007/978-88-470-5295-6_68, © Springer-Verlag Italia 2014

Fig. 68.2 The PET and axial MIP reconstruction image showed right ventricular hypertrophy and secondary pulmonary hypertension to the atria. No injuries to report a recurrence

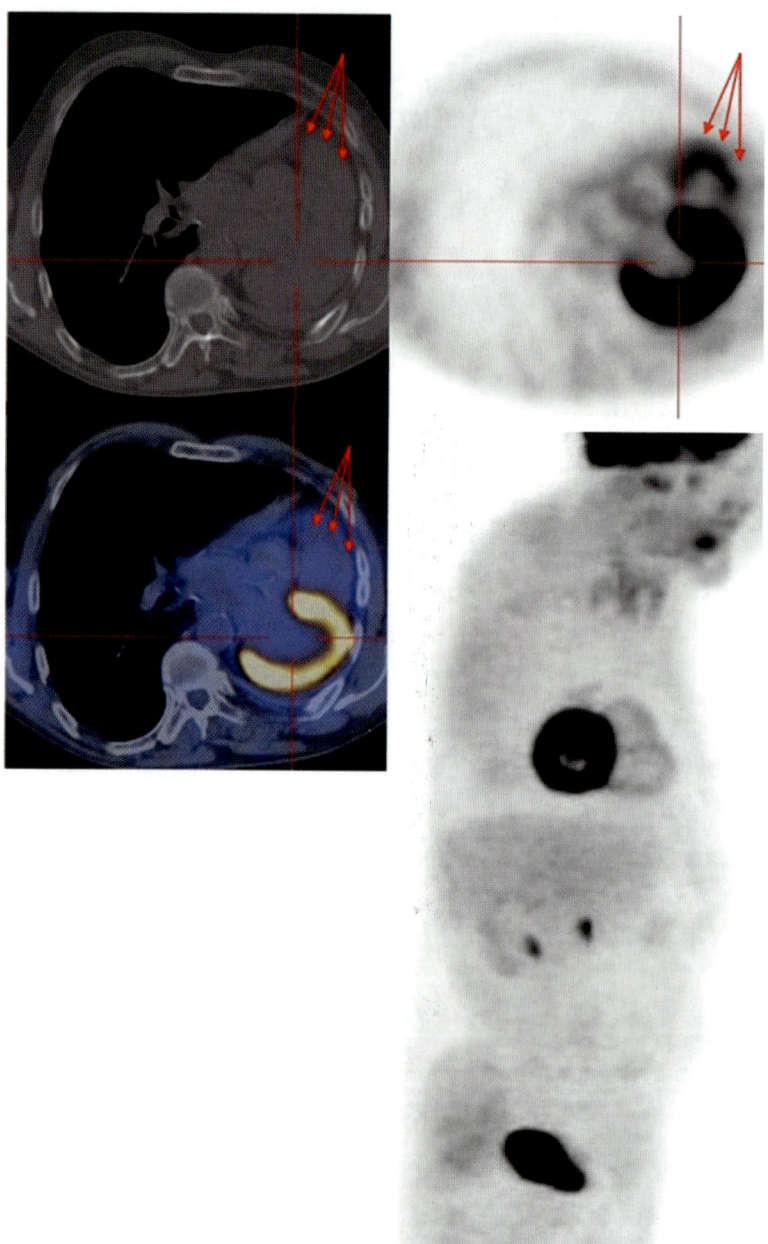

• Chest X-ray: no evidence of parenchymal right lesions in a patient with massive left hemithorax opacification and mediastinal hemithorax attraction.

68.2 Diagnostic Question

Search for focal lesions with high glucose metabolism in patient with previous lung cancer: follow-up.

68.3 Report

The PET does not show focal areas of abnormal glucose consumption indicating a metabolic recovery of lung cancer, in the context of massive left hemithorax opacification shown by previous scans.

Absence of repetitive injuries with high consumption of glucose in the remaining parts of the body examined.

68.4 Conclusions

The PET scan shows no focal lesions characterized by pathological FDG metabolism in the body areas examined indicating a recurrence of disease within the resolving and biological limits. See Fig. 68.1, 68.2.

68.5 Key Points

- In patients with NSCLC in clinical remission after surgery, CT-PET is indicated in the follow-up, especially when other diagnostic techniques provide doubtful or indeterminate answers.
- Nuclear medicine identifies the presence of locoregional recurrence, nodal mediastinal involvement, and distant metastases with high accuracy.
- Patients undergoing extended pulmonary resections may develop pulmonary hypertension secondary to hemodynamic overload of the small circle and a distortion of the mediastinal structures. In these cases, it detects an increased concentration of glucose for the secondary hypertrophy of the right heart, due to the high pressures of the small circle.

Pulmonary Solitary Nodule in Patient with Prostatic Adenocarcinoma in Follow-Up

69

69.1 Clinical History

75-year-old patient with prostatic adenocarcinoma, Gleason score 6 (3 + 3), in medical therapy, shows left pulmonary nodule, recently evaluated with biopsy and still waiting for cyto-histological report.

- Bone scan: negative for focal lesions.
- Chest CT: presence in the left upper lobe of a 27 mm lesion with irregular margins, which infiltrates the parietal pleura.

69.2 Diagnostic Question

Pulmonary nodule of nature to be determined in patient with prostate cancer: search for focal lesions with a high metabolism of glucose.

69.3 Report

Pulmonary nodule in the posterior segment of the left upper lobe, characterized by modest FDG metabolism, SUV max 3.

Absence of significant areas of pathological glucose consumption in the remaining parts of the body examined.

69.4 Conclusions

The PET scan shows a left pulmonary nodule that has modest increase in glucose metabolism, in part caused by secondary reactive inflammation to recent FNAB (Figs. 69.1, 69.2). In case of negative cyto-histological result, CT follow-up at 3 months will have to be performed, to define the volumetric evolution.

69.5 Key Points

In patients without a known malignancy, the presence of multiple pulmonary nodules ≥ 1 cm in diameter is most commonly due to metastatic lesions, and nodules < 5 mm in diameter, which overlap the visceral pleura or interlobular septa and are detected incidentally, are most commonly benign lesions.

In contrast, in patients with known cancer, the multiple pulmonary nodules ≥ 5 mm in diameter are more likely to be malignant.

The lung metastases generally have rounded appearance with sharply demarcated edges. Cavitation phenomena are found in less than 5 % of malignant lesions and are found mainly in squamous carcinomas.

P. F. Rambaldi, *Whole-Body FDG PET Imaging in Oncology*,
DOI: 10.1007/978-88-470-5295-6_69, © Springer-Verlag Italia 2014

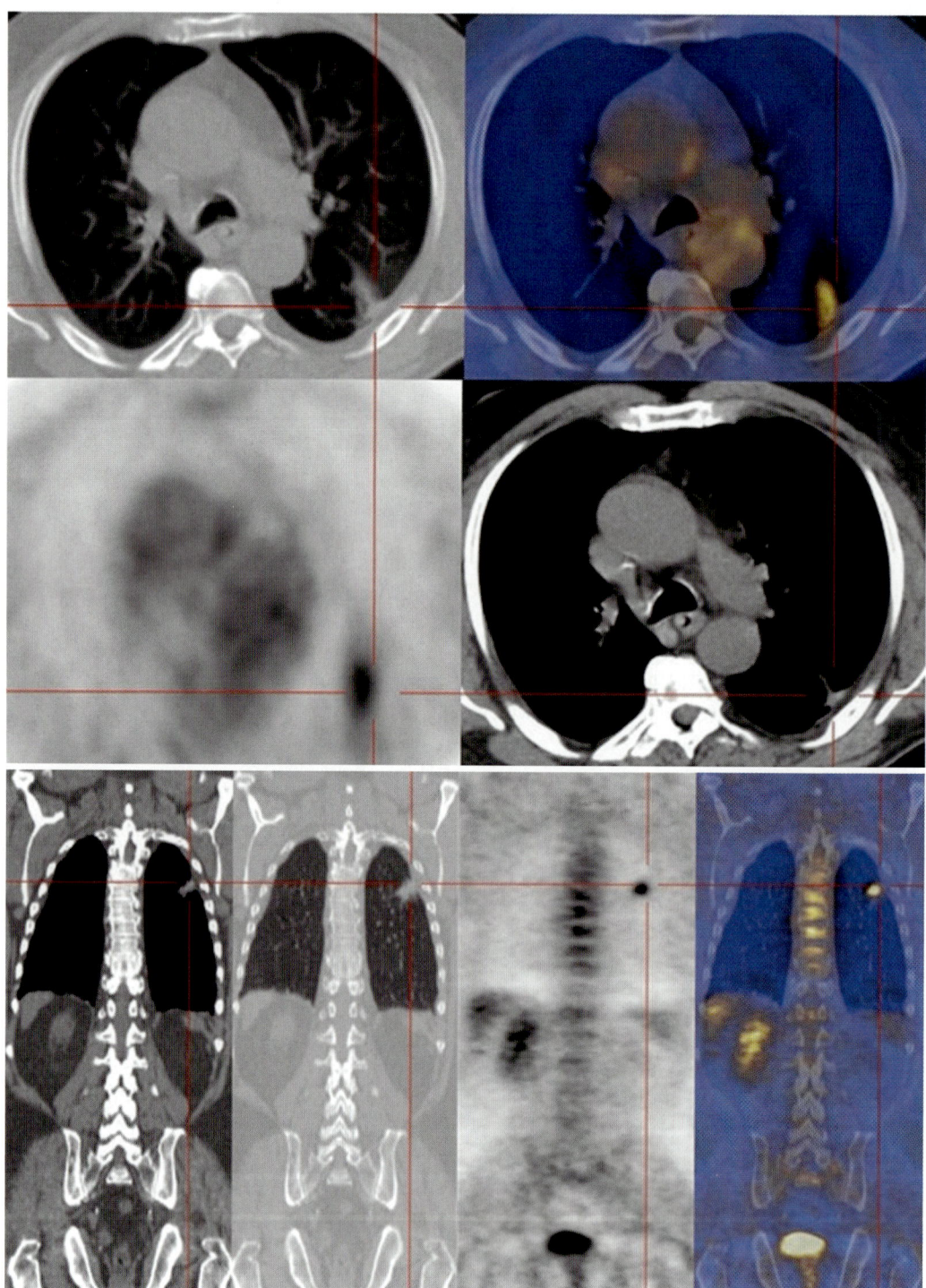

Fig. 69.1 At the posterior segment of the upper lobe of the left lung, CT-PET shows a parenchymal nodule with ill-defined margins, at the basis of the parietal pleura, that seems to infiltrate adjacent tissues due the presence of spikes. The biological activity of the lesion is low

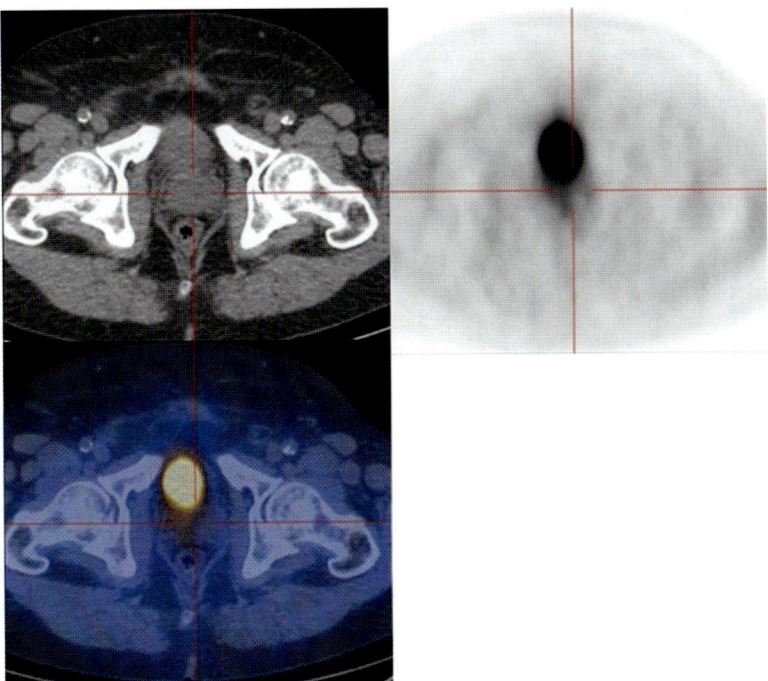

Fig. 69.2 The PET-CT scan shows a slightly increased prostate in size, with inhomogeneous density. There were no focal lesions characterized by high metabolism because prostatic adenocarcinomas have little affinity for FDG

A pulmonary condensation can be determined by
- bronchopneumonic or outbreak,
- bronchioloalveolar carcinoma.
  - A pulmonary nodule measuring 27 mm cannot be justified by an infectious episode and must be considered doubtful, therefore it was typed.
  - The transthoracic needle aspiration is the technique that has good sensitivity when a lesion is peripheral, while the bronchoscopy has higher accuracy in the definition of lesions adjacent to the bronchi.
  - The fine-needle aspiration may result in glucose uptake by nonspecific reactive inflammatory reaction.

As the previously performed cytologic examination did not show malignant cells, therefore a follow-up at three months with high-resolution CT was suggested.

In patients with solitary pulmonary nodules already evaluated with FNAB, CT-PET allows not only the metabolic lesional characterization but also allows you to exclude the presence of metastatic mediastinal lymph nodes and secondary lesions in any other organs and systems.

This should be emphasized in the report.

Bronchial Chemotreated Carcinoid: Progression of Disease

70.1 Clinical History

73-year-old man with left lung carcinoid and liver and bone metastases. Patient undergoes chemotherapy.

- PET study performed during chemotherapy: pathological increase of glucose metabolism in the posterior segment of the left upper lobe; rib, back and hepatic hilum injuries are negative.
- CT study after chemotherapy: The size of the expansive solid mass occupying the posterior segment of the left upper lobe is slightly reduced, measuring 38 × 28 mm in the axial plane. "Ground glass" of the adjacent paren- chyma. Presence of subcentimetric lymph nodes in the prevascular, left hilar, Barety space and in the aortopulmonary window. Small osteolytic areas to the body of the sternum (11 mm) and in correspondence of some dorsal vertebrae. Small liver hypodense formations (<1 cm), numerically increased when compared to the previous control.

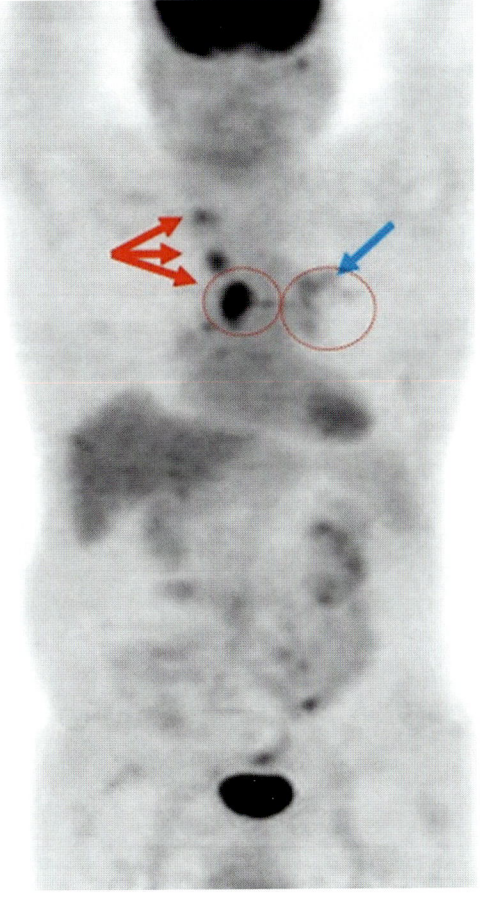

70.2 Diagnostic Question

Search for focal lesions with high glucose metabolism: restaging after chemotherapy for lung carcinoid.

Fig. 70.1 MIP image: bone metastases have a metabolic activity higher than that of the primary tumor, that probably has a contextual internal colliquation

P. F. Rambaldi, *Whole-Body FDG PET Imaging in Oncology*,
DOI: 10.1007/978-88-470-5295-6_70, © Springer-Verlag Italia 2014

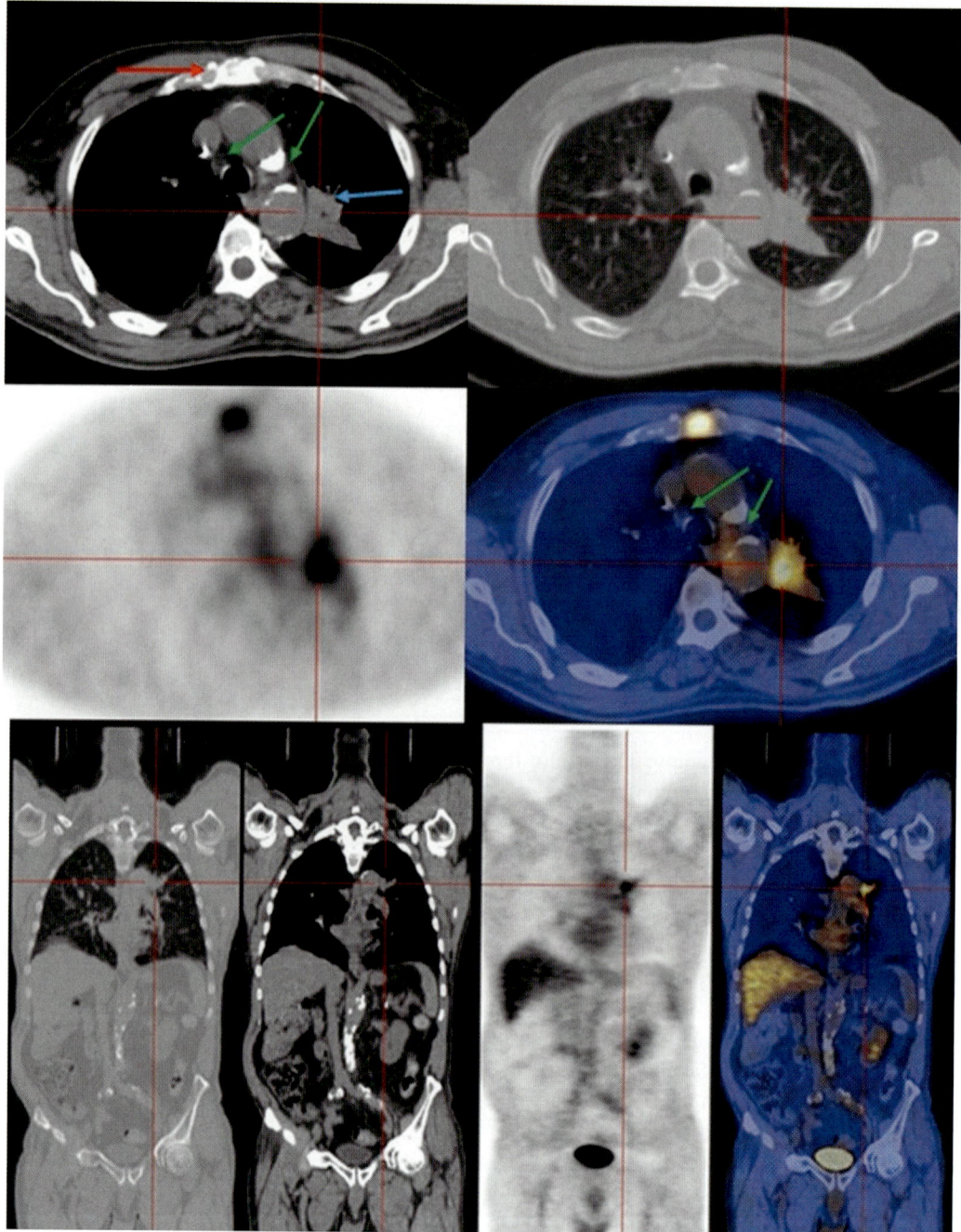

Fig. 70.2 The PET-CT scan shows a solid mass characterized by pathological metabolism at the posterior segment of the left upper lobe. This mass is spiculated, infiltrating the surrounding tissues, is inseparable from the mediastinal vascular structures and determines modest atelectasis of the parenchyma. The body of the sternum presents a lytic lesion with high metabolism. At the aortopulmonary window and the Barety space, CT shows some subcentimetric lymph nodes that do not have abnormal glucose consumption

Fig. 70.3 At CT, the posterior segment of the sixth right costal arch appears dysmorphic, swollen, with morphostructural alterations. In the same section at the body of the sternum another sub-centimeter lytic lesion with sclerotic margins can be seen. Both have high carbohydrate consumption

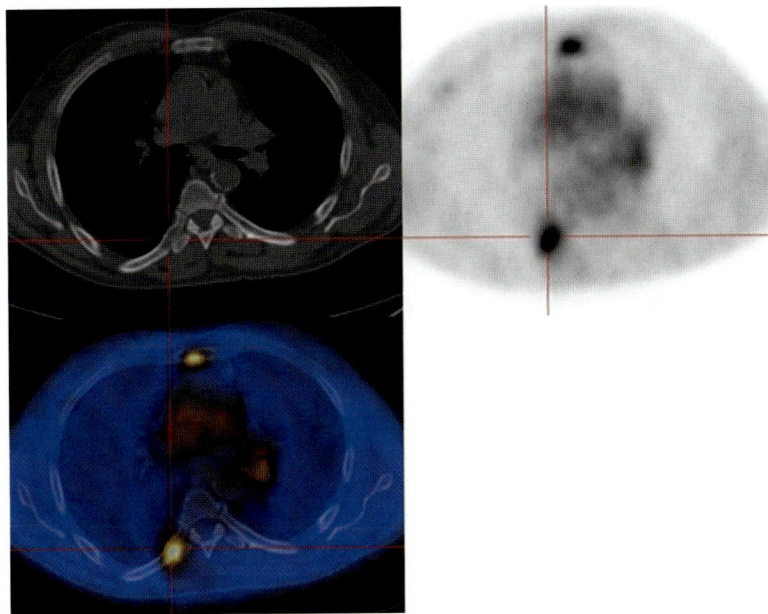

70.3   Report

The PET scan shows a lung mass characterized by a modest increase in the consumption of glucose to the posterior segment of the upper lobe of the left lung, SUV max 3.8.

Presence of metastatic bone lesions with a high metabolism at the sternum, the right clavicle, the soma of D8, the left transverse process of the fifth and sixth dorsal soma, sixth rib either on the anterior and posterior arches, SUV max 7.

The subcentimetric hepatic nodules reported by CT do not show pathological metabolism due to resolving limits.

70.4   Conclusions

The PET scan shows pathological metabolism of FDG in the left lung cancer and bone metastases as in a recurrent disease. See Figs. 70.1, 70.2, 70.3.

70.5   Key Points

The FDG-PET gives conflicting results when it comes to identify tumors of the APUD system, probably because of their small size and the limited metabolism of FDG. The use of other tracers, such as 11C-L-DOPA and 11C-5-hydroxytryptophan (11C-5-HT), could improve the sensitivity of imaging of neuroendocrine tumors, but the need for a cyclotron adjacent to nuclear medicine limits its clinical use.

- Consequently, in APUD neoplasms, the use of PET-FDG is controversial for the high incidence of false-negatives.
- In these cases, a careful evaluation of CT images acquired in co-registration is always important, because they help to morphologically identify lesions characterized by low metabolism.

Some authors believe that FDG-PET is still useful in the study of APUD tumors because the high consumption of glucose suggests

- intense cellular metabolism,
- increased aggressiveness,
- lesser differentiation.

We can say that when the FDG-PET performed during staging or restaging shows a high consumption of glucose:

- the prognosis is worse,
- a more aggressive therapeutic approach is suggested,
- PET can be used in the follow-up to determine the therapeutic response.

Pulmonary Actinomycosis in Dialysis Patient

71

71.1 Clinical History

45-year-old woman with chemo-treated NHL, clinical and in remission for 3 years documented as seen on both CT and CT-PET.

Comorbidity: Chronic renal failure, secondary to polycystic kidney disease on dialysis for a year.

Follow-up at 4 years, ten months after the start of dialysis.

- CT: symmetric lung fields with visibility of multiple small nodules bilaterally. Liver density inhomogeneous due to the presence of different hypodense nodules, some of cystic appearance.

Follow-up at 4 years and 3 months.

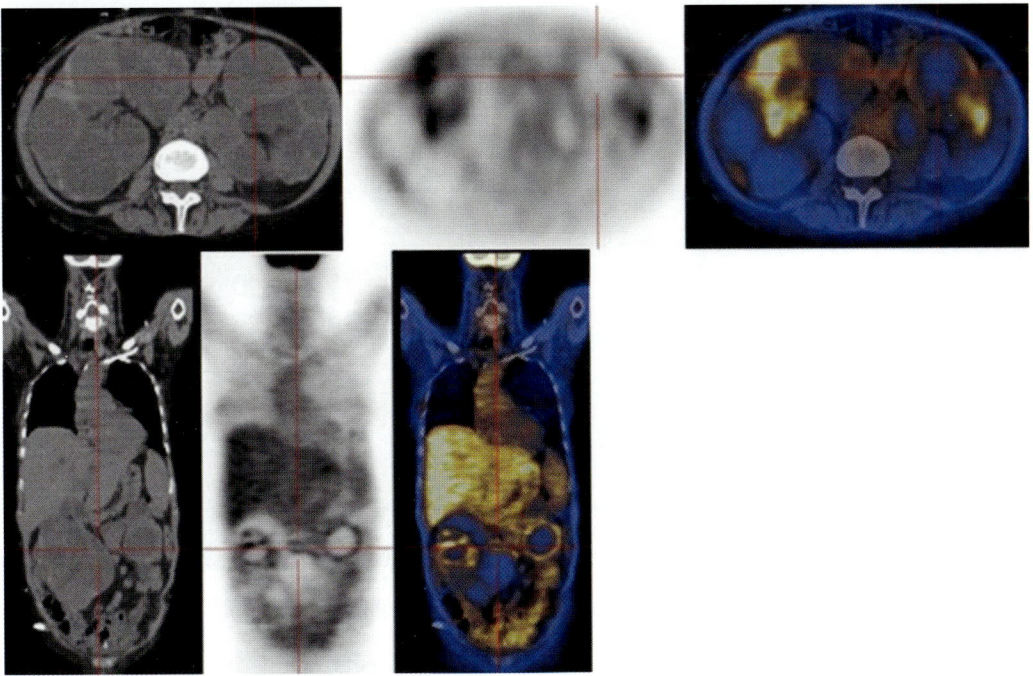

Fig. 71.1 CT shows dysmorphic kidneys, sharply increased in size, structure subverted by numerous coarse parenchymal cysts that have abnormal deposition of the tracer at the PET scan. Absence of focal lesions

P. F. Rambaldi, *Whole-Body FDG PET Imaging in Oncology*,
DOI: 10.1007/978-88-470-5295-6_71, © Springer-Verlag Italia 2014

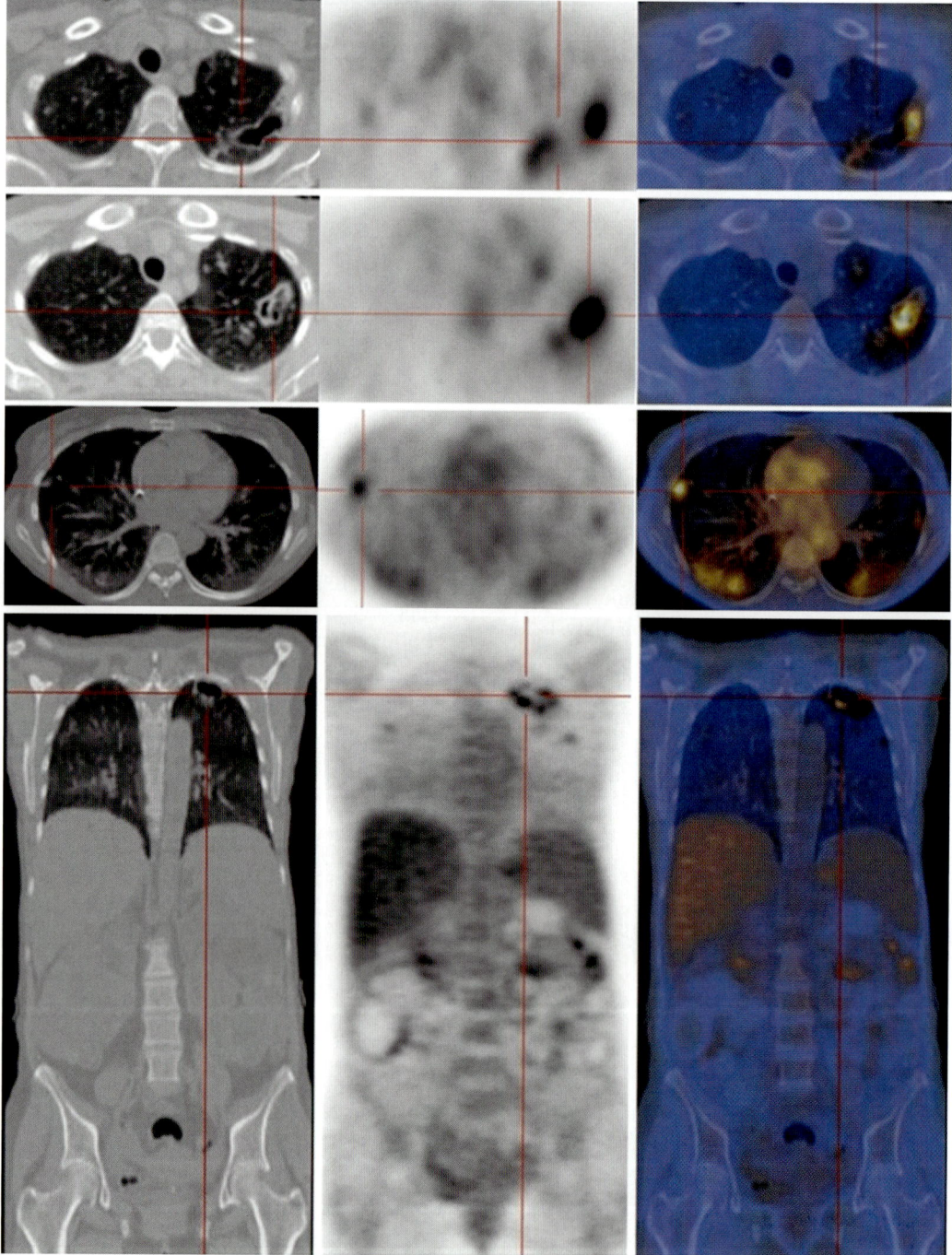

Fig. 71.2 At the apical segment of the left upper lobe, CT-PET image shows an oval lesion with air inside, with unevenly thickened margins that express low metabolic activity. Multiple bilateral pulmonary nodules of various sizes, some measuring more than a centimeter, other millimetric, can be seen

- CT: lung fields with multiple parenchymal symmetrical pseudonodules bilaterally. Subcentimetric nodal elements in the ilo-mediastinal region.
- PET-FDG: presence of some areas of hyperaccumulation bilaterally within the lung and mediastinum, the most evident with SUV max 4.6

71.2 Diagnostic Question

Woman with previous NHL in follow-up and concomitant bilateral nodular lung disease to be defined: search for lesions with a high metabolism of glucose, 6 months after the previous CT-PET scan.

71.3 Report

Multiple pulmonary nodules characterized by a modest increase in the consumption of glucose, the most evident at the upper lobe of the left lung, SUV max 5.5.

No focal areas of abnormal metabolism in the remaining parts of the body examined.

71.4 Conclusions

The PET scan shows multiple pulmonary nodules of dubious nature that show increased metabolic activity, slightly comparable with the previous examination. It seems useful to rule out an opportunistic infectious disease in dialyzed patient. Cytohistological determination was subsequently performed. See Figs. 71.1, 71.2, 71.3.

71.5 Key Points

- The patient was scanned because suffering from NHL in clinical remission. In this new evaluation, the metabolic activity of the concomitant pulmonary disease came out.

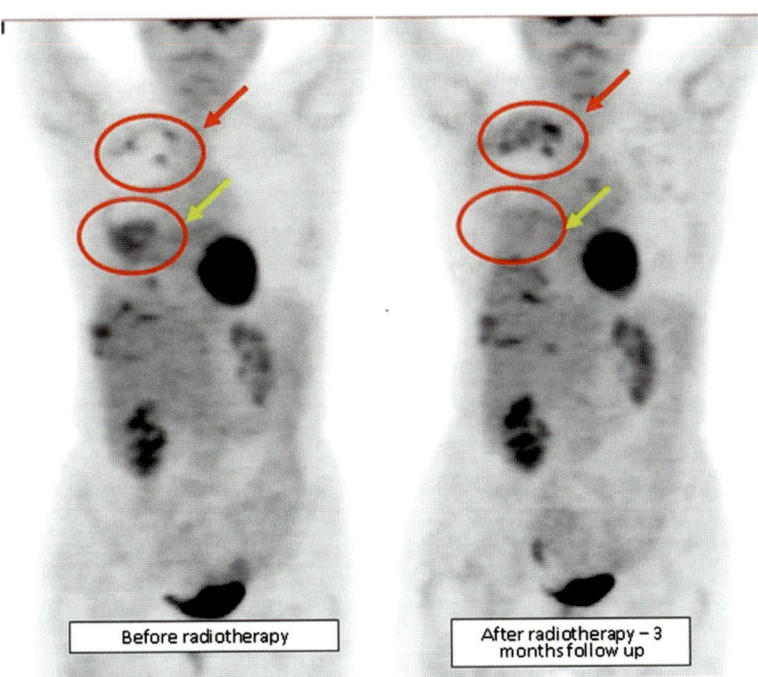

Before radiotherapy

After radiotherapy – 3 months follow up

Fig. 71.3 The MIP image, printed with double window. The spread and extent of the disease within the chest due to multiple nodules of different sizes, ranging from a few millimeters to centimeters, also documented by CT; high background abdominal activity which depends on the dysmetabolic condition of the patient who has: severe CRF on dialysis, secondary to polycystic disease, impaired function of the liver (hepatomegaly)

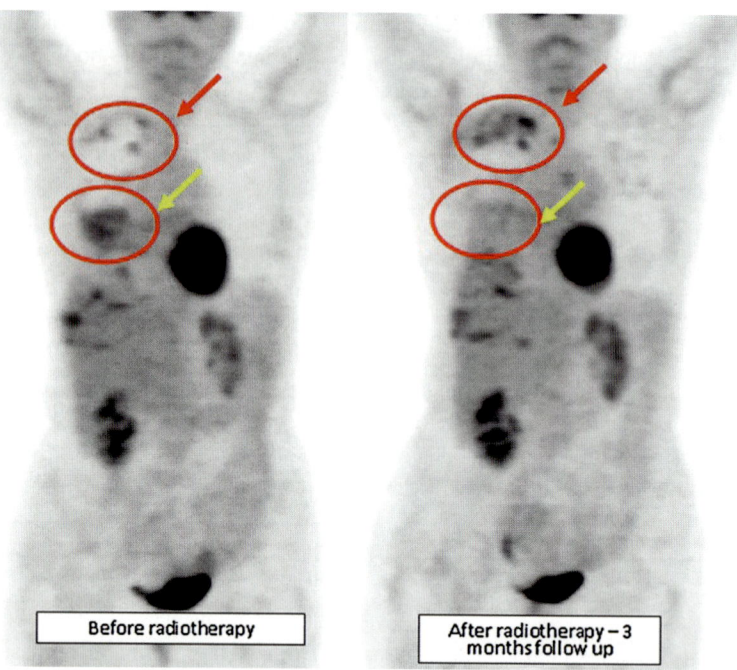

Fig. 71.4 Before and after radiotherapy

- Presence of multiple lung lesions in slight progression compared to previous controls, suggests a benign, even though rapidly evolving disease, which requires a more aggressive diagnostic approach.

Definitive diagnosis: pulmonary actinomycosis.

The nodules of actinomycosis may occur in any location and can mimic malignancy. Lung lesions are distinct from those of TB and metastatic conditions (Fig. 71.4).

Pulmonary Adenocarcinoma with Pleural Metastases: Restaging After Radiotherapy and Pleural Talcage

72

72.1 Clinical History

68-year-old woman with lung adenocarcinoma and metastases to the right parietal pleura.
- CT: 32 × 24 mm solid lesion in the lower lobe of the right lung, with spikes that reach both the pleura and the hilum; centimetric lymph nodes along the vascular-bronchial interstitium can be seen. Volumetric pseudonodular expansion of the right adrenal gland (23 × 12 mm). At the lower pole of the ipsilateral kidney there is a 18 mm solid, vascularized nodule.

Talcage of the right pleural cavity due to pleural effusion from metastatic ipsilateral lung cancer.

Stereotactic radiotherapy (SRT) of the right pulmonary hilar-basal mass.

Chemotherapy was then performed.
- CT (study performed in the course of chemotherapy): the size of the pulmonary right hilar-basal mass is stable (35 mm), with hypodense contextual colliquation. The lesional spikes towards the parietal pleura and the hilum through the vascular-bronchial tree persist. Stable the solid, vascularized lump at the lower pole of the right kidney (18 mm), on the other hand the lump at the ipsilateral adrenal gland is not visible, the adrenal gland being of normal size.

72.2 Diagnostic Question

Restaging of right lung adenocarcinoma after chemotherapy, ended by 16 days: search for focal lesions with a high metabolism of glucose.

72.3 Report

The PET scan shows a pulmonary right hilar-basal nodule, characterized by restricted carbohydrate consumption, SUV max 2.6, associated with widespread metabolic disorder caused by inflammatory and fibrotic-disventilatory postactinic phenomena in the ipsilateral lower lobar region, SUV max 2.1 (Fig. 72.1).

Increased FDG deposition in multiple nodules at the parietal, mediastinal and diaphragmatic right pleura, SUV max 4.

Absent glucose consumption of the renal right lower polar and ipsilateral adrenal mass. No focal areas of abnormal metabolism in the remaining parts of the body examined.

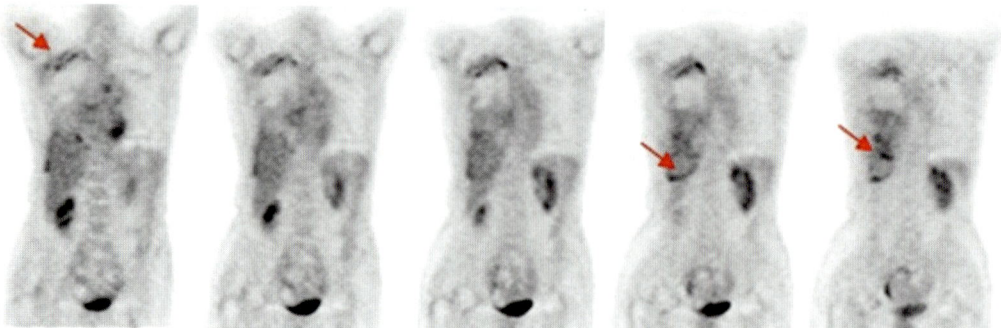

Fig. 72.1 The PET scan shows high metabolic activity secondary to post actinic reaction at the pulmonary hilum and right basal pleural granulomatous reaction secondary to ipsilateral talcage

72.4   Conclusions

The PET scan shows high metabolic activity secondary to post actinic reaction at the pulmonary hilum and right basal pleural granulomatous reaction secondary to ipsilateral talcage (Figs. 72.1, 72.2).

72.5   Key Points

In the treatment for lung cancer, radiotherapy determines an actinic reaction, sometimes so intense that decreases substantially only over time. The volume of lung irradiated, which is expected to be limited (as small as possible), the total administered dose, fractionation, and the combination with chemotherapy and concomitant respiratory diseases are all risk factors that contribute to a stabilized parenchymal damage: actinic fibrosis.

In the acute phase of radiation, pneumonitis is generally asymptomatic, and respiratory functional parameters do not undergo significant alterations although the alveolar-capillary diffusion is impaired (Fig. 72.3a). Once the radiation treatment is complete, the acute radiation pneumonitis occurs after 4–12 weeks, but only rarely it is associated with dyspnea, cough, and fever.

The actinic fibrosis is observed 6–12 months after radiotherapy and may be associated with a significant reduction in inspiratory and expiratory volumetric parameters (Fig. 72.3b). Is it possible its appearance without clinical evidence of previous pneumonia. A significant increase in the risk of pulmonary toxicity is related to irradiation of locoregional lymph node stations.

- When the actinic reaction subsides, there is still a slight increase in lesional glucose consumption, which is non-focal and determined by the chronicity of the inflammatory process and fibrosis (Fig. 72.4a). This phenomenon can be protracted over time (months, years) for the triggering of a chronic inflammatory reaction that feeds on itself, supported by immunocompetent cells and fibroblasts.
- After radiotherapy, the guidelines suggest re-evaluation with PET after 3 months (Fig. 72.4b) to reduce the rate of false positives.
- The metabolic activity of a radiation pneumonitis is higher than that of the liver, while that of fibrosis generally is lower.

Even procedures as the talcage lead to the activation of chronic inflammatory processes with formation of granulomas, that heavily

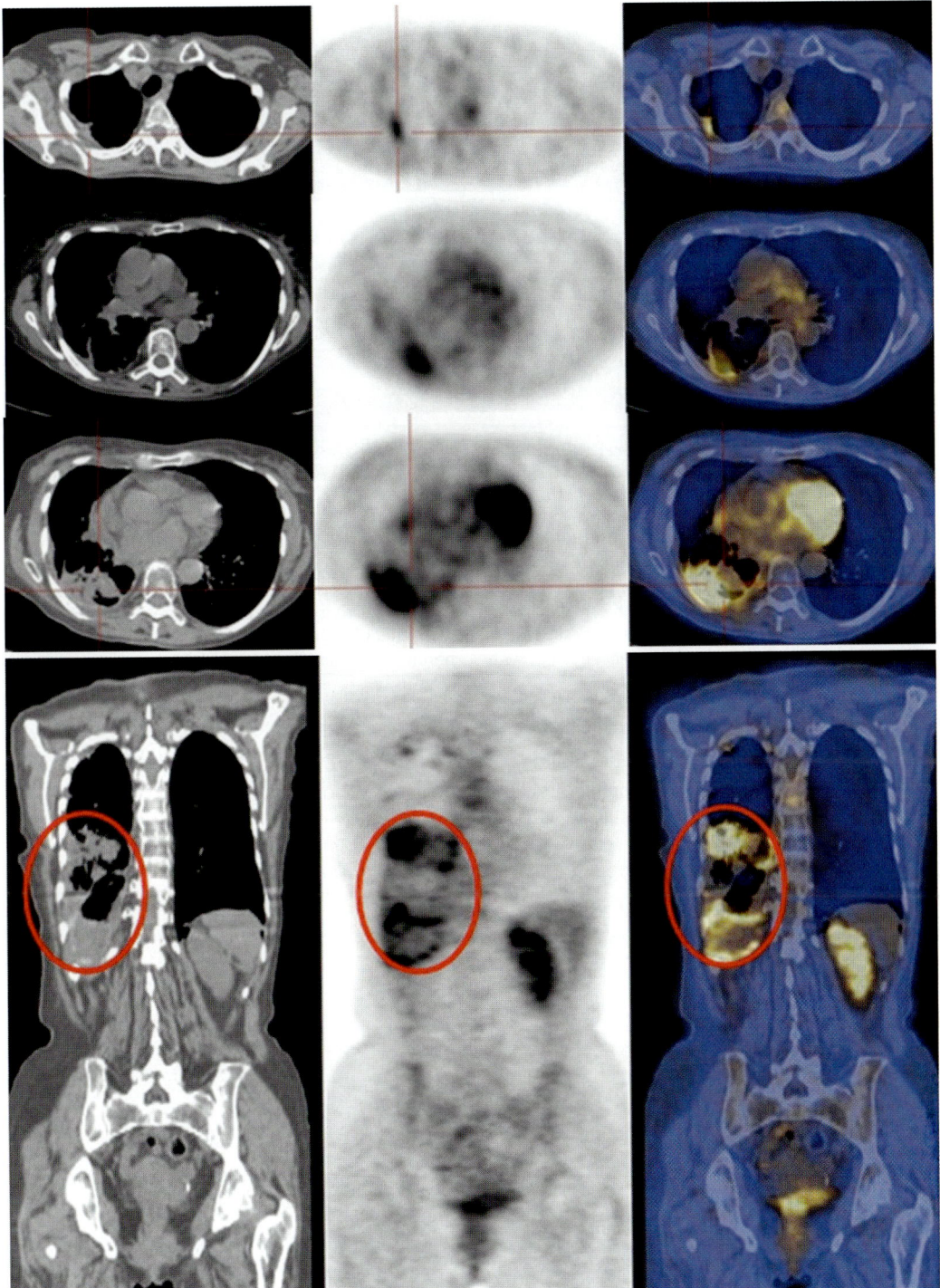

Fig. 72.2 At the posterior basal segment of the right lower lobe, a CT scan shows a large area of consolidation tissue that PET shows to have limited consumption of glucose and is therefore to be correlated with actinic outcomes. There can also be seen multiple pleural high FDG metabolism lumps determined by the granulomatous reaction to the talcage

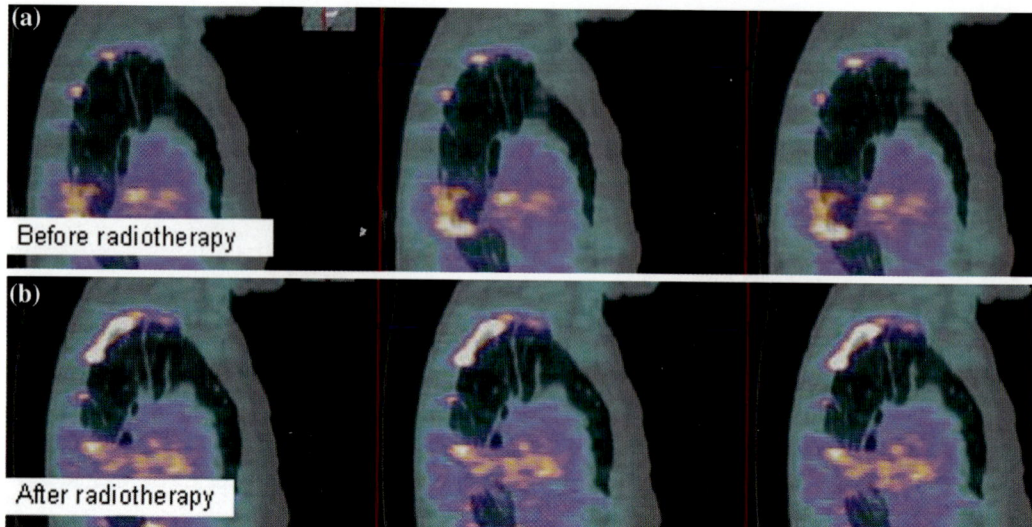

Fig. 72.3 Three months after radiotherapy PET was repeated; the comparison of MIP images and sagittal reconstructions shows: increase in the consumption of carbohydrate in the radiotreated apical pleural nodules and reduction of the deposition of FDG in the lesion ipsilateral basal. A first assessment of the data suggests a progression of the pathology of lesions treated with radiotherapy alone, the others are unchanged, and this is an implausible. In fact the increase of the deposition glucose is determined by the radiation pneumonitis in correspondence of the upper lobe. The reduction of the metabolic activity of the primary tumor is determined by the reduction of the actinic post-inflammatory and fibrotic evolution. See also Fig. 72.4

uptake glucose at PET; in these patients, it is not always easy to assess the actual metabolic state of the disease for the high rate of false positives; therefore:

- the clinical history, correlating with previous diagnostic investigations and the actual patient's clinical condition, helps reduce errors of interpretation;

- in case of doubt, the correct diagnosis is suggested only by volumetric progression of lesions over time.

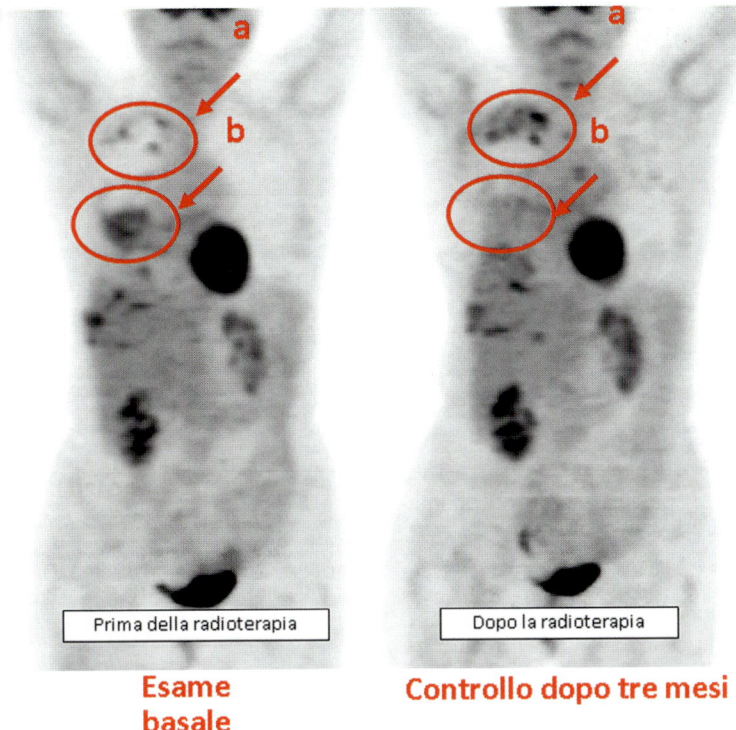

Esame basale — Prima della radioterapia

Controllo dopo tre mesi — Dopo la radioterapia

Fig. 72.4

NSCLC with Bone-Destroying Metastases: Restaging After Chemotherapy

73.1 Clinical History

Bronchopneumonia in 77-year-old man:
- Chest X-ray: parenchymal basal right posterior opacity, with costo-phrenic sinus opacification due to pleural liquid component.
- Chest CT: parenchymal nodule measuring 10 mm, with lobulated margins at the posterior segment of the right upper lobe; another more nuanced nodule in the basal ipsilateral posterior segment. Presence of some hilar-mediastinal subcentimetric lymph nodes.

   Scan performed after three months for onset of chest and pelvic pain.
- Chest CT: heterogeneous parenchymal lung middle lobe; lithic type structural alteration of newly formed solid material element of a right costal element and ipsilateral iliac wing.
- PET: hyperaccumulation of the tracer in the right pulmonary hilar region, SUV max = 15, the postero-lateral wall of the right hemithorax, SUV max = 16, and ipsilateral iliac wing, SUV max 15.6.

   Histological diagnosis of "epidermoid lung cancer" with rib and the iliac wing metastases.

   Chemotherapy and radiotherapy on the right iliac bone lesion.

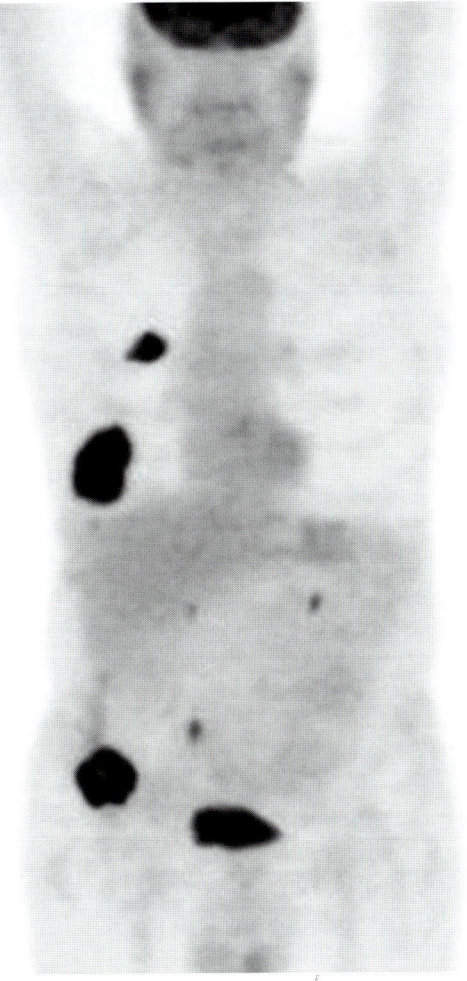

Fig. 73.1 PET scan showed abnormal glucose consumption of the right lung hilar nodule

P. F. Rambaldi, *Whole-Body FDG PET Imaging in Oncology*,
DOI: 10.1007/978-88-470-5295-6_73, © Springer-Verlag Italia 2014

Fig. 73.2 In correspondence of the middle lobe of the right lung, CT-PET shows a solid nodule, uneven, with irregular margins and striae that connect it with the hilum. This mass is characterized by high glucose metabolism

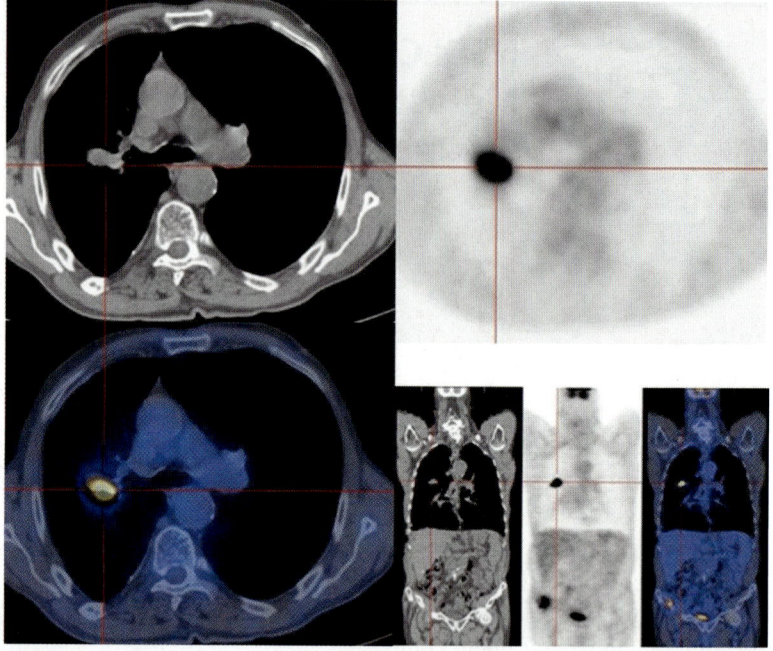

73.2 Diagnostic Question

Search for focal lesions with high glucose metabolism in patient with NSCLC and bone metastases: restaging one month after the end of chemotherapy and three after radiation therapy performed at the right iliac wing. Chest pain persists to the right and to the ipsilateral pelvis, associated with functional limitation.

73.3 Report

The PET scan showed abnormal glucose consumption of the right lung hilar nodule, SUV max 14, bone metastases to the ninth posterolateral right costal arch, SUV max 14, and ipsilateral iliac wing, SUV max 12 (Fig. 73.1).

Softer carbohydrate consumption of the right posterolateral tenth rib, SUV max 2.8.

No areas of abnormal metabolism of the remaining parts of the body examined.

73.4 Conclusions

The PET scan shows poor response to treatment of lung cancer and bone metastases already mentioned in history. See Figs. 73.2, 73.3, 73.4.

73.5 Key Points

The PET-CT scan defines the following:
- poor response to radiotherapy for the persistence of high metabolism of the bone lesion at the right iliac wing,
- poor response to chemotherapy for the persistence of high metabolism and vitality of primary lung nodule and bone metastases;
- no progression of the disease because:

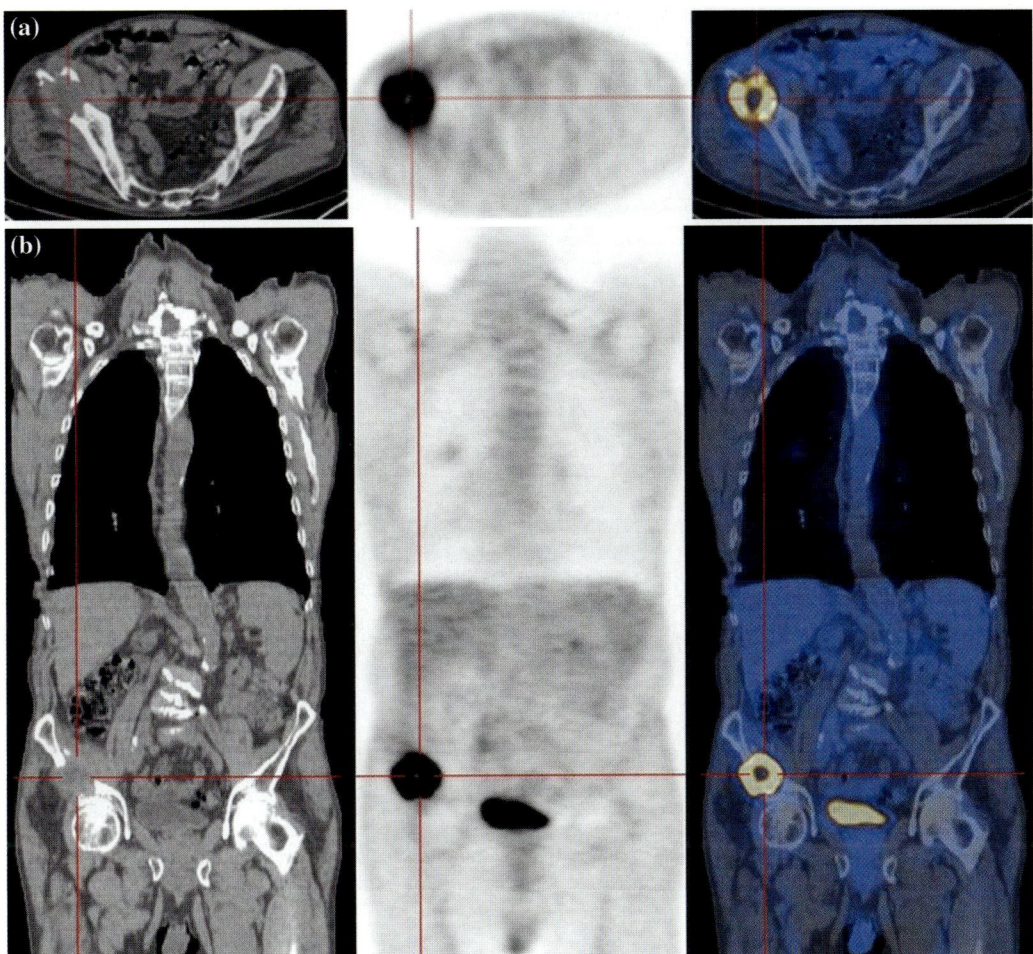

Fig. 73.3 The PET-CT scan shows a gross mass expansion which replaces the right iliac wing (a). The coronal reconstruction documents the involvement of the antero-superior acetabular roof (b). The consumption of glucose in the neoformation is high, even if there is a contextual area with low uptake, due to necrotic-colliquative phenomena, caused at least in part by the radiation treatment performed

– the individual lesions did not increase in volume and metabolic activity
– there are no new metastases.

Characteristic of the morphological and metabolic skeletal injuries is that they cause intense pain because they have rapid progression and marked local invasiveness, demonstrated by:

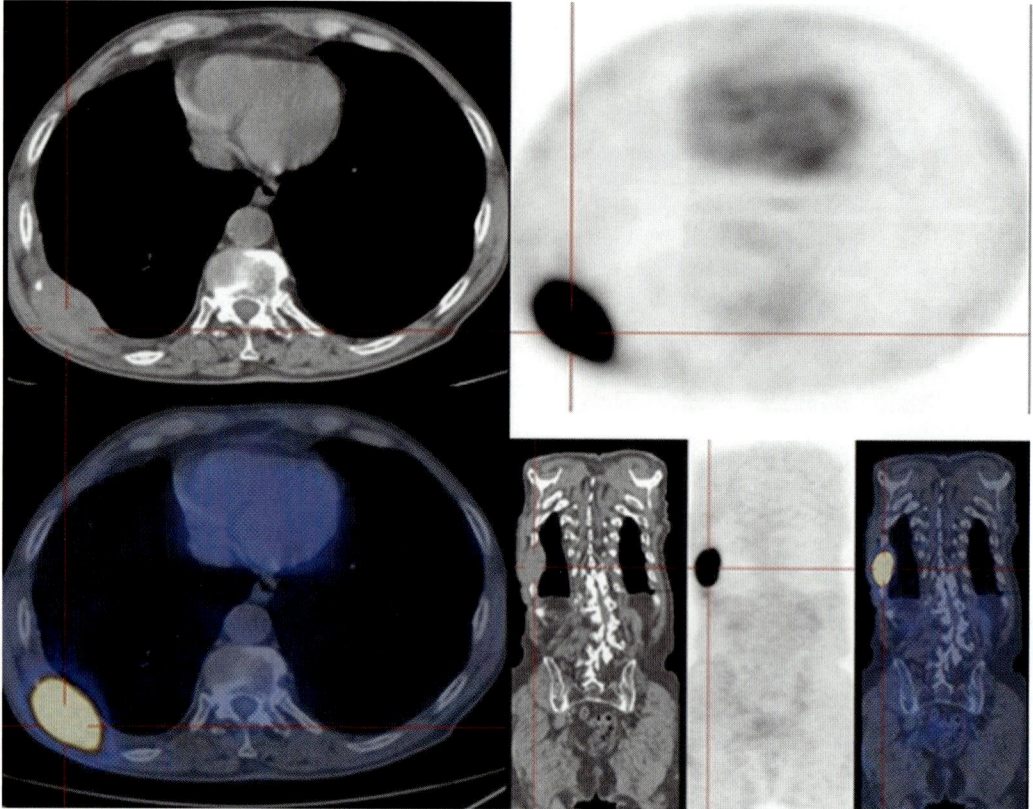

Fig. 73.4 The CT-PET shows the morpho-structural lytic alteration of the posterolateral right IX costal arch, that is no longer recognizable because replaced by a coarse solid mass with a high metabolism

- size of metastases that exceed the margins of the district involved,
- no reparative response of bone, whose margins are not recognizable,
- presence of lesional colliquation,
- complete destruction and replacement of the bone that is no longer recognizable.

Undifferentiated Gastric Adenocarcinoma with Peritoneal Carcinosis

74

74.1 Clinical History

74-year-old man who already underwent gast-roresection for benign gastric ulcer at age 44, admitted for recurrent abdominal pain and disorders of the alvus.

- EGD: 7 cm-long gastric stump with stromal congested mucosa.
- Endoscopic polypectomy of the transverse colon: adenomatous mostly hairy polyp, with characters of moderate dysplasia. At the level of the tunica propria, in the axis of the polyp, there are images of a suspicious focal infiltrative glandular growth.

 Follow-up at 6 months:

- Sense of abdominal distension and ascites.
- Colonoscopy with biopsy and histological diagnosis of "infiltration of the mucosa by undifferentiated carcinoma."
- Removal of peritoneal fluid "positive for malignant cells" with cytologic pattern of poorly differentiated adenocarcinoma

74.2 Diagnostic Question

Search for the primary tumor in patient with peritoneal carcinomatosis: definition of the metabolism of glucose.

74.3 Report

Focal pathological increase of the consumption of glucose in the front wall of the gastric stump, SUV max 14.

In the abdomen and pelvis are some solid nodules characterized by modest increase in carbohydrate consumption to be referred to peritoneal carcinomatosis, SUV max 5.4. At the CT scan, conspicuous ascites is evident.

No areas of abnormal increase in glucose metabolism in the remaining parts of the body examined.

74.4 Conclusions

The PET scan shows pathological glucose consumption in a suspected focal lesion at the anterior wall of the gastric stump (Fig. 74.1, yellow arrow). Endoscopic re-evaluation and subsequent cyto-histological determination is useful. Presence of peritoneal carcinomatosis and secondary ascites (Fig. 74.1, red arrows).

EGDS was repeated and the biopsy showed an undifferentiated adenocarcinoma.

Definitive diagnosis: 30 years after gastrectomy, this patient developed a tumor on the stump of the stomach that has infiltrated the transverse colon and resulted in a peritoneal carcinomatosis.

P. F. Rambaldi, *Whole-Body FDG PET Imaging in Oncology*,
DOI: 10.1007/978-88-470-5295-6_74, © Springer-Verlag Italia 2014

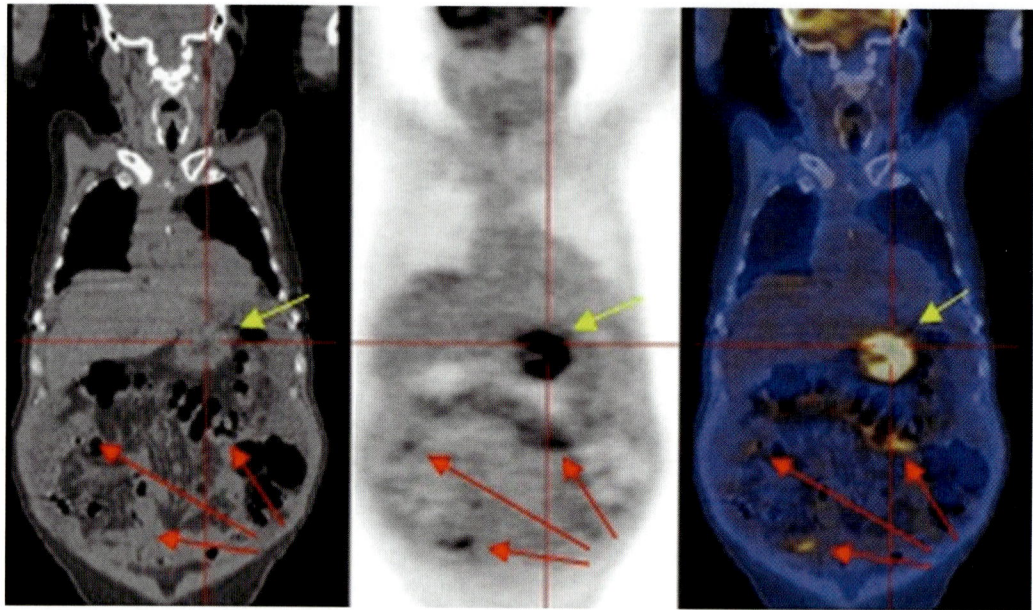

Fig. 74.1 The PET scan shows pathological glucose consumption in a suspected focal lesion at the anterior wall of the gastric stump

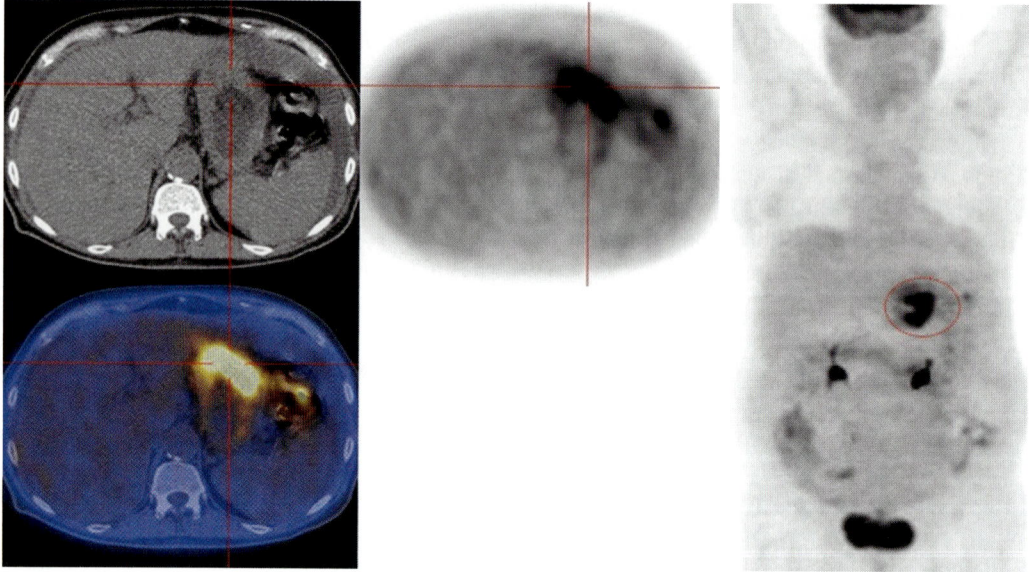

Fig. 74.2 CT shows marked thickening of the anterior wall of the gastric stump, not dissociable from the transverse colon, that appears relaxed. PET shows metabolic enhancement of the stump of the stomach and some small abdominal solid nodules that cannot be dissociated from the walls of the intestinal loops

74.5 Key Points

The walls of the stomach have intrinsic glucose consumption related to the physiological peristalsis (Fig. 74.2). Benign pathological conditions such as gastritis or ulcer can lead to an increased gastric metabolism due to the presence of a nonspecific inflammatory component.

- This finding has not a very high SUV max, and it is rarely higher than 5.
- In this patient, the SUV max of 14 definitely suggests a tumor.
- The correct etiopathogenetic diagnosis is endoscopic.
- The endoscopy is essential because it allows you to perform a biopsy.

Gastric cancer can cause peritoneal carcinomatosis, but the accuracy of contrast-enhanced CT and CT-PET is not very high when the lesions are subcentimetric. Sometimes you need a diagnostic laparoscopy.

- A peritoneal carcinomatosis should always be suspected when the patient complains of abdominal pain and bloating.
- In the presence of carcinomatosis, it is not always possible to determine the location of the primary tumor.
- Laparoscopy is not indicated when the CT-PET identifies the location of the primary tumor and demonstrates peritoneal carcinomatosis.

Infiltrating Gastric Adenocarcinoma: Follow-Up After Neoadjuvant Chemotherapy

75

75.1 Clinical History

60-year-old woman with gastric infiltrating adenocarcinoma, not surgically treated for the presence of lymph node metastases.

Follow up after chemotherapy.

- Markers: CEA = 247 ng/ml (nv < 10), CA19-9 = 85 U/ml (nv < 33).
- CT: marked thickening of the stomach wall with uneven impregnation of the contrast medium at the fundus and the body. The stomach is not well separable from the pancreas. Multiple lymph node metastases adjacent to the stomach, the largest measuring 25 mm.

75.2 Diagnostic Question

Restaging after chemotherapy in patient with gastric adenocarcinoma: search for focal lesions with a high metabolism of glucose.

75.3 Report

Intense, pathological glucose consumption of the gastric wall, more intense at the body and the fundus, SUV max 16 (Fig. 75.1).

Gross perigastric lymph node with high metabolism, SUV max 12. Another lymph node is evident in the intercavo—aortic region, SUV max 6 (Fig. 75.2).

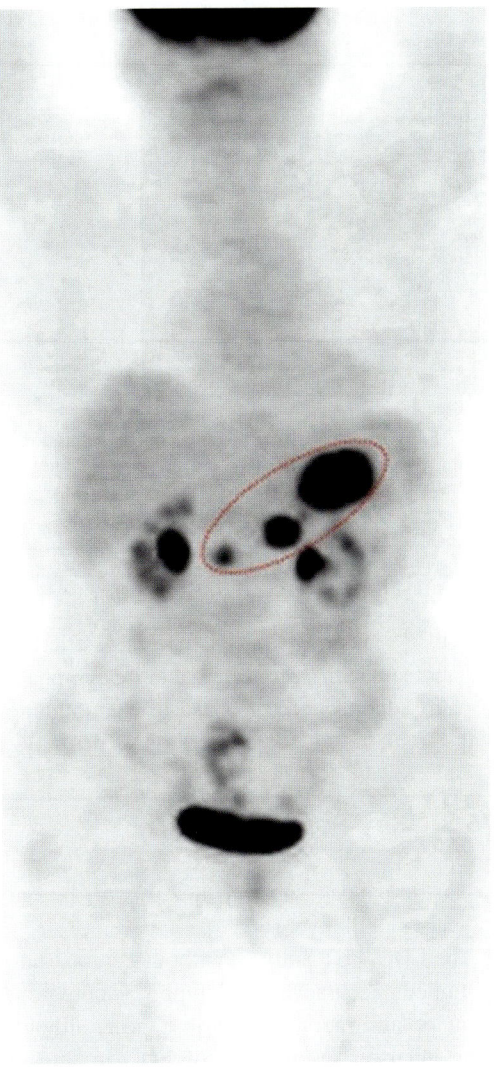

Fig. 75.1 Intense, pathological glucose consumption of the gastric wall, more intense at the body and the fundus, SUV max 16

P. F. Rambaldi, *Whole-Body FDG PET Imaging in Oncology*,
DOI: 10.1007/978-88-470-5295-6_75, © Springer-Verlag Italia 2014

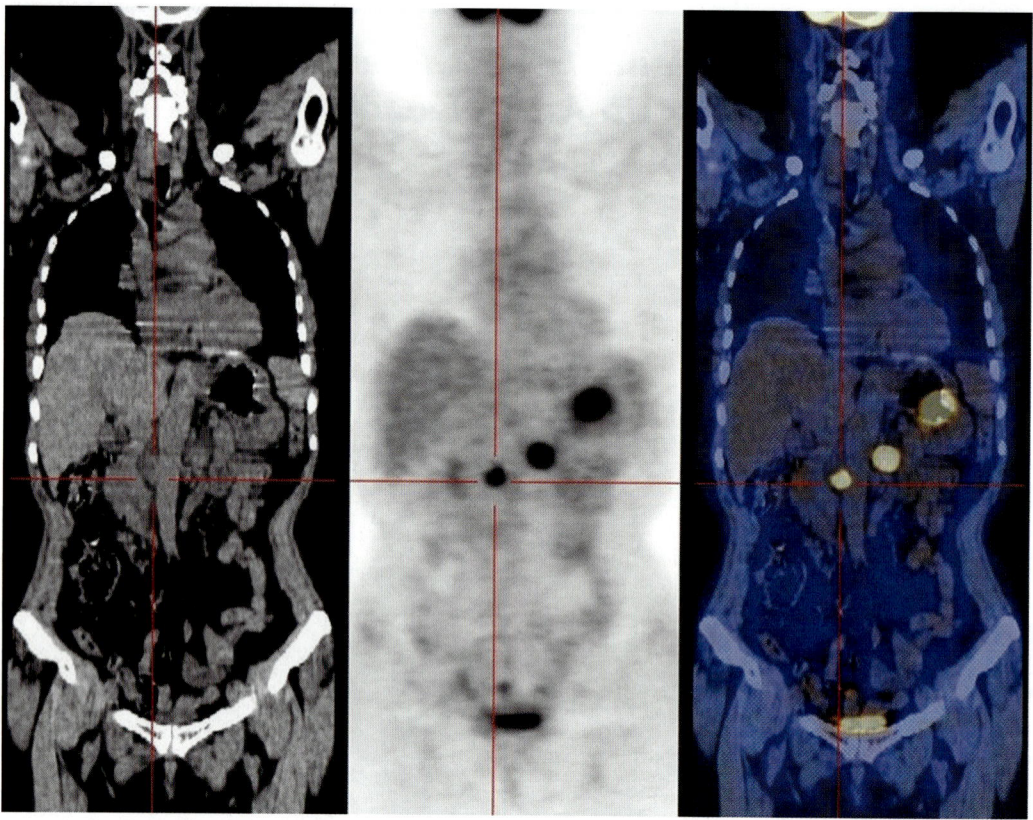

Fig. 75.2 Gross perigastric lymph node with high metabolism, SUV max 12. Another lymph node is evident in the intercavo—aortic region, SUV max 6

75.4   Conclusions

The PET scan shows persistence of gastric high metabolism with secondary satellite lymphadenopathy, due to poor response to chemotherapy (Fig. 75.3).

75.5   Key Points

In gastric cancer, surgical therapy will be only radical or palliative.

- The FDG-PET and CT without contrast have limited accuracy in defining locoregional tumor infiltration of gastric cancer, although an intense concentration of FDG in a lesion suggests a transmural organ involvement and thus a worse prognosis.

- A reduction in the metabolic activity of 25–35 % demonstrated by PET performed after the first and second cycles of neoadjuvant chemotherapy (interim PET), suggests a response to treatment and a group of patients with better prognosis.

- Some histological types of gastric cancer, such as the mucinous type, have a low uptake of FDG, and in these cases, a PET scan has limited accuracy.

In this patient, the persistence of disease with high metabolic activity shows little response to chemotherapy, so a different approach might have to be suggested.

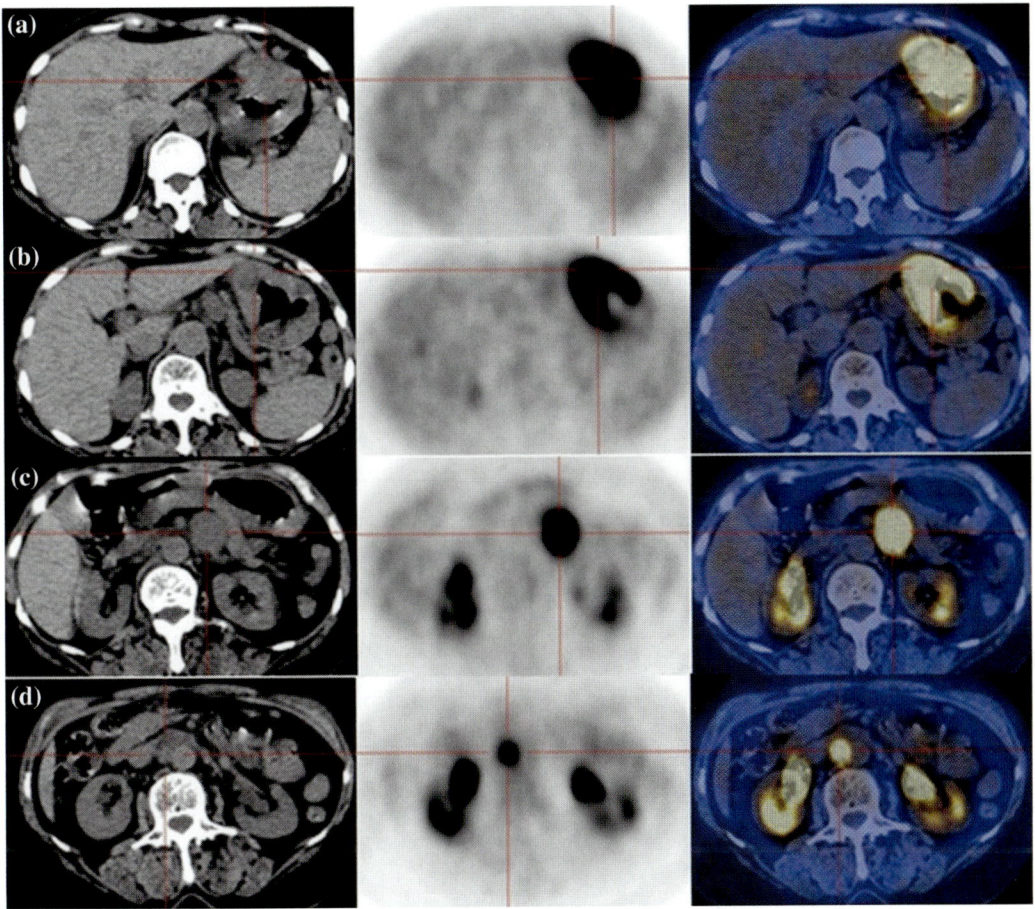

Fig. 75.3 At CT-PET it is evident a marked thickening of the gastric wall with a hypodense focal area at the fundus (a, b). Presence of two hypodense lymph nodes, the largest, perigastric, measuring 37 mm (c), the other pericentimetric node lies in the intercavo-aortic region (d). All of these lesions have a high metabolism

76.1 Clinical History

69-year-old man with a diagnosis of adenocarcinoma of the stomach (G2 pT2, pN1, PM0), underwent total gastrectomy with esophago-jejunal Roux anastomosis.

Follow-up at 18 months.

- PET: pathological uptake in a nodal spot at the hepatic hilum. Hyperaccumulation near the right scapula, some dorsal vertebrae and pelvis, extending, in a more nuanced fashion, to the proximal epiphysis of the left femur.
- CT of the pelvis: structural alteration of the left acetabular roof and femoral head, where a small erosion of the cortical and the remodeling of the underlying spongiosa, due to a repetitive focal lesion, can be seen.
- FNAB of an axillary lymph node with cytology is negative for malignant cells.

Reassessment after chemotherapy (3 months).

- Chest CT: Conspicuous bilateral pleural effusion characterized by inhomogeneous density. Air bronchogram can be seen in the right lung but is absent in the lower lobe of the left lung. Bilateral hilar and rear mediastinal micro nodal metastases.

Chemotherapy protocol goes on.

76.2 Diagnostic Question

Evaluation of response after chemotherapy, completed 3 weeks before in patient with

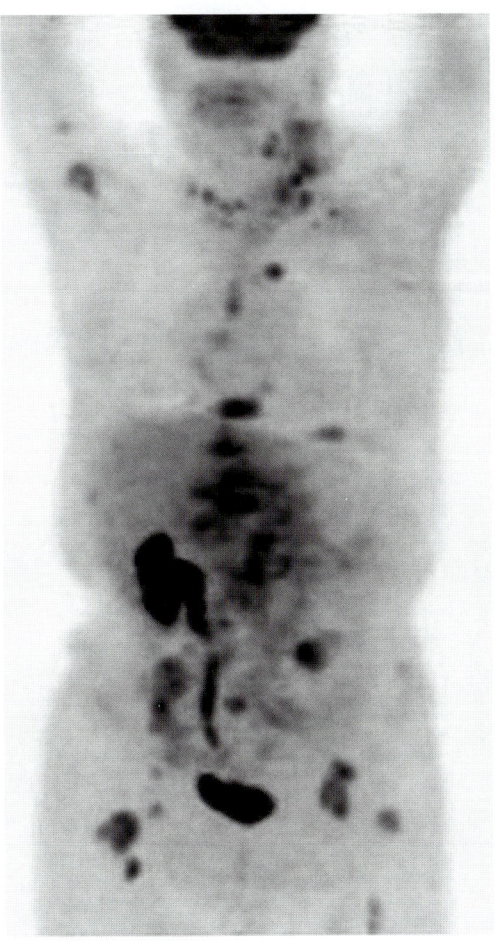

Fig. 76.1 The PET scan shows multiple enlarged lymph nodes with high glucose metabolism in the celiac-mesenteric-aortic, left lumbo-aortic regions; bilaterally in the iliac region, even though more pronounced on the left side, SUVmax 14

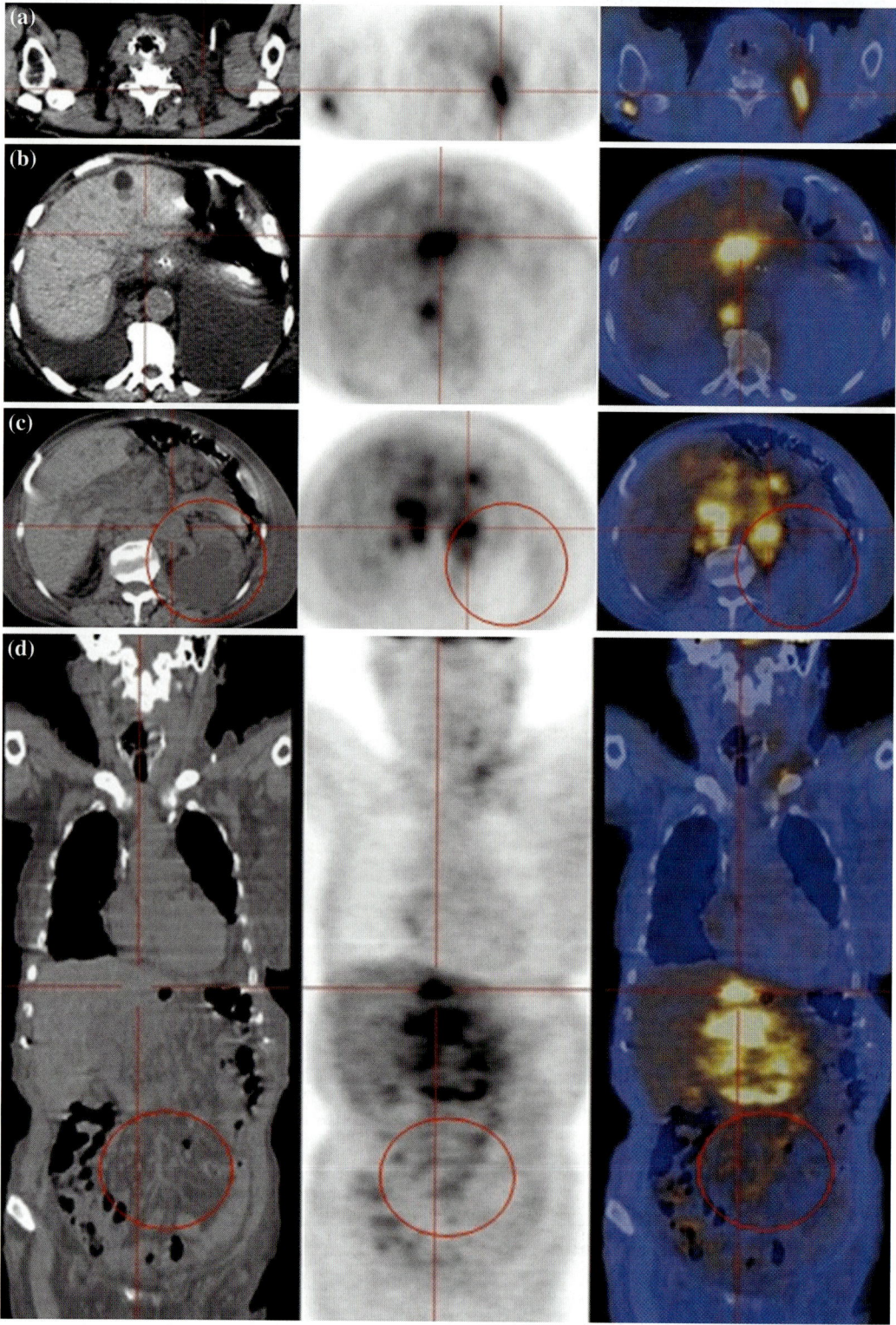

◄   **Fig. 76.2** A CT scan shows subcentimetric lymph nodes in the left latero-cervical region that extend towards the ipsilateral clavicular fossa (a). Multiple formations nodes measuring more than a centimeter each, tending to confluence and "casting" the celiac-mesenteric, paracaval, intercavo—lumbo-aortic and left aortic stations (b, c). The coronal reconstruction documents the mesenteric distension, with multiple subcentimetric lymph nodes involved (d). PET shows the remarkable metabolism of lymph node and bone metastases. The left kidney is excluded for significant obstructive hydronephrosis (c)

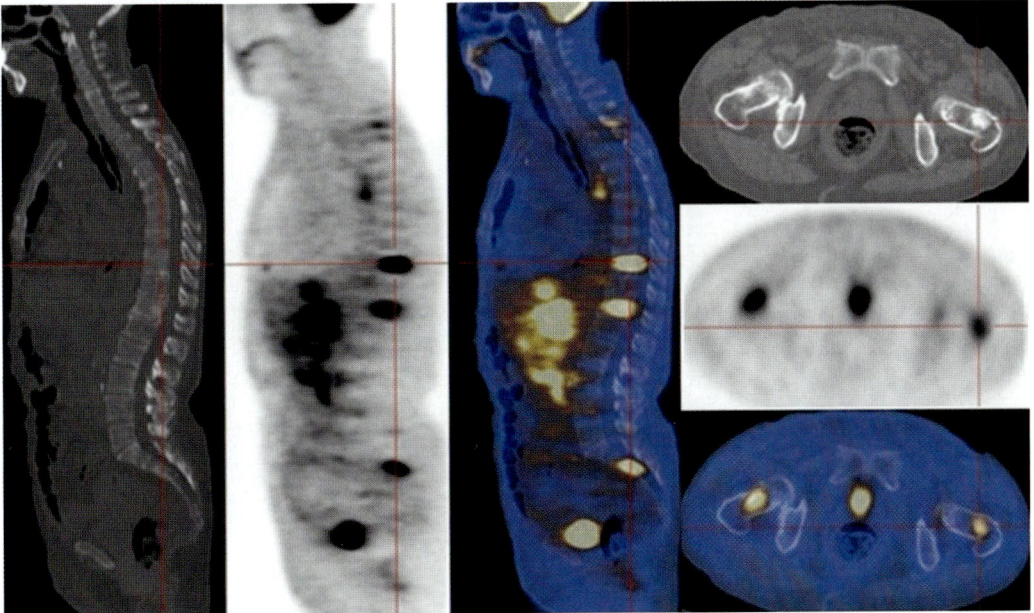

Fig. 76.3 PET-CT showed multiple bone metastases, some thickening, the most evident in the left femur. The sagittal reconstruction confirms the involvement of some vertebrae in the spine and the sacrum. Glucose metabolism is intense

metastatic gastric cancer: search for lesions with a high metabolism of glucose.

76.3   Report

The PET scan shows multiple enlarged lymph nodes with high glucose metabolism in the celiac-mesenteric-aortic, left lumbo-aortic regions; bilaterally in the iliac region, even though more pronounced on the left side, SUVmax 14 (Fig. 76.1).

Presence of numerous mediastinal anterior and posterior nodes with high metabolism, SUVmax 7.5; nodes can be found in the clavicular fossa and the latero-cervical region on both sides, with greater involvement on the left, SUVmax 7.

Multiple skeletal lesions with a high FDG uptake, with involvement of the right scapula, some dorso-lumbar vertebrae, femurs and pelvis, more pronounced in the sacrum and the sacro-iliac articulation, SUVmax 10.

The left kidney is excluded for severe obstructive hydronephrosis due to the infiltration of the ureter. The right pielo-ureteral region shows a lesser dilatation that does not reflect obstructive component.

76.4   Conclusions

The PET scan shows a progression of disease with various skeletal metastasis and lymph node diffuse involvement, due to poor response to chemotherapy. See Figs. 76.2, 76.3, 76.4.

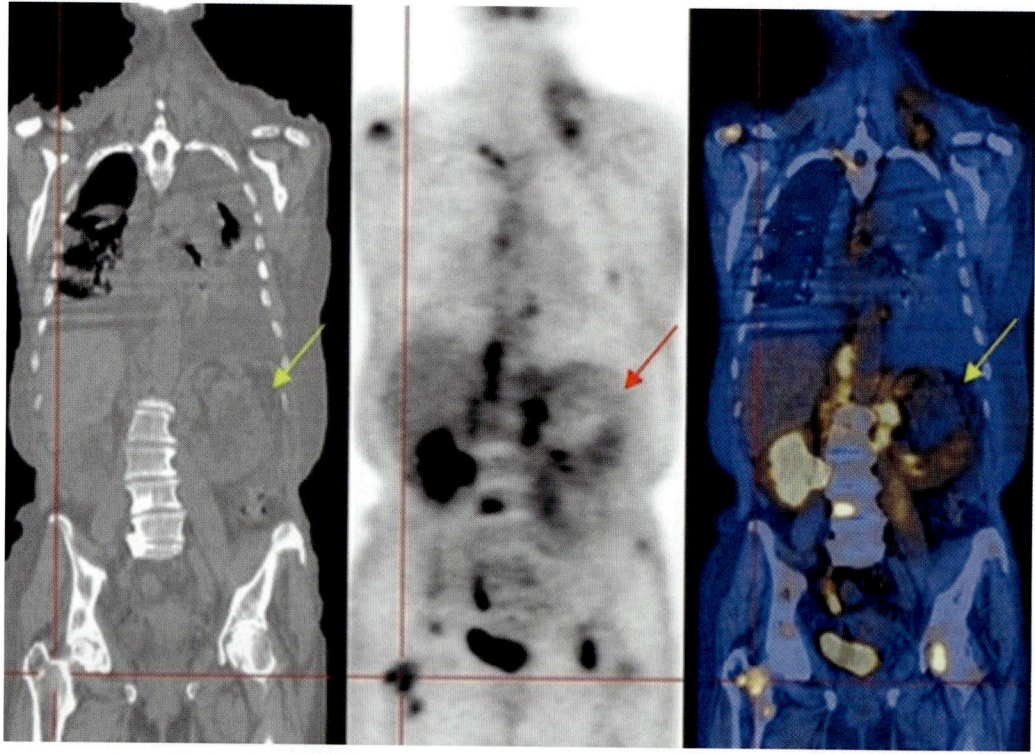

Fig. 76.4 The left kidney is excluded for significant obstructive hydronephrosis

76.5   Key Points

- The PET-CT has high accuracy both in the staging of gastric carcinomas than in restaging after chemotherapy.
- The intensity of the concentration of FDG correlates with the grade of biological aggressiveness of the tumor.
- Bone metastases are frequent in advanced stages of disease, rare in the early stages.

In restaging, PET has the role of defining the response to chemotherapy even when the images of the previous examination are not available and you only have a report of the previous scans.

Follow-Up of Bladder Carcinoma: Incidental Diagnosis of Metachronous Pulmonary Cancer

77

77.1 Clinical History

74-year-old man who underwent TUR for transitional cell bladder carcinoma (GII-III WHO). A year after, he underwent TUR for transitional non-invasive carcinoma of the bladder (GII WHO). After 6 months, the bladder was removed due to recurrence.

Subsequently he underwent chemotherapy.
Follow-up after 1 year:

- CT: 50 mm solid mass of the basal-posterior segment of the lower lobe of the right lung. A FNAB was then performed and it came out indeterminate, for the presence of "blood and inflammatory elements." Absence of malignant cells.
- Bone scintigraphy: negative for focal lesions.

77.2 Diagnostic Question

Search for focal lesions with high glucose metabolism in patient with bladder cancer and right lung mass, with origin yet to be determined.

77.3 Report

The solid lung mass in the right postero-basal segment, which was already examined with a FNAB, shows pathological increase in the consumption of glucose, SUV max 11.5 (Fig. 77.1).

No areas of abnormal metabolism in other parts of the body examined.

77.4 Conclusions

The PET scan confirms the presence of a right lung mass characterized by high metabolism, compatible with NSCLC, however, to be studied histologically. See Figs. 77.2, 77.3.

77.5 Key Points

There is not an established role of FDG-PET in the study of bladder cancer:

nuclear medicine allows characterization of metabolic lesions seen at CT, but does not define the histology, which is the diagnostic element

P. F. Rambaldi, *Whole-Body FDG PET Imaging in Oncology*,
DOI: 10.1007/978-88-470-5295-6_77, © Springer-Verlag Italia 2014

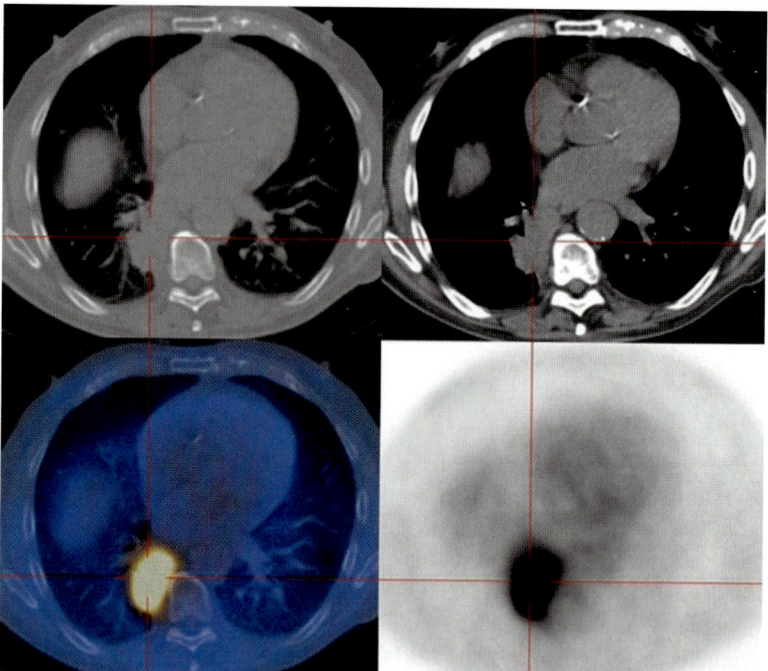

Fig. 77.1 The solid lung mass in the right postero-basal segment, which was already examined with a FNAB, shows pathological increase in the consumption of glucose, SUV max 11.5

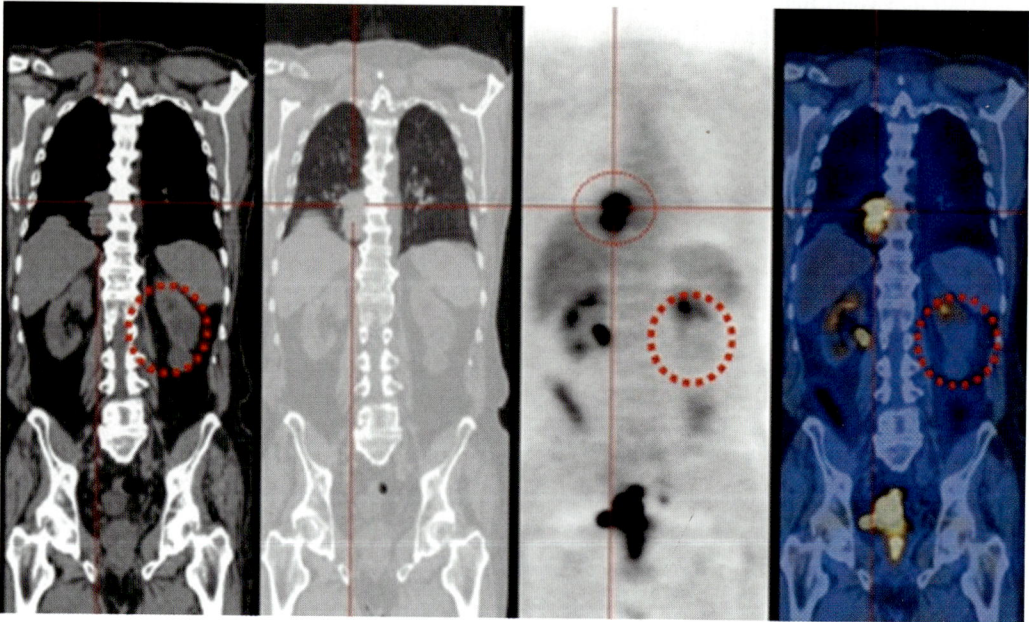

Fig. 77.2 The PET-CT scan shows a heterogeneous mass in the posterior basal segment of the right lung that invades surrounding tissues and appears inseparable from the hilum. The metabolism of glucose of the lesion is high. At the CT scan it is evident a cystic dysplasia of the left lower renal district, characterized by reduced parenchymal function

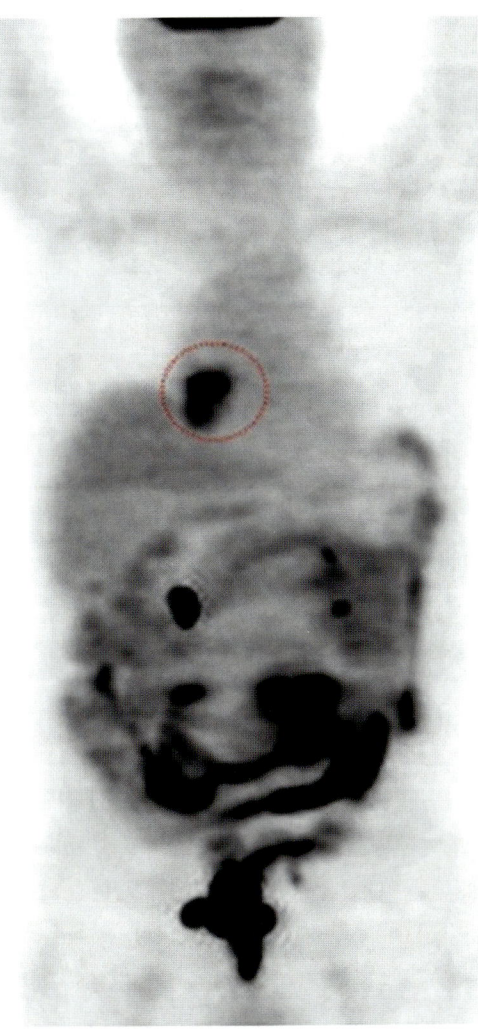

needed for the subsequent medical or surgical therapeutic approach;

the presence of a solitary lung mass suggests a metachronous neoplasm, vice versa metastases are multiple, have regular margins, and settle in the mantlar area;

in patients at high risk for lung cancer in which the primary or secondary CT does not define the nature of nodules and masses, it is useful to perform a PET scan to:

• quantify glucose metabolism;
• exclude metastases in other organs and systems.

A positive PET scan suggests the malignancy of the lesion; therefore, the histological characterization is necessary.

The patient has repeated FNAB which allowed the definitive histological diagnosis of lung adenocarcinoma.

Fig. 77.3 MIP image: clear increase in the metabolism of the right lung mass. In the abdomen and pelvis there are artifacts from altered urinary washout of the tracer due to previous cystectomy

78.1 Clinical History

A 72-year-old man underwent surgery for a poorly differentiated urothelial carcinoma of the bladder infiltrating the muscular deep tunic (G3-pT2b, pN2, PMX) associated with prostatic adenocarcinoma Gleason score 6 (3 + 3), located in both lobes.

- Did not undergo chemoradiotherapy.
  Follow-up at 6 months.
- Bone scintigraphy: negative for focal lesions.
- Cancer markers: CEA = 19.0 ng/mL (nv < 10).
- CXR: left fibrotic outcomes with wall "casting" calcifications and obliteration of the left costo-phrenic sinus, patchy parenchymal opacities with the based at the pleural wall in the lung left middle lobe. Right scissural thickening.

- Chest CT: bilateral pleural thickening with calcified plaques in the context, more explicit in the anterior basal segments bilaterally. Pleural effusion on the right. Expansive solid, uneven, irregular mass with spiculated profiles in the anterior segment of the left upper lobe (40 mm).

  Cyto-histological examination of the mass in the left lung: presence of malignant cells consistent with metastatic poorly differentiated urothelial carcinoma.

78.2 Diagnostic Question

Search for focal lesions with high glucose metabolism in patient with a history of double cancer and solitary lung metastasis: pre-surgical restaging.

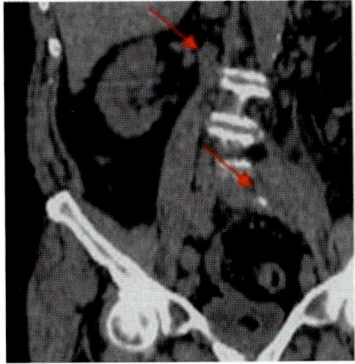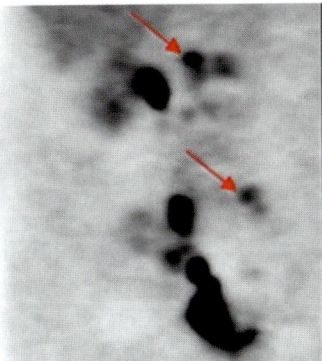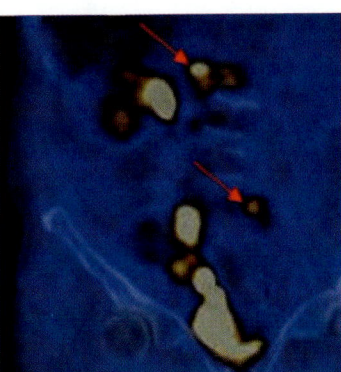

Fig. 78.1 The PET shows progression of disease due to the presence of a lung metastasis and lymph nodes characterized by increased deposition of FDG

P. F. Rambaldi, *Whole-Body FDG PET Imaging in Oncology*,
DOI: 10.1007/978-88-470-5295-6_78, © Springer-Verlag Italia 2014

Fig. 78.2 The CT shows a *solid* mass, uneven, with irregular spiculated profiles in the anterior segment of the *upper* lobe of the *left* lung invading the parietal pleura

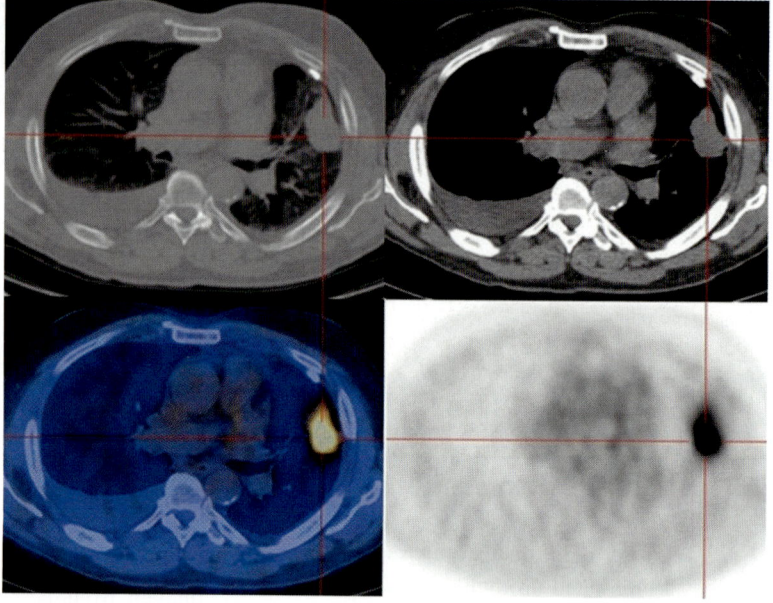

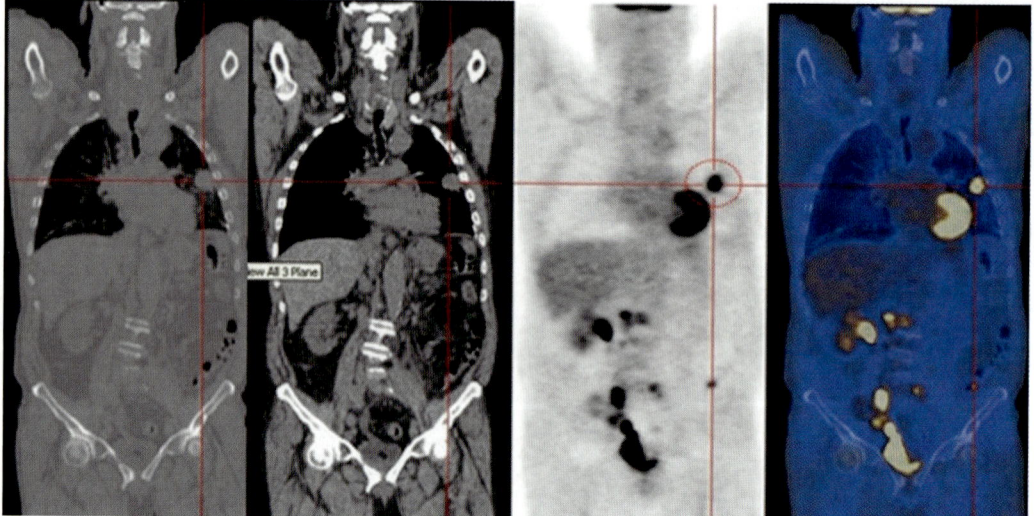

Fig. 78.3 PET shows *high* glucose consumption lesion. Presence of pleural effusion on the *right* contralateral to the mass

78.3   Report

Lung mass in the anterior segment of the left upper lobe, characterized by intense consumption of glucose, SUVmax 8.

Presence of some lymph nodes increased in size, with a high FDG metabolism in the para-aortic right region, near the renal artery and the left common iliac nodal station, with infiltration of the ureter. These masses show a SUVmax of 6.7 and 5 respectively.

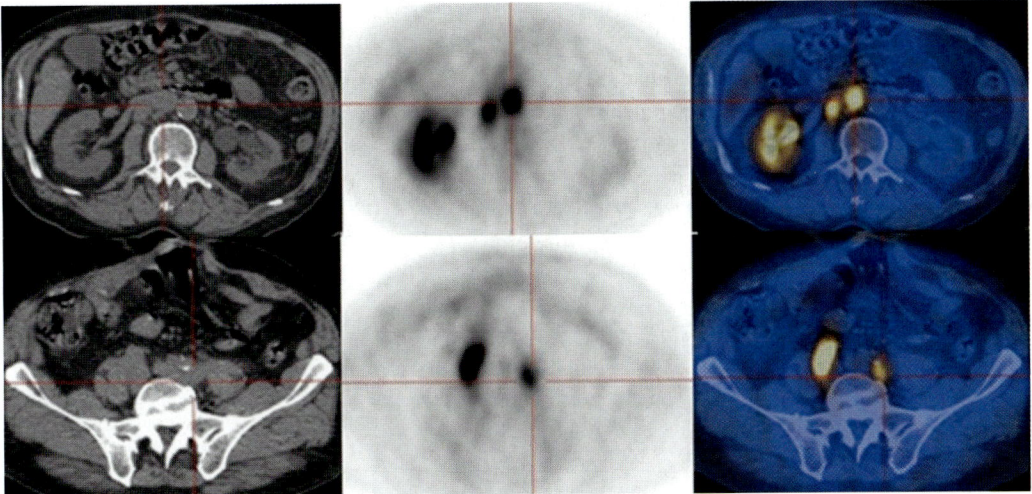

Fig. 78.4 The TC-PET demonstrates some lymph nodes of increased size, *high* metabolism within the paraortic *right* region, in proximity of the renal artery and the *left* common iliac artery

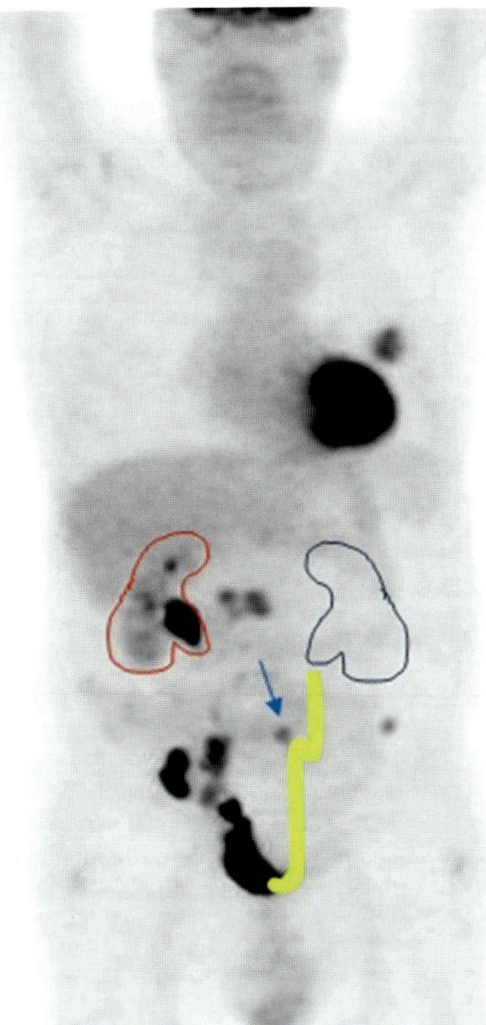

The left kidney shows negligible parenchymal function for ipsilateral obstructive secondary hydronephrosis.

No areas of abnormal increase in glucose consumption in the remaining parts of the body examined.

78.4   Conclusions

The PET shows progression of disease due to the presence of a lung metastasis and lymph nodes characterized by increased deposition of FDG (Figs. 78.1, 78.2, 78.3, 78.4, 78.5).

78.5   Key Points

In patients with a neobladder, urinary stasis caused by loss of the physiological peristalsis and by the pielo-ureteral hypotonia is frequent.

- The dynamic assessment MIP image allows to better define the status of the urinary tract as a whole. This element is sometimes useful to

◀ **Fig. 78.5** In the MIP reconstruction, there is no concentration in the left kidney that is, thus, excluded. The right kidney appears normal in morphology, size and parenchymal function. Modest activity appears in the right ureter, dilated until the distal third, due to atony determined by loss of the physiological ureteral peristalsis, characteristic of patients with neobladder. Absence of obstruction on the same side distinguish metastatic lesions from nonspecific accumulation.

- The right kidney has a good function (red ROI), it is evident a secondary parenchymal to low-ureteral dilatation, more evident at the distal end, at the mouth in the neobladder.
- To the left renal filtration of the tracer is not seen. Lymphadenopathy in the common iliac artery (blue arrow) probably infiltrated the ureter (yellow line) determining an obstructive stenosis, so the kidney is functionally excluded.

The presence of pulmonary metastases and lymph node involvement excludes the surgical option.

79.1   Clinical History

68-year-old treated with cysto-prostato-vesciculectomy and pelvic lymphadenectomy with ileal conduit urinary diversion (Bricker conduit) for a high-grade urothelial carcinoma (G3). Histological examination demonstrated benign prostatic hypertrophy with rare foci of intraepithelial neoplasia of low and high degree.

The patient did not undergo neither radio- nor chemotherapy-treatment.

Revaluation four months after surgery.

- MRI of the abdomen and pelvis: absence of focal lesions.
- Ultrasound: absence of clear focal lesions.
- Pelvis XR: a large area of cortical osteolysis of the right ischio-pubic branch compatible with metastatic lesions.

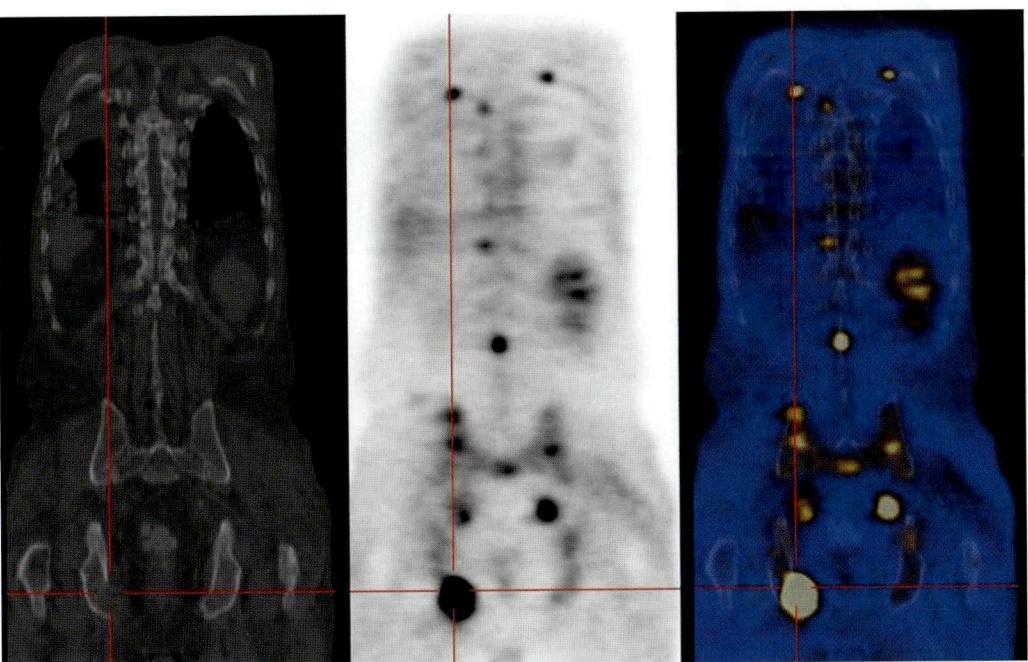

Fig. 79.1 The PET scan shows bone, lung and lymph node secondary disease due to disseminated urothelial carcinoma

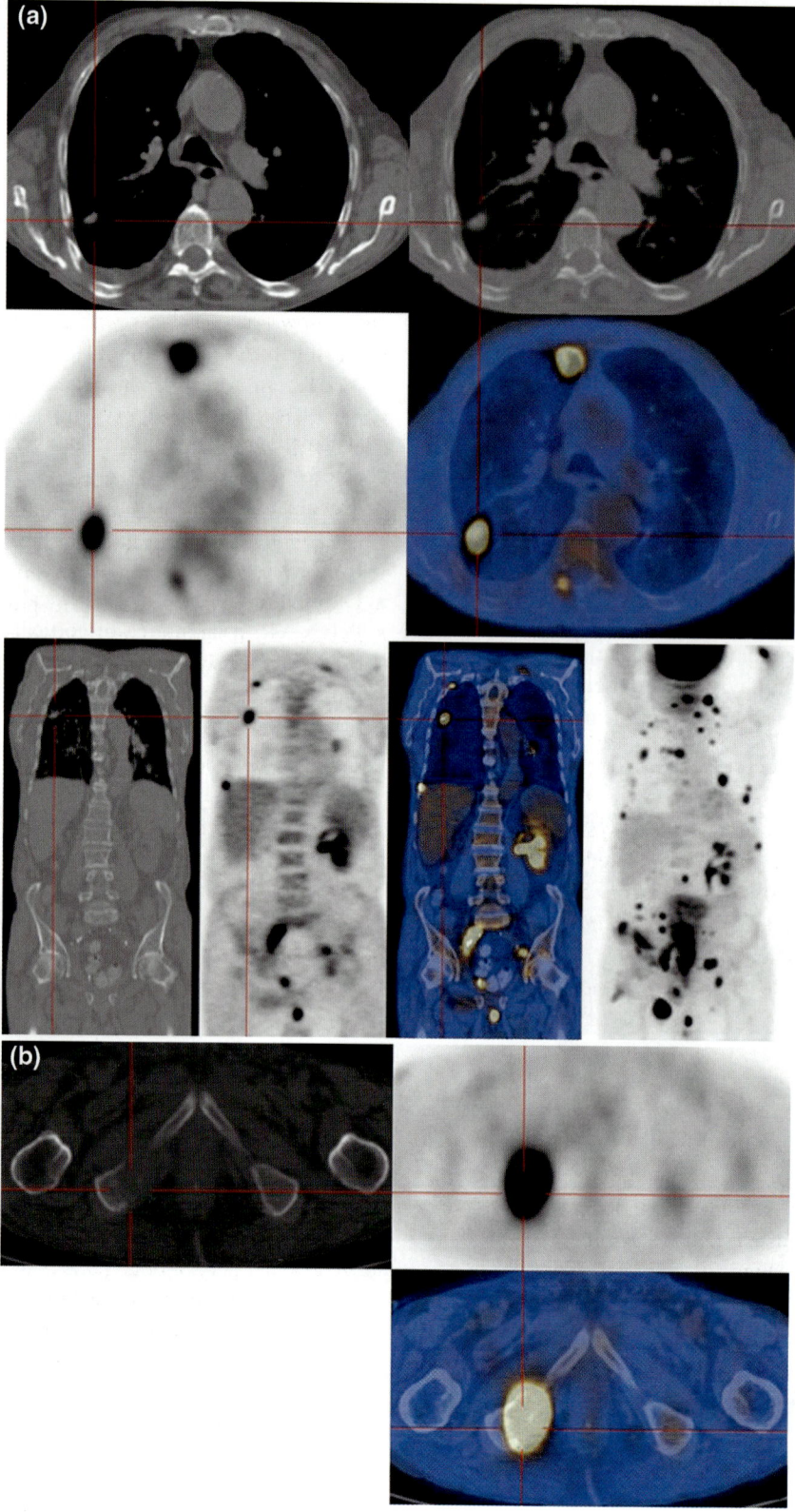

◄ **Fig. 79.2** The CT-PET shows multiple pulmonary solid metastatic nodules (a); only two have high concentration of FDG, the other subcentimetric nodules are below the resolving power of the technique. Presence of numerous metastatic bone lesions with extensive metabolism, most of which are not seen on CT because they have not yet determined enough demineralization and destruction, an element that occurs only belatedly (b)

- CT: Large hypodense area of intraspongious osteolysis with infiltration of the cortical branch of the right ischio-pubic branch, expression of metastatic disease.

  The patient complains of pain in the pelvis, with important functional limitation. Poor general conditions.

79.2   Diagnostic Question

Urothelial carcinoma of high-grade (G3), surgically treated, now with bone metastases: restaging.

79.3   Report

Multiple bone and lung lesions characterized by abnormal glucose consumption compatible with metastatic disease, SUVmax 16.

The wide area of osteolysis in the ischio-pubic branch right documented by X-ray, shows intense glucose consumption, SUVmax 14, and its likely to be a bone-destroying lesion at risk of pathologic fracture.

Lymphadenopathy of the iliac-obturator bilateral stations with high metabolism, SUV-max 10.

79.4   Conclusions

The PET scan shows bone, lung and lymph node secondary disease due to disseminated urothelial carcinoma (Figs. 79.1, 79.2).

79.5   Key Points

Prostate cancer with normal PSA after surgery rarely develops lytic bone metastases with a high metabolism of glucose. It is clear that the skeletal, lung, and lymph nodal lesions are secondary to the high-grade urothelial neoplasm.

Numerous studies in the literature assert the limited sensitivity of FDG-PET in the staging and follow-up of patients with urothelial carcinoma for its low consumption of glucose, so a CT-PET scan is recommended:
- in patients with carcinomas with a high degree of malignancy;
- in patients with double cancer;
- when a metabolic characterization of questionable lesions is necessary.

When a large number of secondary lesions in multiple organs and systems are present, it is dispersive to describe every single metastasis: the nuclear physician must always carefully observe the PET images and the CT ones because the report should not be just an aseptic list of secondary lesions.

You should identify metastases which, if not promptly treated, may lead to a deterioration in the quality of life of the patient, so the report is necessary not only to highlight the critical injuries, but also specify the clinical relevance of the regions which:
- are at risk of pathologic fracture and to be stabilized;
- are responsible for pain, thus requiring analgesic therapy (radiotherapy or specific medical treatment);
- cause renal or biliary obstruction.

In the report, it is possible to make an explicit reference to the CT images obtained with coregistration technique to identify and better characterize a bone injury or other parts of the body that have clinical relevance and it determines a change in the therapeutic strategy and/or prognosis.
- The most significant images can be printed in detail.
- In case of doubt, radiological examinations aimed to clarify the diagnostic picture can be requested.

- When the risk of pathologic fracture is high, nuclear medicine can and should suggest the timing of the subsequent process of surgical stabilization.
- In these cases, the law suggests a direct conversation with the prescriber to accelerate therapeutic procedures. For example, in the presence of incipient collapse of a vertebral body, hospitalization and a subsequent stabilization by the administration of cement can be suggested.

Urothelial Carcinoma: Follow-Up After Surgery

80

80.1 Clinical History

Cystectomy, hysterectomy, oophorectomy and ureterostomy in the right iliac fossa for urothelial carcinoma of the bladder infiltrating the uterus in a 47-year-old woman. Chemotherapy was then performed.

Follow-up after two years

- CT: in the left iliac fossa, close to the iliac vessels and the clips within the previous lymphadenectomy, a mass measuring 6 × 5 cm is detected, cystic type, with multiple sepimentations, unchanged when compared to previous scans. Intercavo-aortic and paracaval subcentimetric lymph nodes, unchanged from previous scans. Right iliac-obturator (17 × 15 mm) and ipsilateral inguinal (22 × 15 mm) adenopathies.

80.2 Diagnostic Question

Search for lesions with a high carbohydrate metabolism in woman undergoing cystectomy for urothelial carcinoma.

80.3 Report

No areas of abnormal glucose consumption in the parts of the body examined.

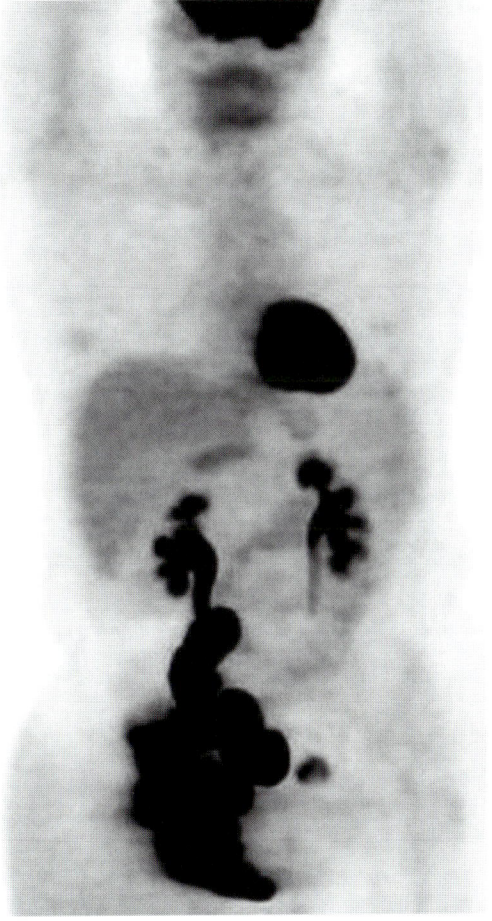

Fig. 80.1 MIP IMAGE: abnormal urinary activity that is projected in the pelvic area. It is associated with bilateral nonobstructive hydronephrosis

The lymph nodes reported previously in the CT and reported in history, do not show pathological concentration of FDG. Follow-up to determine any increase in volume could be useful in the future. See Fig. 80.1.

80.4 Conclusions

The PET scan shows no areas of abnormal glucose consumption within the resolving limits and biological technology.

80.5 Key Points

The physiological renal excretion of FDG makes it difficult to evaluate the renal district in patients with pelvic neobladder or stomas, especially in the presence of marked hydroureteronephrosis. In these cases, PET has limited accuracy in the search for locoregional recurrence.

- It is useful to know the exact reconstructive surgery technique used in the specific case, for proper reporting.
- CT allows to identify lymph nodes increased in size, on which to determine consumption of glucose with a PET scan, avoiding false positives.

In case of doubt, it is recommended a follow-up with contrast-enhanced CT to determine the increase in volume of the lesions.

Printing and Binding: Stürtz GmbH, Würzburg